SPARKS & TAYLOR'S ℮R
Nursing Diagnosis Pocket Guide

Second Edition

Sheila Sparks Ralph, RN, PhD, FAAN
Professor, Division of Nursing (Ret.)
Shenandoah University
Winchester, Virginia

Cynthia M. Taylor, RN, MS
Nurse Consultant
Coordinator, Parish Nurse Program
St. Michael's Church
Kailua Kona, Hawaii

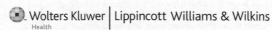
. Wolters Kluwer | Lippincott Williams & Wilkins
Health
Philadelphia · Baltimore · New York · London
Buenos Aires · Hong Kong · Sydney · Tokyo

Acquisitions Editor: Patrick Barbera
Product Manager: Katherine Burland
Production Project Manager: Cynthia Rudy
Editorial Assistant: Dan Reilly
Design Coordinator: Joan Wendt
Manufacturing Coordinator: Karin Duffield
Prepress Vendor: S4 Carlisle

2nd edition

9 8 7 6 5 4 3 2

Printed in China

Library of Congress Cataloging-in-Publication Data
Ralph, Sheila Sparks.
  Sparks and Taylor's nursing diagnosis pocket guide / Sheila Sparks Ralph, Cynthia M. Taylor.—2nd ed.
      p. ; cm.
  Nursing diagnosis pocket guide
  Includes bibliographical references and index.
  ISBN 978-1-4511-8746-5 (alk. paper)
  I. Taylor, Cynthia M.   II. Title.   III. Title: Nursing diagnosis pocket guide.
  [DNLM: 1. Nursing Diagnosis—methods—Handbooks.   2. Patient Care Planning—Handbooks. WY 49]
  610.73—dc23

                                                                    2012051592

Care has been taken to confirm the accuracy of the information presented and to describe generally accepted practices. However, the author(s), editors, and publisher are not responsible for errors or omissions or for any consequences from application of the information in this book and make no warranty, expressed or implied, with respect to the currency, completeness, or accuracy of the contents of the publication. Application of this information in a particular situation remains the professional responsibility of the practitioner; the clinical treatments described and recommended may not be considered absolute and universal recommendations.

  The author(s), editors, and publisher have exerted every effort to ensure that drug selection and dosage set forth in this text are in accordance with the current recommendations and practice at the time of publication. However, in view of ongoing research, changes in government regulations, and the constant flow of information relating to drug therapy and drug reactions, the reader is urged to check the package insert for each drug for any change in indications and dosage and for added warnings and precautions. This is particularly important when the recommended agent is a new or infrequently employed drug.

  Some drugs and medical devices presented in this publication have Food and Drug Administration (FDA) clearance for limited use in restricted research settings. It is the responsibility of the health care provider to ascertain the FDA status of each drug or device planned for use in his or her clinical practice.

CONTRIBUTORS

Anne Z. Cockerham, PhD, CNM, WHNP
Course Coordinator/Clinical Bound Team Leader
Frontier Nursing University
Hyden, Kentucky

Jennifer Matthews, PhD, RN, CNS, CNE, FAAN
Professor, School of Nursing
Clinical Nurse Specialist-Adult Health
Certified Nurse Educator
Lead Nurse Planner, Continuing Education
Shenandoah University
Winchester, Virginia

Helen H. Mautner, MSN, RN, CNE, FCN
Assistant Professor, School of Nursing
Shenandoah University
Winchester, Virginia

Marian Newton, PhD, RN
Professor, School of Nursing
Shenandoah University
Winchester, Virginia

Sherry Rawls-Bryce, MSN, RN
Assistant Professor, School of Nursing
Shenandoah University
Winchester, Virginia

Janice Smith, PhD, RN
Associate Professor, School of Nursing
Shenandoah University
Winchester, Virginia

Rosalie Tapia, MSN, RN
Adjunct Clinical Instructor, School of Nursing
Shenandoah University
Winchester, Virginia

For student nurses as well as expert clinicians, *Sparks and Taylor's Nursing Diagnosis Pocket Guide,* second edition, offers a clearly written, authoritative care plan for each of the NANDA International (NANDA-I) approved nursing diagnoses to help meet patients' health care needs. The guide is organized using a unique assessment framework based on the *NNN Taxonomy of Nursing Practice: A Common Unifying Structure for Nursing Language* (Dochterman & Jones, 2003) and the intervention terms from the *International Classification for Nursing Practice* (ICNP® Version 1; International Council of Nurses, 2005). This framework provides a comprehensive yet easy-to-use format for writing plans of care for clients. The book also includes the linkages between NANDA-I and the Nursing Interventions Classification (NIC) and Nursing Outcomes Classification (NOC) labels. You'll find the care plans in this book, which are presented in a consistent, easy to use, full color design, are invaluable in every health care setting you encounter throughout your career.

GUIDELINES FOR USING *SPARKS AND TAYLOR'S NURSING DIAGNOSIS POCKET GUIDE*

All care plans contain the following sections:

- **Diagnostic statement.** Each diagnostic statement includes a NANDA-I-approved diagnosis. The *Sparks and Taylor's Nursing Diagnosis Pocket Guide,* second edition, contains all the diagnoses approved by NANDA-I through 2012.
- **Definition.** Each diagnosis is explained with a NANDA-I approved definition.
- **Defining characteristics.** This section lists clinical findings that confirm the diagnosis. For diagnoses expressing the possibility of a problem, such as "Risk for Injury," this section is labeled Risk Factors.
- **Assessment.** This section suggests parameters to use when collecting data to ensure an accurate diagnosis. Complete assessment parameters are presented in Appendix A. The parameters are based on the NNN Taxonomy of Nursing Practice and include four

domains: functional, physiological, psychosocial, and environmental (see Appendix A). The domains are subdivided into classes; each class includes key subjective and objective data to be assessed. For each plan, the authors have indicated the parameters that are most necessary for that diagnosis.

- **Expected outcomes.** Here you'll find realistic goals for resolving or ameliorating the patient's health problem, written in measurable behavioral terms. You should select outcomes that are appropriate to the condition of your patient. Outcomes are arranged to flow logically from admission to discharge of the patient. Outcomes identified by NOC research are included for your consideration.

- **Interventions and rationales.** This section provides specific activities you carry out to help attain expected outcomes. Interventions are organized using the following terms: determine, perform, inform, attend, and manage. These intervention types use the International Classification of Nursing Practice taxonomy that is explained in more detail later in these guidelines. Each intervention contains a rationale, highlighted in italic. Rationales receive typographic emphasis because they form the premise for every nursing action. You'll find it helpful to consider rationales before intervening. Understanding the why of your actions can help you see that carrying out repetitive or difficult interventions is an essential element of your nursing practice. More importantly, it can improve critical thinking and help you avoid mistakes. Interventions from NIC research are included for your consideration.

- **Reference.** Each plan concludes with a reference that you may find useful if you need further information about the nursing diagnosis.

NURSING PROCESS OVERVIEW

The cornerstone of clinical nursing, the nursing process, is a systematic method for taking independent nursing action. Steps in the nursing process include:

- assessing the patient's problems
- forming a diagnostic statement
- identifying expected outcomes
- creating a plan to achieve expected outcomes
- implementing the plan or assigning steps for implementation to others
- evaluating the plan's effectiveness.

These phases of the nursing process—assessment, nursing diagnosis formation, outcome identification, care planning, implementation, and evaluation—are dynamic and flexible; they commonly overlap.

Becoming familiar with this process has many benefits. It will allow you to apply your knowledge and skills in an organized, goal-oriented manner. It will also enable you to communicate about professional topics with colleagues from all clinical specialties and practice settings. Using the nursing process is essential to documenting nursing's role in the provision of comprehensive, quality patient care.

By clearly defining those problems a nurse may treat independently, the nursing process has helped dispel the notion that nursing practice is based solely on carrying out physician's orders. Nurse researchers and expert practitioners continue to develop a body of knowledge specific to the field. Nursing literature is providing direction to students and seasoned practitioners for evidence-based practice. A strong foundation in the nursing process will enable you to better assimilate emerging concepts and to incorporate these concepts into your practice.

Assessment

The vital first phase in the nursing process—assessment—consists of the patient history, the physical examination, and pertinent diagnostic studies. The other nursing process phases depend on the quality of the assessment data for their effectiveness.

Your initial patient assessment begins with the collection of data (patient history, physical examination findings, and diagnostic study data) and ends with a statement of the patient's nursing diagnosis(es).

Building a Database

The information you collect in taking the patient's history, performing a physical examination, and analyzing test results serves as your assessment database. Your goal is to gather and record information that will be most helpful in assessing your patient. You can't realistically collect—or use—*all* the information that exists about the patient. To limit your database appropriately, ask yourself the following questions:

- What data do I want to collect?
- How should I collect the data?
- How should I organize the data to make care planning decisions?

Your answers will help you be selective in collecting meaningful data during patient assessment.

The well-defined database for a patient may begin with admission signs and symptoms, chief complaint, or medical diagnosis.

It may also center on the type of patient care given in a specific setting, such as the intensive care unit, the emergency department, or an outpatient care center. For example, you wouldn't ask a trauma victim in the emergency department whether she has a family history of breast cancer, nor would you perform a routine breast examination on her. You would, however, do these types of assessment during a comprehensive health checkup in an outpatient care setting.

If you work in a setting where patients with similar diagnoses are treated, choose your database from information pertinent to this specific patient population. Even when addressing patients with similar diagnoses, however, complete a thorough assessment to make sure that unanticipated problems don't go unnoticed.

Collecting Subjective and Objective Data

The assessment data you collect and analyze fall into two important categories: subjective and objective. The patient's *history*, embodying a *personal perspective* of problems and strengths, provides *subjective data*. It's your most important assessment data source. Because it's also the most subjective source of patient information, it must be interpreted carefully.

In the *physical examination* of a patient—involving inspection, palpation, percussion, and auscultation—you collect one form of *objective data* about the patient's health status or about the pathologic processes that may be related to his illness or injury. In addition to adding to the patient's database, this information helps you interpret his history more accurately by providing a basis for comparison. Use it to validate and amplify the historical data. However, don't allow the physical examination to assume undue importance—formulate your nursing diagnosis by considering *all* the elements of your assessment, not just the examination.

Laboratory test results are another objective form of assessment data and the third essential element in developing your assessment. Laboratory values will help you interpret—and usually clarify—your history and physical examination findings. The advanced technology used in laboratory tests enables you to assess anatomic, physiologic, and chemical processes that can't be assessed subjectively or by physical examination alone. For example, if the patient complains of fatigue (history) and you observe conjunctival pallor (physical examination), check his hemoglobin level and hematocrit (laboratory data).

Both subjective (history) and objective (physical examination and laboratory test results) data are essential for comprehensive patient assessment. They validate each other and together provide more data than either can provide alone. By considering history, physical examination, and laboratory data in their appropriate relationships to one another, you'll be able to develop a nursing diagnosis on which to formulate an effective care plan.

A patient may request a complete physical checkup as part of a periodic (perhaps annual) health maintenance routine. Such a patient may not have a chief complaint; therefore, this patient's health history should be comprehensive, with detailed information about lifestyle, self-image, family and other interpersonal relationships, and degree of satisfaction with current health status.

Be sure to record health history data in an organized fashion so that the information will be meaningful to everyone involved in the patient's care. Some health care facilities provide patient questionnaires or computerized checklists. (See assessment parameters based on NNN Taxonomy of Nursing Practice in Appendix A.)

When documenting the health history, be sure to record negative findings as well as positive ones; that is, note the absence of symptoms that other history data indicate might be present. For example, if a patient reports pain and burning in his abdomen, ask him whether he has experienced nausea and vomiting or noticed blood in his stools. Record the presence or absence of these symptoms.

Remember that the information you record will be used by others who will be caring for the patient. It could even be used as a legal document in a liability case, a malpractice suit, or an insurance disability claim. With these considerations in mind, record history data thoroughly and precisely. Continue your questioning until you're satisfied that you've recorded sufficient detail.

Don't be satisfied with inadequate answers, such as "a lot" or "a little"; such subjective terms must be explained within the patient's context to be meaningful. If taking notes seems to make the patient anxious, explain the importance of keeping a written record. To facilitate accurate recording of the patient's answers, familiarize yourself with standard history data abbreviations.

When you complete the patient's health history, it becomes part of the permanent written record. It will serve as a database with which you and other health care professionals can monitor the patient's progress. Remember that history data must be specific and precise. Avoid generalities. Instead, provide pertinent, concise, detailed information that will help determine the direction and sequence of the physical examination—the next phase in your patient assessment.

After taking the patient's health history, the next step in the assessment process is the *physical examination*. During this assessment phase, you obtain objective data that usually confirm or rule out suspicions raised during the health history interview.

Use four basic techniques to perform a physical examination: *inspection, palpation, percussion,* and *auscultation* (IPPA). These skills require you to use your senses of sight, hearing, touch, and smell to formulate an accurate appraisal of the structures and functions of body systems. Using IPPA skills effectively lessens the chances that you'll overlook something important during the physical examination. In addition, each examination technique collects data that validate and amplify data collected through other IPPA techniques.

Accurate and complete physical assessments depend on two interrelated elements. One is the critical act of sensory perception, by which you receive and perceive external stimuli. The other element is the conceptual, or cognitive, process by which you relate these stimuli to your knowledge base. This two-step process gives meaning to your assessment data.

Develop a system for assessing patients that identifies their problem areas in priority order. By performing physical assessments systematically and efficiently instead of in a random or indiscriminate manner, you'll save time and identify priority problems quickly. First, choose an *examination method.* The most commonly used methods for completing a total systematic physical assessment are *head-to-toe* and *major body systems.*

The head-to-toe method is performed by systematically assessing the patient by—as the name suggests—beginning at the head and working toward the toes. Examine all parts of one body region before progressing to the next region to save time and to avoid tiring the patient or yourself. Proceed from left to right within each region so you can make symmetrical comparisons; that is, when examining the head, proceed from the left side of the head to the right side. After completing both sides of one body region, proceed to the next.

The major body systems method of examination involves systematically assessing the patient by examining each body system in priority order or in an established sequence.

Both the head-to-toe and major body systems methods are systematic and provide a logical, organized framework for collecting physical assessment data. They also provide the same information; therefore, neither is more correct than the other. Choose the method (or a variation of it) that works well for you and is appropriate for your patient population. Follow this routine whenever you assess a patient, and try not to deviate from it.

You may want to plan your physical examination around the patient's *chief complaint* or *concern.* To do this, begin by examining the body system or region that corresponds to the chief complaint. This allows you to identify priority problems promptly and reassures the patient that you're paying attention to his chief complaint.

Physical examination findings are crucial to arriving at a nursing diagnosis and, ultimately, to developing a sound nursing care plan. Record your examination results thoroughly, accurately, and clearly. Although some examiners don't like to use a printed form to record physical assessment findings, preferring to work with a blank paper, others believe that standardized data collection forms can make recording physical examination results easier. These forms simplify comprehensive data collection and documentation by providing a concise format for outlining and recording pertinent information. They also remind you to include all essential assessment data.

When documenting, describe exactly what you've inspected, palpated, percussed, or auscultated. Don't use general terms such as *normal, abnormal, good,* or *poor.* Instead, be specific. Include positive and negative findings. Try to document as soon as possible after completing your assessment. Remember that abbreviations aid conciseness.

Nursing Diagnosis

According to NANDA-I, the nursing diagnosis is a "clinical judg-ment about individual, family, or community experiences/responses to actual or potential health problems/life processes. . . and pro-vides the basis for selection of nursing interventions to achieve outcomes for which the nurse is accountable" (Herdman, 2012, p. 515). The nursing diagnosis must be supported by clinical infor-mation obtained during patient assessment.

Each nursing diagnosis describes a patient problem that a nurse can professionally and legally manage. Becoming familiar with nurs-ing diagnoses will enable you to better understand how nursing prac-tice is distinct from medical practice. Although the identification of problems commonly overlaps in nursing and medicine, the approach to treatment clearly differs. Medicine focuses on curing disease; nurs-ing focuses on holistic care that includes care and comfort.

Nurses can independently diagnose and treat the patient's response to illness, certain health problems and risk for health problems, readiness to improve health behaviors, and the need to learn new health information. Nurses comfort, counsel, and care for patients and their families until they're physically, emotionally, and spiritually ready to provide self-care.

The nursing diagnosis expresses your professional judgment of the patient's clinical status, responses to treatment, and nursing care needs. You perform this step so that you can develop your care plan. In ef-fect, the nursing diagnosis *defines* the practice of nursing. Translating the history, physical examination, and laboratory data about a patient into a nursing diagnosis involves organizing the data into clusters and interpreting what the clusters reveal about the patient's ability to meet basic needs. In addition to identifying the patient's needs in coping with the effects of illness, consider what assistance the patient requires to grow and develop to the fullest extent possible. Your nursing diagnosis describes the cluster of signs and symptoms indicating an actual or potential health problem that you can identify—and that your care can resolve. Nursing diagnoses that indicate potential health problems can be identified by the words "risk for" that appear in the diagnostic label. There are also nursing diagnoses that focus on prevention of health problems and enhanced wellness.

Creating your nursing diagnosis is a logical extension of collecting assessment data. In your patient assessment, you asked each history question, performed each physical examination technique, and considered each laboratory test result because it provided evidence of how the patient could be helped by your care or because the data could affect nursing care.

To develop the nursing diagnosis, use the assessment data you've collected to develop a problem list. Less formal in structure than a fully developed nursing diagnosis, this list describes the patient's problems or needs. It's easy to generate such a list if you use a conceptual model or an accepted set of criterion norms. Examples of such norms include normal physical and psychological development and the assessment parameters based on the NNN Taxonomy of Nursing Practice (see Appendix A).

You can identify the patient's problems and needs with simple phrases, such as *poor circulation, high fever,* or *poor hydration.* Next, prioritize the problems on the list and then develop the working nursing diagnosis.

Some nurses are confused about how to document a nursing diagnosis because they think the language is too complex. By remembering the following basic guidelines, however, you can ensure that your diagnostic statement is correct:

- Use proper terminology that reflects the patient's *nursing* needs.
- Make your statement concise so it's easily understood by other health care team members.
- Use the most precise words possible.
- Use a problem-and-cause format, stating the problem and its related cause.

Whenever possible, use the terminology recommended by NANDA-I.

NANDA-I diagnostic headings, when combined with suspected etiology, provide a clear picture of the patient's needs. Thus, for clarity in charting, start with one of the NANDA-I categories as a heading for the diagnostic statement. The category can reflect an actual or potential problem. Consider this sample diagnosis:

- *Heading*: Disturbed Sleep Pattern
- *Etiology*: Select the appropriate "Related To" phrase from the choices in the care plan
- *Signs and symptoms*: "I don't get enough sleep." "My husband wakes me several times during the night to assist him." You note dark circle under her eyes and some jitteriness.

Do not state a direct cause-and-effect relationship (which may be hard to prove). Remember to state only the patient's problems and the probable origin. Omit references to possible solutions. (Your solutions will derive from your nursing diagnosis, but they aren't part of it.) Errors can also occur when nurses take shortcuts in the nursing process, either by omitting or hurrying through assessment or by basing the diagnosis on inaccurate assessment data.

Keep in mind that a nursing diagnosis is a statement of a health problem that a nurse is licensed to treat—a problem for which you'll assume responsibility for therapeutic decisions and accountability for the outcomes. A nursing diagnosis is **not** a:

- diagnostic test ("schedule for cardiac angiography")
- piece of equipment ("set up intermittent suction apparatus")
- problem with equipment ("the patient has trouble using a commode")
- nurse's problem with a patient ("Mr. Jones is a difficult patient; he's rude and won't take his medication.")
- nursing goal ("encourage fluids up to 2,000 mL/day")
- nursing need ("I have to get through to the family that they must accept the fact that their father is dying.")
- medical diagnosis ("cervical cancer")
- treatment ("catheterize after each voiding for residual urine").

At first, these distinctions may not be clear. The following examples should help clarify what a nursing diagnosis is:

- Don't state a need instead of a problem.
  - *Incorrect*: Fluid replacement related to fever
  - *Correct*: Deficient fluid volume related to fever
- Don't reverse the two parts of the statement.
  - *Incorrect*: Lack of understanding related to noncompliance with diabetic diet
  - *Correct*: Noncompliance with diabetic diet related to lack of understanding

- Don't identify an untreatable condition instead of the problem it indicates (which can be treated).
  - *Incorrect*: Inability to speak related to laryngectomy
  - *Correct*: Social isolation related to inability to speak because of laryngectomy
- Don't write a legally inadvisable statement.
  - *Incorrect*: Skin integrity impairment related to improper positioning
  - *Correct*: Impaired skin integrity related to immobility
- Don't identify as unhealthful a response that would be appropriate, allowed for, or culturally acceptable.
  - *Incorrect*: Anger related to terminal illness
  - *Correct*: Ineffective therapeutic regimen management related to anger over terminal illness
- Don't make a tautological statement (one in which both parts of the statement say the same thing).
  - *Incorrect*: Pain related to alteration in comfort
  - *Correct*: Acute pain related to postoperative abdominal distention and anxiety
- Don't identify a nursing problem instead of a patient problem.
  - *Incorrect*: Difficulty suctioning related to thick secretions
  - *Correct*: Ineffective airway clearance related to thick tracheal secretions

Outcome Identification

During this phase of the nursing process, you identify expected outcomes for the patient. Expected outcomes are measurable, patient-focused goals that are derived from the patient's nursing diagnoses. These goals may be short- or long-term. Short-term goals include those of immediate concern that can be achieved quickly. Long-term goals take more time to achieve and usually involve prevention, patient teaching, and rehabilitation.

In many cases, you can identify expected outcomes by converting the nursing diagnosis into a positive statement. For instance, for the nursing diagnosis "impaired physical mobility related to a fracture of the right hip," the expected outcome might be "The patient will ambulate independently before discharge."

When writing the care plan, state expected outcomes in terms of the patient's behavior—for example, "the patient correctly demonstrates turning, coughing, and deep breathing." Also identify a target time or date by which the expected outcomes should be accomplished. The expected outcomes will serve as the basis for evaluating your nursing interventions. Keep in mind that each expected outcome must be stated in measurable terms. If possible, consult with the patient and his family when establishing expected outcomes. As the patient progresses, expected outcomes should be increasingly directed toward planning for discharge and follow-up care.

Outcome statements should be tailored to your practice setting. For example, in the intensive care unit you may focus on maintaining hemodynamic stability, whereas on a rehabilitation unit you would focus on maximizing the patient's independence and preventing complications.

When writing expected outcomes in your care plan, always start with a specific action verb that focuses on the patient's behavior. By telling your reader how the patient should *look, walk, eat, drink, turn, cough, speak,* or *stand,* for example, you give a clear picture of how to evaluate progress.

The expected outcomes in the *Sparks and Taylor's Nursing Diagnosis Pocket Guide,* second edition, all start with the phrase: "The patient will. . ." and list all the appropriate outcomes. You need to choose which ones are needed for this patient. You will have to specify which person the goals refer to when family, friends, or others are directly concerned.

The Expected Outcome section is followed by selected outcomes from the Nursing Outcomes Classification (NOC) list.

Understanding NOC

The NOC is a standardized language of patient–client outcomes that was developed by a nursing research team at the University of Iowa. It contains 385 outcomes organized into 33 classes and 7 domains. Each outcome has a definition, a list of measurable indicators, and references. The outcomes are research-based, and studies are ongoing to evaluate their reliability, validity, and sensitivity (Johnson, Moorhead, Bulechek, Butcher, Maas, & Swanson, 2012). More information about NOC can be found at the Center for Nursing Classification and Clinical Effectiveness (www.nursing.uiowa.edu/cnc).

Planning

The nursing care plan refers to a written plan of action designed to help you deliver quality patient care. It includes relevant nursing diagnoses, expected outcomes, and nursing interventions. Keep in mind that the care plan usually forms a permanent part of the patient's health record and will be used by other members of the nursing team. The care plan may be integrated into an interdisciplinary plan for the patient. In this instance, clear guidelines should outline the role of each member of the health care team in providing care.

A written care plan gives direction by showing colleagues the goals you have set for the patient and giving clear instructions for helping achieve them. If the patient is discharged from your health care facility to another, your care plan can help ease this transition.

Selecting appropriate nursing actions (interventions): Next, you'll select one or more nursing interventions to achieve each of the expected outcomes identified for the patient. For example, if one expected outcome statement reads "The patient will transfer to chair with assistance," the appropriate nursing interventions include placing the wheelchair facing the foot of the bed and assisting the patient to stand and pivot to the chair. If another expected outcome statement reads "The patient will express feelings related to recent injury," appropriate interventions might include spending time with the patient each shift, conveying an open and nonjudgmental attitude, and asking open-ended questions. Interventions used in the *Sparks and Taylor's Nursing Diagnosis Pocket Guide,* second edition, are organized according to the ICNP types (Description of NNN Taxonomy of Nursing Practice and ICNP, 2005). Because all of your activities are based on assessment data, "Determine" is listed first. The intervention types will appear in the following order: Determine, Perform, Inform, Attend, and Manage. To provide comprehensive care, consider each of the intervention types carefully in your selection.

Reviewing the second part of the nursing diagnosis statement (the part describing etiologic factors) may help guide your choice of nursing interventions. For example, for the nursing diagnosis "Impaired individual resistance related to poor impulse control," you would determine the best nursing interventions for learning techniques to manage behavior. Try to think creatively during this step in the nursing process. It's an opportunity to describe exactly what you and your patient would like to have happen and to establish the criteria against which you'll judge further nursing actions.

The planning phase culminates when you write the care plan and document the nursing diagnoses, expected outcomes, and nursing interventions. Write your care plan in concise, specific terms so that other health care team members can follow it. Keep in mind that because the patient's problems and needs will change, you'll have to review your care plan frequently and modify it when necessary.

Implementation

During this phase, you put your care plan into action. Implementation encompasses all nursing interventions directed toward solving the patient's nursing problems and meeting health care needs. While you coordinate implementation, you also seek help from other caregivers, the patient, and the patient's family.

Implementation requires some (or all) of the following types of interventions:

- **Determine:** assessing and monitoring (e.g., recording vital signs)
- **Perform:** providing care
- **Inform:** teaching and counseling
- **Attend:** making the patient more comfortable, giving emotional support
- **Manage:** referring the patient to appropriate agencies or services

Although it may be brief or narrowly focused, reassessment should confirm that the planned interventions remain appropriate.

Implementation isn't complete until you've documented each intervention, the time it occurred, the patient's response, and any other pertinent information. Make sure each entry relates to a nursing diagnosis. Remember that any action not documented may be overlooked during quality assurance monitoring or evaluation of care. *Another good reason for thorough documentation*: It offers a way for you to take rightful credit for your contribution in helping a patient achieve the highest possible level of wellness. After all, nurses use a unique and worthwhile combination of interpersonal, intellectual, and technical skills when providing care.

Understanding Nursing Interventions Classification

The Nursing Interventions Classification (NIC) is a standardized language of treatments that was developed by a nursing research team at the University of Iowa. It contains 542 interventions organized into 30 classes and 7 domains.

Each intervention has a definition, a list of detailed activities, and references. The interventions are research-based and studies are ongoing to evaluate the effectiveness and cost of nursing treatments Bulechek, Butcher, Dochterman, & Wagner, 2013.

Evaluation

In this phase of the nursing process, you assess the effectiveness of the care plan by answering such questions as:

- How has the patient progressed in terms of the plan's projected outcomes?
- Does the patient have new needs?
- Does the care plan need to be revised?

Evaluation also helps you determine whether the patient received high-quality care from the nursing staff and the health care facility. Your facility bases its own nursing quality assurance system on nursing evaluations.

Include the patient, family members, and other health care professionals in the evaluation. Then, follow the following steps:

- *Select evaluation criteria.* The care plan's projected outcomes—the desired effects of nursing interventions—form the basis for evaluation.
- *Compare the patient's response with the evaluation criteria.* Did the patient respond as expected? If not, the care plan may need revision.
- *Analyze your findings.* If your plan wasn't effective, determine why. You may conclude, for example, that several nursing diagnoses were inaccurate.
- *Modify the care plan.* Make revisions (e.g., change inaccurate nursing diagnoses) and implement the new plan.
- *Re-evaluate.* Like all steps in the nursing process, evaluation is ongoing. Continue to assess, plan, implement, and evaluate for as long as you care for the patient.

DESCRIPTION OF NNN TAXONOMY OF NURSING PRACTICE AND ICNP

Two organizing frameworks are used in the *Sparks and Taylor's Nursing Diagnosis Pocket Guide*: The NNN Taxonomy of Nursing Practice and intervention terms from the International Classification of Nursing Practice. Each of the frameworks is described in this section. We recommend that you get more information about these from the references cited.

NNN Taxonomy of Nursing Practice

The NNN Taxonomy of Nursing Practice (NNNTNP) consists of nursing diagnoses, nursing interventions, and nursing outcomes developed as the result of an invitational conference funded by the National Library of Medicine in 2001 (Dochterman & Jones, 2003). Leaders in nursing language development from NANDA-I for nursing diagnoses, the Center for Nursing Classification and Clinical Effectiveness at the University of Iowa for nursing outcomes and nursing interventions, and selected other experts convened to develop a common unifying taxonomy to further the development, testing, and refinement of nursing language. Results of their efforts were published in *Unifying Nursing Languages: The Harmonization of NANDA, NIC, and NOC* (Dochterman & Jones, 2003) and *NANDA International Nursing Diagnoses: Definitions and Classification* 2003–2004 (Ralph, Craft-Rosenberg, Herdman, & Lavin, 2003). Since that time the NANDA Taxonomy Committee has placed new diagnoses in the taxonomy (Herdman, 2009).

The NNNTNP has 4 domains and 28 classes. The domains, classes, and their definitions are depicted in Appendix B. Assessment parameters based on the taxonomy were developed for the *Sparks and Taylor's Nursing Diagnosis Pocket Guide, second edition*.

International Classification for Nursing Practice

There has been universal agreement among nurses about the importance of recognizing our practice parameters since the time of Florence Nightingale. A resolution to establish an International Classification for Nursing Practice (ICNP®) was passed by the International Council of Nurses (ICN) in 1989. The components of the ICNP® describe the elements of nursing practice: "what nurses **do** relative to certain **human needs** to produce certain **results** (nursing interventions, diagnoses, and outcomes)" (ICN, 2005, p. 11).

The ICNP® is a unified nursing language system. It consists of a multiaxial model intended to be a resource in developing information systems for nursing globally. The seven axes include Focus, Judgment, Means, Action, Time, Location, and Client. The *Sparks and Taylor's Nursing Diagnosis Pocket Guide*, second edition, uses the Action Axis for the basis of selecting nursing interventions. The terms used are Determine, Perform, Inform, Attend, and Manage. Each of these terms is further defined in Appendix C. Each care plan in the *Sparks and Taylor's Nursing Diagnosis Pocket Guide*, second edition, uses at least one of each type of intervention and they are always listed in the order above.

References

Bulechek, G.M., Butcher, H.K., Dochterman, J.M., & Wagner, C.M. (Eds.).(2013). *Nursing Interventions Classification* (NIC), 6th edition. St. Louis: Elsevier.

Dochterman, J. M., & Jones, D. A. (Eds.). (2003). *Unifying nursing languages: The harmonization of NANDA, NIC, and NOC*. Washington, DC: NursesBooks. org.

Herdman, T. H. (Ed.). (2012). *NANDA international nursing diagnoses: Definitions and classification 2012–2014*. Oxford, UK: Wiley-Blackwell.

International Council of Nurses. (2005). *International classification for nursing practice*. Geneva, Switzerland: Author.

Johnson, M., Moorhead, S., Bulechek, G., Butcher, H., Maas, M., & Swanson, E. (2012). *NOC and NIC Linkages to NANDA-I and Clinical Conditions: Supporting Critical Reasoning and Quality Care*. St. Louis: Elsevier.

Ralph, S. S., Craft-Rosenberg, M., Herdman, T. H., & Lavin, M. A. (2003). *NANDA nursing diagnoses & classification*. Philadelphia, PA: NANDA International.

ACKNOWLEDGMENTS

We would like to express our sincere appreciation to the nurses who contributed to the *Nursing Diagnosis Pocket Guide*. Their expertise and commitment to quality patient care made this work possible. We are also grateful to Lippincott Williams & Wilkins for their assistance and enthusiastic support of our work.

Finally, we dedicate this book to nursing students and clinicians who are striving to provide quality care in today's challenging health care arena.

SHEILA SPARKS RALPH, RN, PhD, FAAN
CYNTHIA M. TAYLOR, RN, MS

CONTENTS

PART I

Nursing Diagnoses Care Plans

DEFINITION

Insufficient physiological or psychological energy to endure or complete required or desired daily activities

DEFINING CHARACTERISTICS

- Abnormal blood pressure and heart rate response to activity
- Electrocardiographic changes reflecting arrhythmias and/or ischemia
- Exertional discomfort and/or dyspnea
- Verbal report of fatigue and/or weakness

RELATED FACTORS

- Bed rest
- Generalized weakness
- Imbalance between oxygen supply and demand
- Immobility
- Sedentary lifestyle

ASSESSMENT FOCUS

(Refer to comprehensive assessment parameters.)

- Activity/exercise
- Cardiac function
- Respiratory function

EXPECTED OUTCOMES

The patient will

- Regain and maintain muscle mass and strength.
- Maintain maximum joint range of motion (ROM).
- Perform isometric exercises.
- Help perform self-care activities.
- Maintain heart rate, rhythm, and blood pressure within expected range during periods of activity.
- State understanding of and willingness to cooperate in maximizing the activity level.
- Perform self-care activities to tolerance level.

SUGGESTED NOC OUTCOMES

Activity Tolerance; Endurance; Energy Conservation; Self-Care: Activities of Daily Living (ADLs); Self-Care: Instrumental Activities of Daily Living (IADLs)

INTERVENTIONS AND RATIONALES

<u>Determine:</u> Monitor physiologic responses to increased activity level, including respirations, heart rate and rhythm, and blood pressure, *to ensure that these return to normal within 2 to 5 minutes after stopping exercise.*

<u>Perform:</u> Perform active or passive ROM exercises to all extremities every 2 to 4 hours. *These exercises foster muscle strength and tone, maintain joint mobility, and prevent contractures.*

Turn and reposition patient at least every 2 hours. Establish a turning schedule for the dependent patient. Post schedule at bedside and monitor frequency. *Turning and repositioning prevent skin breakdown and improve lung expansion and prevent atelectasis.*

Maintain proper body alignment at all times *to avoid contractures and maintain optimal musculoskeletal balance and physiologic function.*

Encourage active exercise: Provide a trapeze or other assistive device whenever possible. *Such devices simplify moving and turning for many patients and allow them to strengthen some upper-body muscles.*

Inform: Teach about isometric exercises *to allow patients to maintain or increase muscle tone and joint mobility.*

Teach caregivers to assist patients with ADLs in a way that maximizes patients' potential. *This enables caregivers to participate in patients' care and encourages them to support patients' independence.*

Attend: Provide emotional support and encouragement *to help improve patient's self-concept and motivate patient to perform ADLs.*

Involve patient in planning and decision making. *Having the ability to participate will encourage greater compliance with the plan for activity.*

Have patient perform ADLs. Begin slowly and increase daily, as tolerated. *Performing ADLs will assist patient to regain independence and enhance self esteem.*

Manage: Refer to case manager/social worker to ensure that a home assessment has been done and that whatever modifications were needed to accommodate the patient's level of mobility have been made. *Making adjustments in the home will allow the patient a greater degree of independence in performing ADLs, allowing better conservation of energy.*

SUGGESTED NIC INTERVENTIONS

Activity Therapy; Ambulation; Body Mechanics Promotion; Energy Management; Exercise Promotion: Strength Training; Exercise Therapy: Balance, Joint Mobility, Muscle Control

REFERENCE

Rodrigues, C. G., et al. (2011, July–September). Nursing diagnosis of activity intolerance: Clinical validation in patients with refractory angina. *International Journal of Nursing Terminology Classification, 22*(3), 117–122.

DEFINITION

At risk for experiencing insufficient physiological or psychological energy to endure or complete required or desired activity

RISK FACTORS

- Circulatory or respiratory problems
- History of previous intolerance
- Inexperience with a particular activity
- Deconditioned status

ASSESSMENT FOCUS

(Refer to comprehensive assessment parameters.)
- Activity/exercise
- Cardiac function
- Respiratory function

EXPECTED OUTCOMES

The patient will
- Maintain muscle strength and joint range of motion (ROM).
- Carry out isometric exercise regimen.
- Communicate understanding of rationale for maintaining activity level.
- Avoid risk factors that may lead to activity intolerance.
- Perform self-care activities to tolerance level.
- Maintain blood pressure, pulse, and respiratory rate within prescribed range during periods of activity (specify).

SUGGESTED NOC OUTCOMES

Activity Tolerance; Endurance; Energy Conservation; Self-Care: ADLs; Self-Care: IADLs

INTERVENTIONS AND RATIONALES

Determine: Assess patient's level of functioning using the functional mobility scale *to determine patient's capabilities.*

Assess patient's physiologic response to increased activity (blood pressure, respirations, heart rate, and rhythm). *Monitoring vital signs helps assess tolerance for increased exertion and activity.*

Perform: Position patient *to maintain proper body alignment.* Use assistive devices as needed *to maintain joint function and prevent musculoskeletal deformities.*

Turn and position patient at least every 2 hours. Establish turning schedule for the dependent patient. Post at bedside and monitor frequency. *Turning helps prevent skin breakdown by relieving pressure.*

Unless contraindicated, perform ROM exercises every 2 to 4 hours. Progress from passive to active, according to patient tolerance. *ROM exercises prevent joint contractures and muscular atrophy.*

Encourage active movement by helping patient use trapeze or other assistive devices *to improve muscle tone and enhance self-esteem.*

<u>Inform:</u> Teach patient how to perform isometric exercises *to maintain and improve muscle tone and joint mobility.*

Teach patient, family member, or other caregiver skills such as placing joints in proper body alignment or correct positioning *to maximize patient's participation in self-care. Informed caregivers can encourage patient to become more independent.*

Teach patient symptoms of overexertion, such as dizziness, chest pain, and dyspnea, *to help him or her take responsibility for monitoring his or her own activity level.*

Assist patient in carrying out self-care activities. Increase patient's participation in self-care, as tolerated, *to foster independence and improve mobility.*

<u>Attend:</u> Encourage patient to become involved in planning care and making decisions related to treatment. *Participation in planning enhances patient compliance.*

Explain rationale for maintaining or improving activity level. Discuss factors that increase the risk of activity intolerance. *Education helps patient avoid activity intolerance.*

Encourage patient to carry out ADLs. Provide emotional support, and offer positive feedback when the patient displays initiative. *Offering emotional support enhances patient's self-esteem and motivation.*

<u>Manage:</u> Communicate patient's level of functioning to all staff. *Communication among staff members ensures continuity of care and enables patient to preserve the identified level of independence.*

SUGGESTED NIC INTERVENTIONS

Activity Therapy; Ambulation; Body Mechanics Promotion; Energy Management; Exercise Promotion: Strength Training; Exercise Therapy: Balance, Joint Mobility, Muscle Control

REFERENCE

Turner, S., Eastwood, P., Cook, A., & Jenkins, S. (2011). Improvements in symptoms and quality of life following exercise training in older adults with moderate/severe persistent asthma. *Respiration, 81*(4), 302–310.

DEFINITION
Inability to prepare for a set of actions fixed in time and under certain conditions

DEFINING CHARACTERISTICS
- Verbalization of fear toward a task to be undertaken
- Verbalization of worries toward a task to be undertaken
- Excessive anxieties toward a task to be undertaken
- Failure pattern of behavior
- Procrastination
- Unmet goals for chosen activity
- Lack of sequential organization
- Lack of plan or resources

RELATED FACTORS
- Lack of family support
- Lack of friend support
- Unrealistic perception of events or personal competence
- Defensive flight behavior when faced with proposed solution
- Hedonism
- Compromised ability to process information

ASSESSMENT FOCUS
(Refer to comprehensive assessment parameters.)
- Behavior
- Communication
- Roles/relationships
- Self-perception

EXPECTED OUTCOMES
The patient will
- Demonstrate improved self-confidence to accomplish tasks.
- Demonstrate improved concentration in task planning and execution.
- Minimize procrastination.
- Articulate personal goals for activity planning and completion.
- Verbalize diminished fear and anxiety concerning task planning and execution.

SUGGESTED NOC OUTCOMES
Cognition; Cognition Orientation; Concentration; Decision Making; Information Processing; Memory

INTERVENTIONS AND RATIONALES
<u>Determine:</u> Assess patient's concerns related to activity planning and execution *to be able to suggest strategies to overcome challenges.*
<u>Perform:</u> Model effective techniques for planning and executing activities. *Patients who are challenged by planning and executing activities often find*

it helpful to observe practical approaches instead of solely hearing theoretical information.

<u>Inform:</u> Teach behavior management strategies *to help the person minimize fears of failure.*

<u>Attend:</u> Praise successes in any steps of planning or executing activities; *positive reinforcement enhances self confidence.*

<u>Manage:</u> Refer or collaborate with physical and/or occupational therapists in managing the patient's activity. *Colleagues in related disciplines bring valuable additional perspectives to these complex clinical situations.*

SUGGESTED NIC INTERVENTIONS

Anxiety Reduction; Behavior Management; Behavior Modification; Calming Technique; Memory Training; Activity Therapy

REFERENCE

Hendrie, G. A., et al. (2012, April). Combined home and school obesity prevention interventions for children: What behavior change strategies and intervention characteristics are associated with effectiveness? *Health Education Behavior,* 39(2), 159–171.

DEFINITION
At risk for any noxious or unintended reaction associated with the use of iodinated contrast media that can occur within 7 days after agent injection

RISK FACTORS
- History of previous adverse effect from iodinated contrast media
- History of allergies
- Extremes of age
- Dehydration
- Concurrent use of medications (e.g., ß-blockers, interlukin-2, metformin, nephrotoxic medications)
- Fragile veins
- Underlying disease (e.g., heart disease, pulmonary disease, blood dyscrasias, endocrine disease, renal disease, pheochromocytoma, autoimmune disease)
- General debilitation

ASSESSMENT FOCUS
(Refer to comprehensive assessment parameters.)
- Risk management
- Pharmacological function
- Physical regulation
- Knowledge

EXPECTED OUTCOMES
The patient will
- Not experience an adverse reaction to iodinated contrast media.
- Recognize personal risk factors for adverse reaction.
- Ask questions if new information requires clarification.

SUGGESTED NOC OUTCOMES
Risk Control; Risk Detection; Knowledge: Treatment Procedure(s); Immune Hypersensitivity Response; Allergic Response: Systemic or Localized

INTERVENTIONS AND RATIONALES
<u>Determine:</u> Assess for any previous adverse reaction to contrast media.

Identify preexisting disease states and current medications history that may trigger reaction to iodinated contrast media. *This is essential for the safe administration of contrast media and prevention of adverse effects.*

Assess for history of asthma food allergies, or other allergies *which may increase likelihood of an adverse reaction.* Assess for presence of other medical conditions including heart failures and renal insufficiency *which may increase risk of adverse reaction.*

<u>Perform:</u> Consider prehydration with normal saline solution *to decrease risk of renal damage.*

Withhold metformin before any administration of contrast media and resume after 48 hours once renal function has been evaluated. *This will reduce any medication-associated renal tissue damage due to contrast media.*

Premedication with corticosteroids or antihistamines may be indicated *to reduce incidence of reaction in patients with known risk factors.*

Inform: Educate patient regarding risk factors associated with adverse reaction to iodinated contrast media. *Knowledge of risk factors is essential in preventing adverse reaction and possible organ damage.*

Ensure patient is aware of personal risk factors to share with future providers. *This will promote continued safe administration of iodinated contrast media.*

Attend: Encourage patient to share concerns about procedures requiring use of iodinated contrast media *to reduce anxiety.*

Manage: Collaborate with other members of the health care team regarding presence of risk factors associated with adverse reaction to iodinated contrast media. *This will allow for modifications in the preparation for the procedure and prevent complications.*

SUGGESTED NIC INTERVENTIONS

Risk Identification; Teaching: Individual; Allergy Management

REFERENCES

Radwan, M. A., et al. (2011). Monitoring metformin in cardiac patients exposed to contrast media using ultra-high-performance liquid chromatography tandem mass-spectrometry. *Therapeutic Drug Monitoring, 33*(6), 742–749.

Valente, S., et al. (2011). Creative strategies to improve patient safety: Allergies and adverse drug reactions. *Journal for Nurses in Staff Development, 27*(1), 1–5.

DEFINITION

Inability to clear secretions or obstructions from the respiratory tract to maintain a clear airway

DEFINING CHARACTERISTICS

- Adventitious breath sounds, such as crackles, rhonchi, and wheezes
- Changes in respiratory rate and rhythm
- Cyanosis
- Diminished breath sounds
- Difficulty vocalizing
- Dyspnea
- Ineffective or absent cough
- Orthopnea
- Restlessness
- Sputum production
- Wide-eyed

RELATED FACTORS

- *Environmental*: Second-hand smoke, smoke inhalation, smoking
- *Physiological*: Allergic airways, asthma, chronic obstructive pulmonary disease, infection, neuromuscular dysfunction, and hyperplasia of the bronchial walls
- *Obstructed airway*: Airway spasm, excessive mucus, exudate in the alveoli, foreign body in airway, presence of artificial airway, retained secretions, secretions in the bronchi

ASSESSMENT FOCUS

(Refer to comprehensive assessment parameters.)
- Activity/exercise
- Cardiac function
- Respiratory function

EXPECTED OUTCOMES

The patient will
- Maintain patent airway.
- Have no adventitious breath sounds.
- Have a normal chest x-ray.
- Have an oxygen level in normal range.
- Breathe deeply and cough to remove secretions.
- Expectorate sputum.
- Demonstrate controlled coughing techniques.
- Have adequate ventilation.
- Demonstrate skill in conserving energy while attempting to clear airway.
- State understanding of changes needed to diminish oxygen demands.

SUGGESTED NOC OUTCOMES

Aspiration Prevention; Respiratory Status: Airway Patency; Respiratory Status: Ventilation

INTERVENTIONS AND RATIONALES

<u>Determine:</u> Assess respiratory status at least every 4 hours or according to established standards. *Obstruction in the airway leads to atelectasis, pneumonia, or respiratory failure.* Monitor arterial blood gases values

and hemoglobin levels *to assess oxygenation and ventilatory status.* Report deviations from baseline levels; oxygen saturation should be higher than 90%.

Monitor sputum, noting amount, odor, and consistency. *Sputum amount and consistency may indicate hydration status and effectiveness of therapy. Foul-smelling sputum may indicate respiratory infection.*

Perform: Turn patient every 2 hours; place the patient in lateral, sitting, prone, and upright positions as much as possible *for maximal aeration of lung fields and mobilization of secretions.*

Mobilize patient to full capabilities *to facilitate chest expansion and ventilation.*

Suction, as ordered, *to stimulate cough and clear airways.* Be alert for progression of airway compromise. Perform postural drainage, percussion, and vibration *to facilitate secretion movement.*

Provide adequate humidification *to loosen secretions.* Administer expectorants, bronchodilators, and other drugs, as ordered, and monitor effectiveness. Provide bronchodilator treatments before chest physiotherapy *to optimize results of the treatment.* Administer oxygen, as ordered, *to promote oxygenation of cells throughout the body.*

Inform: Teach patient an easily performed cough technique *to clear airway without fatigue.*

Attend: Avoid placing patient in a supine position for extended periods *to prevent atelectasis.*

When helping the patient cough and deep-breathe, use whatever position best ensures cooperation and minimizes energy expenditure, such as high Fowler's position or sitting on side of bed. *Such positions promote chest expansion and ventilation of basilar lung fields.*

Encourage adequate water intake (3 to 4 L/day) *to ensure optimal hydration and loosening of secretions,* unless contraindicated. Encourage sputum expectoration *to remove pathogens and prevent spread of infection.* Provide tissues and paper bags for hygienic disposal *to prevent spreading infection.*

Manage: If conservative measures fail to maintain partial pressure of arterial oxygen (PaO_2) within an acceptable range, prepare for endotracheal intubation, as ordered, *to maintain artificial airway and optimize PaO_2 level.*

SUGGESTED NIC INTERVENTIONS

Airway Management; Aspiration Precautions; Cough Enhancement; Oxygen Therapy; Respiratory Monitoring; Ventilation Assistance

REFERENCE

Nemeth, J., Maghraby, N., & Kazim, S. (2012). Emergency airway management: The difficult airway. *Emergency Medical Clinics of North America, 30*(2), 401–420.

DEFINITION

Vague uneasy feeling of discomfort or dread accompanied by an autonomic response (the source often nonspecific or unknown to the individual); a feeling of apprehension caused by anticipation of danger. It is an alerting signal that warns of impeding danger and enables the individual to take measures to deal with threat.

DEFINING CHARACTERISTICS

- *Behavioral*: Diminished productivity, fidgeting, restlessness, scanning and vigilance, poor eye contact, insomnia
- *Affective*: Apprehensive, distressed, fearful, jittery, uncertain, wary, regretful
- *Physiological*: Facial tension, hand tremors, increased perspiration, quivering voice
- *Sympathetic*: Anorexia, cardiovascular excitation, diarrhea, facial flushing, increased blood pressure and/or pulse, dilated pupils
- *Parasympathetic*: Abdominal pain, decreased blood pressure and/or pulse, fatigue, nausea, urinary frequency, hesitancy, or urgency
- *Cognitive*: Blocking of thoughts, confusion, impaired attention, forgetfulness, tendency to blame others

RELATED FACTORS

- Threat to self-concept
- Situational crises
- Maturational crises
- Stress
- Unmet needs
- Change in economic status, environment, health, role
- Familial association
- Substance abuse
- Unconscious conflict about goals or values; unmet needs

ASSESSMENT FOCUS

(Refer to comprehensive assessment parameters.)
- Communication
- Coping
- Emotional status
- Psychological status

EXPECTED OUTCOMES

The patient will
- Identify factors that elicit anxious behaviors.
- Participate in activities that decrease feelings of anxious behaviors.
- Practice relaxation techniques at specific intervals each day.
- Cope with current medical situation without demonstrating severe signs of anxiety.
- Demonstrate observable signs of reduced anxiety.
- State that the level of anxiety has decreased.

SUGGESTED NOC OUTCOMES

Anxiety Level; Coping; Anxiety Self-Control; Hyperactivity Level; Impulse Self-Control; Psychosocial Adjustment: Life Change; Social Interaction Skills; Stress Level; Symptom Control

INTERVENTIONS AND RATIONALES

<u>Determine:</u> Listen attentively to patient to determine exactly what he or she is feeling. *Listening on the part of the nurse helps the patient identify anxious behaviors more easily and discover the source of anxiety.*

Assess types of activities *that help reduce patient's stress levels.*

Monitor physiologic responses including respirations, heart rate and rhythm, and blood pressure.

<u>Perform:</u> Reduce environmental stressors (including people), and remain with patient during severe anxiety. *Anxiety often results from lack of trust in the environment and/or fear of being alone.*

Offer relaxing types of music for quiet listening periods. *Listening to relaxing music may have a calming effect.*

Promote proper body alignment *to avoid contractures and maintain optimal musculoskeletal balance and physiologic function.* Encourage active exercise to promote *a sense of well-being.*

<u>Inform:</u> Teach patient relaxation techniques (guided imagery, progressive muscle relaxation, and meditation) to be performed at least every 4 hours *to restore psychological and physical equilibrium by decreasing autonomic response to anxiety.*

<u>Attend:</u> Provide emotional support and encouragement *to improve self-concept and encourage frequent use of relaxation techniques.*

Allow extra visiting times with family *if this seems to allay patient's anxiety about activities of daily living.*

Involve patient in planning and decision making to encourage interest and compliance. Encourage patient to talk about the kinds of activities that promote feelings of comfort. Assist patient to create a plan to try engaging in at least one of these activities each day. *This gives the patient a sense of control.*

Make sure that patient has clear explanations for everything that will happen to him or her. Ask for feedback to ensure that the patient understands. *Anxiety may impair patient's cognitive abilities.*

<u>Manage:</u> Refer to case manager/social worker or professional mental health caretaker to provide mental health assistance. *Encouraging the use of community mental health resources reinforces the fact that anxiety reduction is a long-term process.*

SUGGESTED NIC INTERVENTIONS

Anger Control Assistance; Anticipatory Guidance; Anxiety Reduction; Behavior Modification: Social Skills; Calming Technique; Coping Enhancement; Simple Guided Imagery; Support Group; Active Listening

REFERENCE

Lo, Y. (2012). The importance of transcultural nursing in cancer care. *British Journal of Nursing, 21*(4), S32–S37.

DEFINITION

At risk for entry of gastrointestinal (GI) secretions, oropharyngeal secretions, solids, or fluids into the tracheobronchial passages

RISK FACTORS

- Decreased GI motility
- Delayed gastric emptying
- Depressed cough and gag reflexes
- Feeding or GI tubes
- Impaired swallowing
- Incompetent lower esophageal sphincter
- Increased gastric residual or intragastric pressure
- Reduced level of consciousness
- Situations hindering elevation of upper body
- Surgery or trauma to face, mouth, or neck
- Tracheotomy or endotracheal tube
- Wired jaws

ASSESSMENT FOCUS

(Refer to comprehensive assessment parameters.)

- Elimination
- Neurocognition
- Respiratory function

EXPECTED OUTCOMES

The patients will

- Have clear breath sounds on auscultation.
- Have normal bowel sounds.
- Maintain patent airway.
- Breathe easily, cough effectively, and show no signs of respiratory distress or infection.
- Demonstrate measures to prevent aspiration.
- Maintain respiratory rate within normal limits for age.
- Describe plan for home care.

SUGGESTED NOC OUTCOMES

Aspiration Prevention; Knowledge: Treatment Procedure(s); Respiratory Status: Ventilation; Risk Control; Swallowing Status

INTERVENTIONS AND RATIONALES

Determine: Assess for gag and swallowing reflexes. *Impaired reflexes may cause aspiration.*

Assess respiratory status at least every 4 hours or according to established standards; begin cardiopulmonary monitoring *to detect signs of possible aspiration* (increased respiratory rate, cough, sputum production, and diminished breath sounds).

Auscultate bowel sounds every 4 hours and report changes. *Delayed gastric emptying may cause regurgitation of stomach contents.*

Elevate the head of the bed or place the patient in Fowler's position *to aid breathing.*

Recognize the progression of airway compromise and report your findings *to detect complications early.*

<u>Perform:</u> Help patient turn, cough, and deep breathe every 2 to 4 hours. Perform postural drainage, percussion, and vibration every 4 hours, or as ordered. Suction, as needed, to stimulate cough and clear upper and lower airways. *These measures promote drainage of secretions and full expansion of lungs.*

Perform chest physiotherapy before feeding *to decrease the risk of emesis leading to aspiration.*

Elevate patient during feeding, and use an upright position after feeding. *Such positioning uses gravity to prevent regurgitation of stomach contents and promotes lung expansion.*

Place patient in the lateral or prone position and change position at least every 2 hours *to reduce the potential for aspiration by allowing secretions to drain.*

<u>Inform:</u> Instruct patient and family members in home care plan. They must demonstrate the ability to carry out measures to prevent or respond to aspiration events *to ensure adequate home care before discharge.*

<u>Attend:</u> Encourage fluids within prescribed restrictions. Provide humidification, as ordered (such as a nebulizer). *Fluids and humidification liquefy secretions.*

SUGGESTED NIC INTERVENTIONS

Airway Management; Aspiration Precautions; Feeding; Positioning; Respiratory Monitoring; Vital Signs Monitoring; Vomiting Management; Airway Suctioning

REFERENCE

Metheny, N. A., Davis-Jackson, J., & Stewart, B. J. (2010). Effectiveness of an aspiration risk-reduction protocol. *Nursing Research, 59*(1), 18–25.

DEFINITION

Disruption of the interactive process between parent/significant other and child/infant that fosters the development of a protective and nurturing reciprocal relationship

RISK FACTORS

- Anxiety over parental roles
- Illness in infant that doesn't allow initiation of interaction with parents
- Inability of parents to meet their personal needs
- Lack of privacy, physical barriers, separation, substance abuse, premature infant

ASSESSMENT FOCUS

(Refer to comprehensive assessment parameters.)

- Communication
- Coping
- Emotional status
- Role/relationships
- Sleep and rest
- Values and beliefs

EXPECTED OUTCOMES

The parents will

- Initiate positive interaction with child.
- Hold child and talk to him or her.
- Express confidence in their ability to respond to child's needs.
- Respond appropriately to child.
- Express positive feelings about child.
- Express confidence in their ability to care for child.
- Recognize when they need assistance.

The child will

- Respond positively to parents.
- Show interest in parents' faces.
- Become calm when soothed by parents.

SUGGESTED NOC OUTCOMES

Parenting Performance; Role Performance

INTERVENTIONS AND RATIONALES

<u>Determine:</u> Assess composition of family and ages of members; ability of family to meet physical and emotional needs of its members; knowledge of growth and development patterns; energy levels of parents; recent life changes; child's neurological and sensory status, including vision and hearing; sleep patterns of parents and child. *This information will assist in establishing appropriate interventions.*

<u>Perform:</u> Reduce environmental stressors (including people) where it is possible *to observe whether the parents' responses to the child are appropriate.*

Provide parents and child with periods of privacy *to promote attachment.*

Provide physical care to child when appropriate. This may be to demonstrate to the family *the appropriate way to perform ADLs.*

<u>Inform:</u> Teach parents to observe and understand behavioral cues from the child. For example, the child may become fussy when he or she is ready for a nap or may pull his or her ear if he or she has an earache. Explain the range of options for responding to these cues positively. *It is important that the parents have a variety of options made available to them.*

Teach parents to give physical care when the needs exist *to increase their self-confidence and self-competence.*

Teach relaxation techniques (guided imagery, progressive muscle relaxation, and meditation) that can be done by the parents *to restore psychological and physical equilibrium by decreasing autonomic response to anxiety.*

<u>Attend:</u> Provide emotional support and encouragement *to help improve parents' self-concept and self-confidence in parental roles.*

Initiate discussions with parents on life changes precipitated by the birth of the child. *Parents are often confused and blame themselves because the stress of birth causes frustration and anger.*

Encourage parents to talk about the kinds of activities that promote feelings of comfort. Assist parents to create a plan to engage in at least one of these activities each day. *This provides parents with a sense of control over their own lives.*

Make sure parents have clear explanations for everything that is expected of them. Ask for feedback to ensure parents understand. *Anxiety may impair their cognitive abilities.*

<u>Manage:</u> Provide the name of professionals and/or agencies where parents can receive assistance *to continue developing attachment skills and/or ongoing support.* Refer to case manager/social worker to assess the home environment *to enable the parents to make modifications that will be needed.*

SUGGESTED NIC INTERVENTIONS

Abuse Protection Support: Child; Child Coping Enhancement; Developmental Enhancement; Parenting Promotion; Guided Imagery

REFERENCE

Spurr, S., et al. (2011, November/December). A wellness framework for pediatric nursing clinical practice. *Holistic Nursing Practice, 25*(6), 298–308.

DEFINITION

Life-threatening, uninhibited sympathetic response of nervous system to noxious stimulus after spinal cord injury at T7 or above

DEFINING CHARACTERISTICS

- Paroxysmal hypertension (sudden periodic elevated blood pressure, systolic over 140 mm Hg and diastolic over 90 mm Hg)
- Bradycardia or tachycardia (pulse <60 or more than 100 beats/minute) Diaphoresis above injury
- Red splotches (vasodilation) on skin above injury
- Pallor below injury
- Diffuse headache not confined to any nerve distribution area
- Bladder or bowel distention
- Chilling
- Conjunctival congestion
- Horner's syndrome (contracted pupils, partial ptosis, enophthalmos, loss of sweating on affected side of face [sometimes])
- Paresthesia
- Pilomotor reflex
- Blurred vision
- Chest pain
- Metallic taste
- Nasal congestion

RELATED FACTORS

- Bladder distension
- Bowel distension
- Deficient caregiver knowledge
- Deficient patient knowledge
- Skin irritation

ASSESSMENT FOCUS

(Refer to comprehensive assessment parameters.)
- Cardiac function
- Elimination
- Neurocognition
- Risk management

EXPECTED OUTCOMES

The patient will
- Have cause of dysreflexia identified and corrected.
- Experience cardiovascular stability as evidenced by _____ systolic range, _____ diastolic range, and _____ heart rate range.
- Avoid bladder distention and urinary tract infection (UTI).
- Have no fecal impaction.
- Have no noxious stimuli in environment.
- State relief from symptoms of dysreflexia.
- Have few, if any, complications.
- Maintain normal bladder elimination pattern.
- Maintain normal bowel elimination pattern.
- Demonstrate knowledge and understanding of dysreflexia and will describe care measures.
- Experience few or no dysreflexic episodes.

SUGGESTED NOC OUTCOMES

Neurologic Status; Neurologic Status: Autonomic; Sensory Function Status; Vital Signs Status

INTERVENTIONS AND RATIONALES

Determine: Assess for signs of dysreflexia (especially severe hypertension) *to detect condition so that prompt treatment may be initiated.* Take vital signs frequently *to monitor effectiveness of prescribed medications.*

Perform: Place patient in a sitting position or elevate the head of bed *to aid venous drainage from brain, lower intracranial pressure, and temporarily reduce blood pressure.*

Ascertain and correct probable cause of dysreflexia. Check for bladder distention and patency of catheter. If necessary, irrigate catheter with small amount of solution, or insert a new catheter immediately. *A blocked urinary catheter can trigger dysreflexia.*

Check for fecal mass in rectum. Apply dibucaine ointment (Nupercainal) or another product, as ordered, to anus and 1 in. (2.5 cm) into rectum 10 to 15 minutes before removing impaction. *Failure to use ointment may aggravate autonomic response.*

Check environment for cold drafts and objects putting pressure on patient's skin, *which could act as dysreflexia stimuli.* Send urine for culture if no other cause becomes apparent *to detect possible UTI.*

Implement and maintain bowel and bladder elimination programs *to avoid stimuli that could trigger dysreflexia.*

Inform: Instruct patient, family members, or caregiver about dysreflexia, including its causes, signs and symptoms, and care measures *to prepare them to handle possible emergencies related to condition.* Suggest patient carry an AD emergency card such as the one from www.sci-info-pages.com *to provide information quickly for responders unfamiliar with autonomic dysreflexia.*

Attend: Reassure patient that everyone involved in his or her care will be instructed in management of this problem *to relieve anxiety.*

Manage: If hypertension persists despite other measures, administer ganglionic blocking agent, vasodilator, or other medication as ordered. *Drugs may be required if hypertension persists or if noxious stimuli can't be removed.*

SUGGESTED NIC INTERVENTIONS

Dysreflexia Management; Neurologic Monitoring; Surveillance; Temperature Management; Vital Signs Monitoring

REFERENCE

Krassioudov, A. (2012). Autonomic dysreflexia: Current evidence related to unstable arterial blood pressure control among athletes with spinal cord injury. *Clinical Journal of Sports Medicine, 22*(1), 39–45.

DEFINITION

At risk for life-threatening, uninhibited response of the sympathetic nervous system, post spinal shock, in an individual with spinal cord injury or lesion at T6 or above (has been demonstrated in patients with injuries at T7 and T8)

RISK FACTORS

An injury or lesion at T6 or above and at least one of the following noxious stimuli:

Cardiac/pulmonary problems
- Deep vein thrombosis
- Pulmonary emboli

Gastrointestinal stimuli
- Bowel distension
- Constipation or fecal impaction
- Digital stimulation
- Enemas
- Esophageal reflux
- Gallstones
- Gastric ulcers
- Gastrointestinal (GI) system pathology
- Musculoskeletal–integumentary stimulation
- Cutaneous stimulation (e.g., pressure ulcer, ingrown toenail, dressings, burns, rash)
- Fractures
- Heterotrophic bone
- Pressure over bony prominences
- Pressure over genitalia
- Range of motion exercises
- Spasm
- Sunburns
- Wounds

Neurological stimuli
- Irritating stimuli below level of injury

Regulatory stimuli
- Extreme environmental temperatures
- Temperature fluctuations

Reproductive stimuli
- Ejaculation
- Labor and delivery
- Menstruation

- Ovarian cyst
- Pregnancy
- Sexual intercourse

Situational Stimuli
- Constrictive clothing (e.g., straps, stockings, shoes)
- Narcotic/opiate withdrawal
- Positioning
- Reactions to pharmaceutical agents (e.g., decongestants)
- Surgical procedure

Urological stimuli
- Bladder distension or spasm
- Calculi, catheterization, epididymitis, urethritis, urinary tract infection
- Detrusor sphincter dyssynergia

ASSESSMENT FOCUS
(Refer to comprehensive assessment parameters.)
- Cardiac function
- Elimination
- Neurocognition
- Risk management

EXPECTED OUTCOMES
The patient will
- Identify and reduce risk factors for dysreflexia.
- Avoid bladder distention.
- Not experience a urinary tract infection.
- Maintain normal urinary and bowel elimination patterns.
- Be free from fecal impaction.
- Have an environment free from noxious stimuli that may cause dysreflexia.
- Express understanding of causes of dysreflexia.
- Demonstrate understanding of measures to prevent dysreflexia.

SUGGESTED NOC OUTCOMES
Neurologic Status: Autonomic; Symptom Severity; Vital Signs Status

INTERVENTIONS AND RATIONALES
<u>Determine:</u> Assess for risk factors of dysreflexia, such as constipation, fecal impaction, distended bladder, and presence of noxious stimuli. *Identifying risk factors can prevent or minimize dysreflexic episodes.*

Monitor and record intake and output accurately *to ensure adequate fluid replacement, thereby helping to prevent constipation.*

Monitor vital signs frequently *to ensure effectiveness of preventive measures. Severe hypertension may indicate dysreflexia.*

<u>Perform:</u> Check for bladder distention and patency of catheter. *A blocked catheter can trigger dysreflexia.*

Check for abdominal distention and assess bowel sounds. Monitor and record characteristics and frequency of stools. *Fecal impaction may lead to dysreflexia.*

Administer laxative, enema, or suppositories, as prescribed, *to promote elimination of solids and gases from GI tract.* Monitor effectiveness.

Implement and maintain bowel and bladder programs *to avoid stimuli that could trigger dysreflexia.*

<u>Inform:</u> Instruct patient, family member, or caregiver about risk factors, signs and symptoms, and care measures for dysreflexia *to help prevent a possible dysreflexic episode and help him or her respond appropriately should dysreflexia occur.* Suggest patient carry an AD emergency card such as the one from www.sci-info-pages.com *to provide information quickly for responders unfamiliar with autonomic dysreflexia.*

<u>Attend:</u> Encourage fluid intake of 2.5 L daily, unless contraindicated. *Adequate fluid intake helps maintain patency of catheter and aids bowel elimination.*

<u>Manage:</u> Consult with dietitian about increasing fiber and bulk in diet to maximum prescribed by physician *to improve intestinal muscle tone and promote comfortable elimination.*

SUGGESTED NIC INTERVENTIONS

Dysreflexia Management; Neurologic Monitoring; Vital Signs Monitoring

REFERENCE

Rabchevsky, A. G., & Kitzman, P. H. (2011). Latest approaches for the treatment of spasticity and autonomic dysreflexia in chronic spinal cord injury. *Neurotherapeutics, 8*(2), 274–282.

DEFINITION

Disintegrated physiological and neurobehavioral responses of infant to the environment

DEFINING CHARACTERISTICS

- *Attention–interaction system*—abnormal response to sensory stimuli (e.g., difficulty soothing, inability to sustain alert status)
- *Motor system*—altered primitive reflexes; finger splaying; jittery, uncoordinated movement; increased or decreased tone; startles, tremors, or twitches
- *Physiological*—arrhythmias, bradycardia, or tachycardia; desaturation; feeding intolerances; skin color changes
- *Regulatory problems*—inability to inhibit startle; irritability
- *State-organizational system*—active or quiet awake; diffuse sleep

RELATED FACTORS

- *Caregiver*—Cue knowledge deficit; cue misreading; environmental stimulation contribution
- *Environmental*—physical environment inappropriateness; sensory deprivation, inappropriateness, or overstimulation
- *Individual*—gestational or postconceptual age; illness; immature neurological system
- *Postnatal*—feeding intolerance; invasive procedures; malnutrition; motor and/or oral problems; pain; prematurity
- *Prenatal*—congenital or genetic disorders; teratogenic exposure

ASSESSMENT FOCUS

(Refer to comprehensive assessment parameters.)
- Elimination
- Neurocognition
- Nutrition
- Physical regulation
- Role/relationships
- Sensation/perception
- Sleep/rest

EXPECTED OUTCOMES

The parents will
- Learn to identify and understand infant's behavioral cues
- Identify their own emotional responses to infant's behavior
- Identify means to help infant overcome behavioral disturbance
- Identify ways to improve their ability to cope with infant's responses
- Express positive feelings about their ability to care for infant
- Identify resources for help with infant.

The infant will
- Begin to show appropriate signs of maturation.

SUGGESTED NOC OUTCOMES

Knowledge: Infant Care; Neurological Status; Preterm Infant Organization; Sleep; Child Development: 1 Month; Family Coping; Family Functioning; Parenting Performance

INTERVENTIONS AND RATIONALES

<u>Determine:</u> Monitor infant's responses *to ensure effectiveness of preventive measures.*

<u>Inform:</u> Explain to parents that infant maturation is a developmental process. *Their participation is crucial to help them understand the importance of nurturing the infant.*

Explain to parents that their actions can help modify some of infant's behavior; however, make it clear that infant maturation isn't completely within their control. *This explanation may help decrease the parents' feelings of incompetence.*

Explain to parents that infant gives behavioral cues that indicate needs. Discuss appropriate ways to respond to behavioral cues—for example, providing stimulation that doesn't overwhelm the infant; stopping stimulation when the infant gives behavioral cues (such as yawning, looking away, or becoming agitated); and finding methods to calm the infant if she becomes agitated (such as swaddling, gentle rocking, and quiet vocalizations). *Monitoring responses aids in gauging effectiveness of meeting needs.*

Help parents identify and cope with their responses to infant's behavioral disturbance *to help them recognize and adjust their response patterns. When the infant doesn't respond positively, the parents may feel inadequate or become frustrated. They need to understand that these reactions are normal.*

<u>Attend:</u> Explore with parents ways to cope with stress imposed by infant's behavior *to help them develop better coping skills.*

Praise parents when they demonstrate appropriate methods of interacting with the infant *to provide positive reinforcement.*

<u>Manage:</u> Provide parents with information on sources of support and special infant services *to promote coping with infant's long-term needs.*

SUGGESTED NIC INTERVENTIONS

Environmental Management; Neurologic Monitoring; Newborn Care; Parent Education: Infant; Positioning; Sleep Enhancement; Attachment Promotion; Developmental Care; Family Integrity Promotion; Teaching: Infant Stimulation 0–12 Months

REFERENCE

Moore, E. R., et al. (2012, May). Early skin-to-skin contact for mothers and their healthy newborn infants. *Cochrane Database Systematic Reviews, 16*(5), CD003519.

DEFINITION
Risk for alteration in integration and modulation of the physiological and behavioral systems of functioning (such as autonomic, motor, state-organizational, self-regulatory, and attentional–interactional systems)

RISK FACTORS
- Environmental overstimulation
- Invasive or painful procedures
- Lack of containment or boundaries
- Oral or motor problems
- Pain
- Prematurity

ASSESSMENT FOCUS
(Refer to comprehensive assessment parameters.)
- Elimination
- Neurocognition
- Nutrition
- Physical regulation
- Role/relationships
- Sensation/perception
- Sleep/rest

EXPECTED OUTCOMES
The parents will
- Identify factors that place infant at risk for behavioral disturbance.
- Identify potential signs of behavioral disturbance in infant.
- Identify appropriate ways to interact with infant.
- Identify their reactions to infant (including ways of coping with occasional frustration and anger).
- Express positive feelings about their ability to care for infant.
- Identify resources for help with infant.

The infant will
- Maintain physiologic stability
- Maintain an organized motor system
- Respond to sensory information in an adaptive way.

SUGGESTED NOC OUTCOMES
Knowledge: Child Development: 1 Month, 2 Months, 4 Months, 6 Months, and 12 Months; Knowledge: Infant Care; Neurological Status; Child Development: 1 Month; Family Coping; Family Functioning; Parenting Performance; Knowledge: Parenting; Preterm Infant Organization; Sleep

INTERVENTIONS AND RATIONALES
<u>Determine:</u> Monitor infant's responses *to ensure effectiveness of preventive measures.*

<u>Perform:</u> Demonstrate appropriate ways of interacting with the infant *to help parents identify and interpret the infant's behavioral cues and respond appropriately.* For example, help them recognize when the infant is awake and alert, and help them understand when the infant needs more stimulation, such as being spoken to or held.

Inform: Explain to parents that infant maturation is a developmental process and that their participation is crucial to their understanding of the importance of nurturing the infant. *Participation in the process by the parents will both stimulate the developmental process and alert to delays in development.*

Explain to parents that their actions can help modify some of their infant's behavior; however, make it clear that infant maturation isn't completely within their control. *This explanation may decrease the parent's feelings of incompetence.*

Explain to parents that certain risk factors may interfere with the infant's ability to achieve optimal development. These risk factors include overstimulation, lack of stimulation, lack of physical contact, and painful medical procedures. *Educating the parents will help them understand their role in interpreting the infant's behavioral cues and providing appropriate stimulation.*

Describe to the parents the potential signs of a behavioral disturbance in the infant: inappropriate responses to stimuli, such as the failure to respond to human contact or tendency to become agitated with human contact; physiologic regulatory problems, such as a breathing disturbance in a premature infant; and apparent inability to interact with the environment. *Education will help the parents recognize if the infant has a problem in behavioral development.*

Attend: Explore with parents ways to cope with the stress imposed by the infant's behavior *to increase their coping skills.*

Help parents identify their emotional responses to the infant's behavior *to help them recognize and adjust their response patterns.* Explain that it is normal for parents to experience feelings of inadequacy, frustration, or anger if the infant does not respond positively to them.

Praise the parents when they demonstrate appropriate methods of interacting with the infant *to provide positive reinforcement.*

Manage: Provide the parents with information on sources of support and special infant services *to help them cope with the infant's long-term needs.*

SUGGESTED NIC INTERVENTIONS

Infant Care; Newborn Monitoring; Parent Education: Infant; Positioning; Surveillance; Attachment Promotion; Developmental Care; Family Integrity Promotion; Teaching: Infant Stimulation 0–12 Months

REFERENCE

Schmid, G., et al. (2011, April). Predictors of crying, feeding and sleeping problems: A prospective study. *Child: Care, Health and Development, 37*(4), 493–502.

DEFINITION

A pattern of modulation of the physiologic and behavioral systems of functioning (such as autonomic, motor, state-organizational, self-regulatory, and attentional–interactional systems) in an infant that is sufficient for well-being and can be strengthened

DEFINING CHARACTERISTICS

- Use of some self-regulatory behaviors
- Definite sleep–wake states
- Responsiveness to visual and auditory stimuli
- Stable physiologic measures

RELATED FACTORS

- Pain
- Immaturity

ASSESSMENT FOCUS

(Refer to comprehensive assessment parameters.)

- Elimination
- Neurocognition
- Nutrition
- Physical regulation
- Role/relationships
- Sensation/perception
- Sleep/rest

EXPECTED OUTCOMES

The parents will

- Express understanding of their role in infant's behavioral development
- Express confidence in their ability to interpret infant's behavioral cues
- Identify means to promote infant's behavioral development
- Express positive feelings about their ability to care for infant
- Identify resources for help with infant

The infant will

- Maintain physiologic stability
- Maintain an organized motor system
- Respond to information in an adaptive way.

SUGGESTED NOC OUTCOMES

Knowledge: Child Development: 1, 2, 4, 6, and 12 Months; Infant Care; Neurological Status; Sleep; Family Coping; Family Functioning; Parenting Performance

INTERVENTIONS AND RATIONALES

<u>Determine:</u> Monitor infant's responses *to ensure effectiveness of preventive measures.*

<u>Perform:</u> Demonstrate appropriate ways of interacting with the infant, such as moderate stimulation, gentle rocking, and quiet vocalizations, *to help the parents identify the most effective methods of interacting with their child.*

<u>Inform:</u> Explain to parents that infant maturation is a developmental process. Further explain that infants exhibit three behavioral states: sleeping, crying, and being awake and alert. Also explain that infants provide behavioral cues that indicate their needs. *Education will help parents understand the importance of nurturing the infant and prepare them to respond to the infant's behavioral cues.*

Explain to parents that their actions can help promote infant development. Make it clear; however, that infant maturation isn't completely within their control. *Explanation may decrease feelings of anxiety and incompetence and help prevent unrealistic expectations.*

Help parents interpret behavioral cues from their infant *to foster healthy parent–child interaction.* For example, help them recognize when the infant is awake and alert, and point out to them that this is a good time to provide stimulation.

Help parents identify ways they can promote the infant's development, such as providing stimulation by shaking a rattle in front of the infant, talking to the infant in a gentle voice, and looking at the infant when feeding him. *This encourages practices that promote the infant's development. Sensory experiences promote cognitive development.*

<u>Attend:</u> Explore with parents ways to cope with stress caused by the infant's behavior *to increase their coping skills.*

Praise parents for their attempts to enhance their interaction with the infant *to provide positive reinforcement.*

<u>Manage:</u> Provide parents with information on sources of support and special infant services *to encourage them to continue to foster their infant's development.*

SUGGESTED NIC INTERVENTIONS

Attachment Promotion; Developmental Care; Environmental Management: Attachment Process; Family Integrity Promotion; Infant Care; Sleep Enhancement; Teaching: Infant Stimulation 0–12 Months

REFERENCE

Cepanec, M., et al. (2012, July). Mother–father differences in screening for developmental delay in infants and toddlers. *Journal of Communication Disorders, 45*(4), 255–262.

DEFINITION

At risk for a decrease in blood volume that may compromise health

RISK FACTORS

- Pregnancy-related complications (e.g., placenta praevia or abruptio)
- Postpartum complications (e.g., uterine atony, retained placenta)
- Treatment-related side effects (e.g., surgery, medications, administration of platelet-deficient blood products, chemotherapy)
- Circumcision
- Disseminated intravascular coagulopathy
- Inherent coagulopathies (thrombocytopenia, hemophilia)
- Gastrointestinal disorders (e.g., gastric ulcers, polyps, varices)
- Aneurysm
- Impaired liver function (e.g., cirrhosis, hepatitis)
- Trauma or history of falls
- Lack of knowledge

ASSESSMENT FOCUS

(Refer to comprehensive assessment parameters.)

- Cardiac function
- Fluid and electrolytes
- Pharmacologic function/treat-
- ments
- Reproduction
- Tissue perfusion

EXPECTED OUTCOMES

The patient will

- Receive screening to alert clinicians about existing risk factors for bleeding.
- Receive follow-through intervention.
- Receive appropriate clinician staffing and surveillance for a rapid response to rescue the patient before serious bleeding occurs.
- Maintain heart rate, rhythm, blood pressure, and tissue perfusion within expected ranges during episodes of risk.
- Identify and avoid risk situations with potential for trauma injury.

SUGGESTED NOC OUTCOMES

Maternal Status: Antepartum; Maternal Status: Postpartum; Blood Coagulation; Blood Loss Severity; Circulation Status; Vital Sign; Fluid Balance; Electrolyte & Acid Base Balance; Tissue Perfusion: Cellular

INTERVENTIONS AND RATIONALES

Determine: Interview/screen each individual for risk factors for bleeding; some individuals know of their risks for bleeding, whereas others do not. *Assessment findings may indicate need for protective measures.*

Anticipate conditions and episodes of care that may precipitate bleeding especially in high-risk patient care areas *to provide early intervention.* Monitor physiologic responses for values that exceed expected or normal ranges; *early bleeding compensatory mechanisms alter respirations, pulse, and blood pressure and may be present as subtle changes.* Monitor for

occult and for frank bleeding—urine, feces, wounds, and dressings—by visual inspection or point-of-care testing *to identify need for intervention.*
Perform: Correlate findings, risk factors, and current episode of care and patient condition *to determine the imminent level of risk for bleeding.*

Perform vital signs and basic physical assessments for the patient who is at risk for bleeding until assured the risk is past *to provide data needed for early intervention.* Obtain laboratory tests (hemoglobin, hematocrit, complete blood cell count, thrombin time, prothrombin time, activated partial thromboplastin time, etc.) and point-of-care tests (stool, urine, gastric) as ordered; *these tests provide data that may be indications of a bleed.*

Examine dressings, drainage tubes, and collection canisters for presence of blood; report findings *to support need for changes in therapy.*
Inform: Teach patient about intended and unintended effects of medications (heparin, enoxaparin [Lovenox], warfarin (Coumadin), clopidogrel [Plavix], aspirin) that increase the risk of bleeding or prolong clotting. This enables the patient to avoid bleeding-risk situations.

Discuss patterns of risk management *to promote a lifestyle that focuses on health promotion/injury avoidance to diminish injuries.*

Discuss alternatives in ADLs *to avoid trauma-causing injury and bleeding.*
Attend: Provide care protecting an individual from injury *to prevent bleeding.* Implement interventions that reverse or remove the risk of bleeding or bleeding condition *to prevent bleeding or stabilize the patient's physiologic condition and assist in recovery.*

Provide emotional support to the patient who is bleeding and is experiencing physiologic compensatory responses of anxiety, fear, and a sense of dread *as this support provides assurance and is calming.*

Support participation in decisions about the treatment placing the patient at risk for bleeding. *Active participation encourages fuller understanding of the rationale and compliance with the treatment.*
Manage: Refer to case manager or APN those at risk for bleeding secondary to treatment (i.e., warfarin INR) for monitoring and regime adherence. Monitor the recovery of the individual who experienced a bleeding episode *because weakness causes a safety risk for falls or injury.*

SUGGESTED NIC INTERVENTIONS

Bleeding Precautions; Bleeding Reduction; Blood Products Administration; Circulatory Precautions; Fluid/Electrolyte Management; Risk Identification; Teaching; Prescribed Medications; Vital Sign Monitoring

REFERENCE

Roback, J. D. (2012, May/June). Evidence-based guidelines for blood transfusion. *Journal of Infusion Nursing, 35*(3), 187–190.

DEFINITION
At risk for variation of blood glucose/sugar levels from the normal range that may compromise health

RISK FACTORS
- Deficient knowledge of diabetes management
- Developmental level
- Dietary intake
- Inadequate blood glucose monitoring
- Lack of acceptance of diagnosis
- Lack of adherence to diabetes management
- Physical activity level
- Physical/mental health status
- Pregnancy
- Stress
- Weight gain or loss

ASSESSMENT FOCUS
(Refer to comprehensive assessment parameters.)
- Behavior
- Emotional
- Physical regulation
- Neurocognition
- Nutrition
- Tissue integrity

EXPECTED OUTCOMES
The patient will
- Be free from symptoms of hypoglycemia/hyperglycemia.
- Have serum glucose within the prescribed range.
- Verbalize understanding of how to control blood glucose level.

SUGGESTED NOC OUTCOMES
Blood Glucose Level; Diabetes Self-Management; Knowledge: Diabetes Management, Weight Control; Diabetes Self-Management

INTERVENTIONS AND RATIONALES
<u>Determine:</u> Assess patient for symptoms of low serum glucose level and maintain a patient airway if indicated. *A low serum glucose may not be detected in some patients until moderate to severe central nervous system impairment occurs, which can lead to a compromised airway and cardiac arrest*

Assess for the underlying cause (e.g., inadequate dietary intake; illness such as nausea, vomiting, or diarrhea; and too much insulin) *to help patient prevent future episodes and adapt treatment strategies and lifestyle changes.*

Monitor or instruct patient to monitor glucose levels with a glucometer at regular intervals *to identify and respond early to fluctuations in glucose levels that occur outside normal parameters.*

Assess family understanding of prescribed treatment regimen. *The family plays an important role in supporting the patient.*

Assess patient's knowledge of hypo/hyperglycemia *to ensure adequate management and prevent future episodes.*

Monitor for signs and symptoms of hyperglycemia (polyuria, polydipsia, polyphagia, lethargy, malaise, blurred vision, and headache). *Early detection ensures prompt intervention and management.*

Assess for the underlying cause of elevated serum glucose level, including inadequate dietary intake, illness, and poor medication management *to prevent future episodes and develop treatment strategies such as changes in lifestyle.*

<u>Perform:</u> Perform immediate finger stick with a glucometer to *determine glucose level, which will guide treatment strategies.* Administer insulin, as prescribed, *to treat elevated blood glucose levels.*

Provide patient with glucose tablets or gel if he or she is conscious and has ability to swallow. Administer intravenous glucose if patient is unconscious or cannot swallow. *Immediate treatment in the form of oral or intravenous glucose must be administered to reverse the low serum glucose level.* If patient becomes nauseated, turn patient on side *to prevent aspiration.*

Protect patient from injuries, such as falls. *Symptoms of low serum glucose place patient at risk for injury especially when driving and performing other potentially dangerous activities.*

Evaluate serum electrolyte levels. Administer potassium, as prescribed. *With elevated blood glucose levels, potassium and sodium levels may be low, normal, or high, depending on the amount of water loss.* Consider performing serum testing for HgbA$_{1c}$ (glycosylated hemoglobin A$_{3C}$ level) *to evaluate average blood glucose levels over a period of approximately 2 to 3 months and to assess the adherence and effectiveness of the treatment regimen.*

<u>Inform:</u> Teach patient and family self-management of hypoglycemia and hyperglycemia including glucose monitoring at regular intervals *to treat abnormal glucose levels early* and medication management, nutritional intake, exercise, and regular follow-up visits with the physician *to ensure adequate understanding and management of the treatment regimen to prevent future hyperglycemic events.* Patient and family teaching may include referrals to a diabetic educator, diabetic education classes, and a dietician.

<u>Manage:</u> Consult physician if signs and symptoms persist. *Changes in prescribed medications may be needed, such as with oral hypoglycemic agents or insulin dosing.* Call for emergency medical services if patient is unstable outside the hospital.

SUGGESTED NIC INTERVENTIONS

Bedside Laboratory Testing; Health Education; Health Screening; Nutritional Counseling; Teaching: Disease Process, Prescribed Medications, and Prescribed Diet

REFERENCE

Khalaila, R., et al. (2011). Nurse-led implementation of a safe and effective intravenous insulin protocol in a medical intensive care unit. *Critical Care Nurse, 31*(6), 27–35.

DEFINITION
Confusion in mental picture of one's physical self

DEFINING CHARACTERISTICS
- Physiologic changes, behavioral changes, usual patterns of coping with stress
- Missing body part, not looking or touching a body part, negative feelings about a body part
- Frequent or disparaging comments about aging and its physical manifestations
- Personal rigidity or unwillingness to change
- Actual change in structure or function
- Change in social relationships
- Hiding or overexposing of a body part (intentional or unintentional)
- Depersonalization of loss by using third person pronouns
- Unintentional or intentional overexposing of body part

RELATED FACTORS
- Biophysical
- Cognitive
- Cultural
- Illness
- Surgery
- Trauma

ASSESSMENT FOCUS
(Refer to comprehensive assessment parameters.)
- Behavior
- Knowledge
- Sensory perception
- Sexuality
- Values/beliefs

EXPECTED OUTCOMES
The patient will
- Identify physical changes without making disparaging comments.
- Identify at least one positive aspect of aging.
- Use vision or hearing aids appropriately.
- Demonstrate increased flexibility and willingness to consider lifestyles changes.
- Participate in at least one social activity regularly.
- Exercise and engage in other physical activity at level consistent with desire, ability, and safety.
- Perform self-care activities to tolerance level.

SUGGESTED NOC OUTCOMES
Body Image; Grief Resolution; Self-Esteem; Life Change

INTERVENTIONS AND RATIONALES
<u>Determine:</u> Monitor physiologic responses to increased activity level, including respirations, heart rate and rhythm, and blood pressure. Assess understanding of the current health problem and desire to participate in treatment. *Assessment information is helpful in determining appropriate interventions.*

<u>Perform:</u> Perform activities of daily living (ADLs) measures that the patient is unable to perform for self while *promoting as much independence as possible.*

<u>Inform:</u> Provide patient with information on appropriate self-care activities (e.g., maintaining proper diet; bathing as needed; using alcohol-free skin lotions to combat dryness; exercising appropriately to maintain muscle mass, bone strength, and cardiorespiratory health; avoiding fractures related to osteoporosis) *to ensure that the patient will be able to perform self-care measures.*

Teach patient about isometric exercises *to maintain or increase muscle tone and joint mobility.*

Teach caregivers to assist patient with self-care activities in a way that maximizes patient's potential. *This enables caregivers to participate in patient's care while supporting patient's independence.*

<u>Attend:</u> Provide emotional support and encouragement *to improve patient's self-concept and promote motivation to perform ADLs.*

Assist patient to learn how to perform self-care activities. Begin slowly and increase daily, as tolerated. *Performing self-care activities will assist patient to regain independence and enhance self-esteem.*

Involve patient in planning and decision making. *Having the ability to participate will encourage greater compliance with the plan for activity.*

Focus on patient's strengths and what the patient is able to do for self.

Encourage patient to engage in social activities with people of all age groups. *Participation once a week will help relieve patient's sense of isolation.*

<u>Manage:</u> Refer to case manager/social worker *to ensure patient receives long-term assistance with body image problem.*

Refer patient to a support group. *In the context of a group, the patient may develop a more positive view of present situation.*

Refer for corrective eyewear and hearing aids *to address sensory deficits.*

SUGGESTED NIC INTERVENTIONS

Active Listening; Body Image Enhancement; Grief Work Facilitation; Self-Esteem Enhancement

REFERENCE

Cross, H. H., & Hottenstein, P. (2010, July/August). Ostomy care: Starting and maintaining a hospital-based ostomy support group. *Journal of Wound, Ostomy, and Continence Nursing, 37*(4), 393–396.

DEFINITION
At risk for failure to maintain body temperature within normal range

RISK FACTORS
- Altered metabolic rate
- Dehydration
- Exposure to extreme hot/cold environments
- Inappropriate clothing for temperature
- Sedation
- Extremes of weight or age
- Illness/trauma affecting temperature regulation
- Medications causing vasoconstriction or vasodilation
- Inactivity/vigorous activity

ASSESSMENT FOCUS
(Refer to comprehensive assessment parameters.)
- Fluid and electrolytes
- Neurocognition
- Nutrition
- Respiratory function

EXPECTED OUTCOMES
The patient will
- Maintain body temperature of 98.6°F to 99.5°F (37°C to 37.5°C).
- Maintain weight within 5% of baseline.
- Maintain balanced intake and output within normal limits for age.
- Have a urine-specific gravity between 1.010 and 1.015.
- Express understanding of factors that cause hypothermia and hyperthermia.

SUGGESTED NOC OUTCOMES
Hydration; Risk Control; Risk Detection; Thermoregulation

INTERVENTIONS AND RATIONALES
<u>Determine:</u> Assess temperature every 4 hours. Use a temperature-taking method appropriate for age and size. *Prolonged elevation of temperature above 104°F (40°C) may produce dehydration and harmful central nervous system effects.*

Weigh patient every morning and record results. *A decrease in weight may indicate dehydration.*

Assess the patient's knowledge and lifestyle before teaching about hypothermia and hyperthermia *to gear the teaching plan to the patient's needs.*
<u>Perform:</u> Maintain adequate fluid intake by offering small amounts of flavored fluids at frequent intervals; record intake and output every shift. *Fever increases fluid requirements by increasing the metabolic rate.* Provide high-calorie liquids, such as colas, fruit juices, and flavored water sweetened with corn syrup, *to help prevent dehydration.*

Administer antipyretics, as ordered, and monitor effectiveness. *Antipyretics act on the hypothalamus to regulate body temperature.*

Check and record urine-specific gravity with each voiding. *Urine-specific gravity increases with dehydration. Adequate urine output and urine-specific gravity between 1.010 and 1.015 indicate sufficient hydration.*

Give a tepid sponge bath for increased temperature *to increase vaporization from skin and decrease body temperature.*

Inform: Teach patient to dress in lightweight clothing when experiencing elevated body temperature *to allow perspiration to evaporate, thereby releasing body heat.*

Instruct the patient on the signs and symptoms of imbalanced body temperature:

- *Hypothermia*: Shallow respirations; slow, weak pulse; decreased body temperature; low blood pressure; and pallor
- *Hyperthermia*: Shivering, shaking chill; feeling hot; extreme thirst; elevated body temperature; and high blood pressure.

Listing the signs and symptoms helps the patient learn and identify warning signals of imbalanced body temperature. Large black type is easier for the older patient to read.

Explain to the patient or family member why the patient needs warm clothing in cool climates, even indoors. Suggest socks, nonslip house shoes, and leg warmers *to provide warmth to vulnerable lower extremities, where vascular changes may cause decreased temperature sensation.*

Instruct the patient or family member to label home thermostats with large numbers and to use black or bright contrasting colors to indicate appropriate temperature settings. *Easy-to-read labels will help the patient maintain room temperature.*

Teach the patient or his or her family members about the dangers of too much direct sunlight on warm days *to prevent overheating in an older patient with faulty thermoreceptors.*

Attend: Encourage the patient to remain active when in a cool environment *to keep warm and maintain normal metabolism.*

Manage: Suggest that a friend, family member, or volunteer from a local community organization visit the patient daily *to help ensure the patient's safety.*

SUGGESTED NIC INTERVENTIONS

Fever Treatment; Environmental Management; Temperature Regulation; Vital Signs Monitoring

REFERENCE

Block, J., Lilienthal, M., Cullen, L., & White, A. (2012, January–March). Evidence-based thermoregulation for adult trauma patients. *Critical Care Nursing Quarterly, 35*(1), 50–63.

DEFINITION

Dissatisfaction or difficulty a mother, infant, or child experiences with the breastfeeding process

DEFINING CHARACTERISTICS

- Actual or perceived inadequate milk supply (mother)
- Arching and crying when at the breast (infant)
- Evidence of inadequate intake (infant)
- Fussiness and crying within the first hour of feeding (infant)
- Inability to latch on to nipple correctly (infant)
- Insufficient emptying of each breast
- Unsatisfactory breastfeeding process (mother and infant)
- Sustained infant weight loss

RELATED FACTORS

- Infant anomaly
- Infant receiving supplemental feeding with artificial nipple
- Knowledge deficit
- Maternal ambivalence or anxiety
- Poor infant sucking reflex
- Nonsupportive family or partner
- Previous breast surgery or breastfeeding failure

ASSESSMENT FOCUS

(Refer to comprehensive assessment parameters.)
- Communication
- Roles and relationships
- Values and beliefs

EXPECTED OUTCOMES

The mother will
- Express physical and psychological comfort in breastfeeding practice and techniques.
- Show decreased anxiety and apprehension.
- State at least one resource for breastfeeding support.

The infant will
- Feed successfully on both breasts and appear satisfied for at least 2 hours after feeding.
- Grow and thrive.

SUGGESTED NOC OUTCOMES

Breastfeeding Establishment: Maternal and Infant; Breastfeeding Assistance; Emotional Support; Lactation Counseling; Nutritional Management; Parent Education; Support Group

INTERVENTIONS AND RATIONALES

<u>Determine:</u> Assess factors that influence mother's decision to breastfeed. *Assessment information will be used to develop interventions.*

Monitor condition of breasts and nipples to identify problems that might interfere with feeding *to pinpoint problem areas.*

Assess readiness of mother to breastfeed and ability of infant to feed. Monitor mother's breastfeeding technique. *Improper technique, which impedes feeding, will cause the mother to experience anxiety.*

<u>Perform:</u> Position mother in Fowler's position *to enhance mother's relaxation during feeding.* Place infant in proper position for optimal feeding *to produce proper sucking motion.*

<u>Inform:</u> Teach mother and selected caregiver the techniques for encouraging letdown, *including* warm shower, breast massage, physically caring for the neonate, and holding the neonate close to the breasts. *These measures reduce anxiety and promote the let-down reflex.*

Teach mother techniques (e.g., lying on her side, positioning the infant correctly, holding the nipple with C position, talking to and cuddling the infant) *that will help the infant latch on to the breast.*

Instruct mother to remove infant from the breast to be burped midway during the feeding *to allow for expulsion of air that is swallowed.*

<u>Attend:</u> Ask frequently during hospitalization whether the mother has questions while she is attempting to breastfeed. *This will give her the confidence she needs to continue when she gets home.*

Provide mother and infant with a quiet, private, comfortable environment in which to breastfeed. *Decreasing stressors will help to promote successful breastfeeding experience.*

Encourage expression of fears and anxieties between the mother and the infant *to reduce anxiety and increase the mother's sense of control over the process.*

<u>Manage:</u> Offer written information, a reading list, or a referral to a breastfeeding support group to allow for review of information after discharge:

Refer to home health nurse *for a follow-up visit in the home.*

Refer to a nutritionist *for information on good nutrition and fluid management.*

SUGGESTED NIC INTERVENTIONS

Breastfeeding Assistance; Emotional Support; Lactation Counseling; Infant; Parent Education; Support Group

REFERENCES

Kaunonen, M., Hannula, L., & Tarkka, M. T. (2012, July). A systematic review of peer support interventions for breastfeeding. *Journal of Clinical Nursing, 21*(13–14), 1943–1954.

Lewallen, L. P., et al. (2006, August). Toward a clinically useful method of predicting early breastfeeding attrition. *Applied Nursing Research, 19*(3), 144–148.

DEFINITION
Break in continuity of the breastfeeding process as a result of inability or inadvisability to put baby to breast for feeding

DEFINING CHARACTERISTICS
- Desire to maintain lactation and provide breast milk for infant's nutritional needs (mother)
- Failure to receive nourishment at breast for some or all feedings (infant)
- Lack of knowledge about expressing or storing milk (mother)
- Separation of mother and infant

RELATED FACTORS
- Contraindications to breastfeeding
- Infant illness
- Maternal employment
- Maternal illness
- Need to wean infant abruptly
- Prematurity

ASSESSMENT FOCUS
(Refer to comprehensive assessment parameters.)
- Coping
- Communication
- Knowledge
- Values and beliefs

EXPECTED OUTCOMES
The mother will
- Express her understanding of factors that necessitate interruption in breastfeeding.
- Express comfort with her decision about whether to resume breastfeeding.
- Express and store breast milk appropriately.
- Resume breastfeeding when the interfering factor ceases.
- Have adequate milk supply when breastfeeding resumes.
- Obtain relief from discomfort associated with engorgement.
- Ensure that infant's nutritional needs are met.

SUGGESTED NOC OUTCOMES
Breastfeeding Maintenance; Knowledge: Breastfeeding; Motivation; Parent–Infant Attachment; Parenting Performance; Role Performance

INTERVENTIONS AND RATIONALES
Determine: Assess mother's understanding for interrupting breastfeeding *to evaluate need for further instruction.*

Assess mother's desire to resume breastfeeding when reasons for interruption are no longer a factor. *The mother may not wish to continue breastfeeding.*

Assess mother's emotional reactions to having to interrupt breastfeeding. *Emotional feelings may affect resumption after interruption.*

<u>Perform:</u> Review mother's daily routine to advise her how to incorporate breastfeeding into her schedule. Mother must have a plan in order to carry on usual routine and still make sure the baby is fed on schedule.

<u>Inform:</u> Instruct mother in methods for expressing and storing breast milk. Demonstrate the use of a breast pump utilizing the following guidelines:

*   Initiate pumping 24 to 48 hours after delivery.
*   Pump a minimum of five times a day.
*   Pump a minimum of 100 minutes a day.
*   Pump long enough to soften breasts each time regardless of duration.

Instruct mother in ways to prevent breast engorgement *to prevent discomfort that may keep infant from sucking effectively.* Teach the mother about the use of nipple shield (if appropriate). *The shield is designed to alter flat or inverted nipples.*

<u>Attend:</u> Provide emotional support and encouragement *to help improve patient's confidence and motivation to resume breastfeeding when possible.*

Reassure mother that infant's nutritional needs will be met through other methods *to allay her anxiety.*

If mother must pump for a prolonged period, encourage her to use a piston-style electric pump. *Using an electric pump rather than a hand pump produces milk with a higher fat content.*

Involve patient in planning and decision making. *Having the ability to participate will encourage greater compliance with the plan to resume breastfeeding.*

If mother chooses not to resume breastfeeding, advise her to wear a supportive bra, apply ice, and take a mild analgesic *to alleviate discomfort associated with engorgement.*

<u>Manage:</u> Refer to a lactation support group *for continued assistance in resuming breastfeeding after an interruption.*

Provide appropriate educational home assessment. If possible, have a home health nurse visit the mother and infant *to assess progress.*

SUGGESTED NIC INTERVENTIONS

Attachment Promotion; Bottle Feeding; Emotional Support; Infant; Lactation Counseling; Parent Education; Teaching: Individual

REFERENCE

Brown, A., & Jordan, S. (2012, July 5). Impact of birth complications on breastfeeding duration: An internet survey. *Journal of Advanced Nursing.*

DEFINITION

Low production of maternal breast milk

DEFINING CHARACTERISTICS

Infant

- Constipation
- Refuses to suck, wants to suck often, or does not seem satisfied after sucking
- Long breastfeeding time
- Frequent crying
- Voids small amounts of concentrated urine
- Weight gain is <500 g in a month

Mother

- Milk production does not progress
- No milk appears when nipple is pressed
- Volume of expressed breast milk is less than prescribed amount

ASSESSMENT FOCUS

(Refer to comprehensive assessment parameters.)

- Comfort
- Growth and development
- Nutritional
- Elimination
- Sleep/Rest
- Coping
- Role relationships

EXPECTED OUTCOMES

The patient will

- Produce sufficient milk to satisfy the growth needs of the neonate.
- Perceive that she is producing sufficient milk for her baby.
- Mother and baby will achieve successful and sustained breastfeeding sessions.
- Be free of emotions related to low self-esteem, poor body image, and guilt.

SUGGESTED NOC OUTCOMES

Knowledge: Infant Care; Newborn Adaptation; Breastfeeding Establishment: Infant; Breastfeeding Establishment: Maternal; Nutritional Status: Nutrient Intake; Parent–Infant Attachment; Self-Esteem

INTERVENTIONS AND RATIONALES

Determine: Assess to see if neonate is able to latch properly to the nipple to suckle. *Ensuring the baby has latched to the nipple instead of the areola aids in milk expression.*

Evaluate whether there is adequate milk removal from each breast at each session. *Milk production is stimulated and increases by suckling and milk removal.*

Do a physical examination of the breast every shift; check nipples for inversion and for pore openings, *as anatomical conditions will limit the ability of the milk to flow to the newborn.*

Examine breasts for engorgement, inflammation, infection, or pain. *These conditions cause discomfort and limit the tolerance of the mother to breastfeed; the mother must remain healthy to continue breast-feeding; inflammation and infection needs to be treated.*

Assess exhaustion level and the rest and sleep patterns of mother. *Exhaustion and inability to rejuvenate depresses milk production.*

Assess neonate's mouth to determine normal anatomy of tongue and palate; assess neonate's mouth for Candida infection. *Anatomic imperfections and thrush infection affect the neonate's ability to suckle.*

Assess neonate's nose for patency to allow for breathing during suckling. *Neonates are nose breathers and must have patent nares in order to suckle.*

Monitor neonate's weight gain daily. *Sufficient nutrition from breast milk will allow weight gain.* Weigh neonate before and after breastfeeding session. *When used, this is can provide an indicator that the breast milk is sufficient*

Monitor neonate diaper for urine output (number per day, concentration of urine). *Urine output amount and color are indicators of hydration.* Check fluid-electrolyte status of neonate (urine characteristics and amount; stool output). *These measures guide the health care provider in determining hydration status of the neonate.*

Monitor neonate for clinical presence of jaundice. *Breastfed neonates have lower rates of jaundice; if jaundice develops, it may be an indicator of insufficient milk intake.*

<u>Perform:</u> Position mother/baby properly for baby to latch to nipple and suckle. *The couplet may need direction in assuming the best position of comfort for suckling.*

Provide adequate nourishment and fluid intake to the mother (>150 mL/kg/day). *This is the minimum amount of fluid intake to sustain the mother and provide extra fluid for milk production.*

Provide quiet uninterrupted time for breastfeeding. *Distractions and interruptions interfere with milk production, milk ejection, and the neonate's focus on suckling.*

<u>Inform:</u>

Instruct the mother about the following:

- Milk production may take a week before a sufficient amount is produced. *Understanding expectations improves confidence and reduces anxiety.*

- Suckle the newborn at least 8 times a day to stimulate milk production; goal is 8 to 12 times daily. *Understanding expectations improves confidence and reduces anxiety.*
- Express milk or pump breasts regularly if newborn is unable to suckle. *The breasts must be stimulated frequently to stimulate milk production.*
- Provide mother and family unit nutritional instructions for best foods and fluids for intake to support breast milk production. *Adequate and proper nutrition will aid the mother in recovery from labor and delivery and provide important nutrients to the neonate.*
- Teach mother techniques to keep neonate awake during the feeding sessions. *The neonate often needs stimulation to remain awake at breast to suckle sufficient milk.*

<u>Attend:</u> Encourage mother to talk about emotions including frustration and disappointment. *Allowing other to assist the mother through emotional barriers may assist in creating peaceful emotions that add in milk production and milk let-down.* Listen carefully to mother's concerns for clues to emotions and coping with disappointment and guilt; early signs of depression and stress. *Early intervention allows emotional healing and allows the mother to focus on the neonate and breastfeeding.*

<u>Manage:</u> Check with health care provider about substances and medications that can suppress milk production (i.e., caffeine, tobacco–nicotine, pseudoephedrine, diuretics, contraceptive pills). *To improve and sustain milk production, avoidance of substances that depress or limit milk production is important.*

Use a multidisciplinary team approach to support mother for breast milk production—registered nurse, lactation specialist, certified nurse midwife, pediatrician, registered dietitian, social worker. *A team approach brings expertise to address the needs of the mother and promotes health and well-being for the family unit.*

SUGGESTED NIC INTERVENTIONS

Breastfeeding Assistance; Active Listening; Newborn Care; Parent Education: Infant; Teaching: Infant Nutrition; Lactation Counseling; Sleep Enhancement

REFERENCE

American Academy of Pediatrics. (2012). Breastfeeding and the use of human milk: A policy statement. *Pediatrics, 129*(3), e827–e841. doi: 10.1642/peds.2011–3552.

DEFINITION
Inspiration and/or expiration that does not provide adequate ventilation

DEFINING CHARACTERISTICS
- Accessory muscle use
- Altered chest excursion
- Altered respiratory rate or depth or both
- Assumption of 3-point position
- Decreased minute ventilation, expiratory pressure, vital capacity, or tidal volume
- Orthopnea
- Tachypnea or bradypnea
- Dyspnea
- Nasal flaring
- Prolonged expiratory phase
- Pursed lip breathing

RELATED FACTORS
- Anxiety
- Body position
- Chest wall deformity
- Musculoskeletal, neurologic, or neuromuscular impairment
- Obesity
- Pain
- Respiratory muscle fatigue

ASSESSMENT FOCUS
(Refer to comprehensive assessment parameters.)
- Activity/exercise
- Cardiac function
- Neurologic and mental status
- Respiratory function

EXPECTED OUTCOMES
The patient will
- Maintain respiratory rate within 5 breaths/minute of baseline.
- Regain arterial blood gases to baseline.
- Express feelings of comfort when breathing.
- Demonstrate diaphragmatic pursed-lipped breathing.
- Achieve maximal lung expansion with adequate ventilation.
- Maintain heart rate, rhythm, and blood pressure within expected range during periods of activity.
- Demonstrate skill in conserving energy while carrying out activities of daily living (ADLs).

SUGGESTED NOC OUTCOMES
Mechanical Ventilation Response: Adult; Respiratory Status: Airway Patency; Respiratory Status: Gas Exchange; Respiratory Status: Ventilation; Vital Signs

INTERVENTIONS AND RATIONALES
<u>Determine:</u> Monitor and record respiratory rate and depth at least every 4 hours *to detect early stages of respiratory failure.* Auscultate breath sounds at least every 4 hours *to detect decreased or adventitious breath sounds.* Report changes.
<u>Perform:</u> Administer oxygen, as ordered, *to maintain an acceptable level of oxygen at the tissue level.*

Suction airway as needed *to maintain patent airways.*

Assist patient to Fowler's position, *which will promote expansion of lungs and provide comfort*. Support upper extremities with pillows, providing a table and cover it with a pillow to lean on.

Turn and reposition patient at least every 2 hours. Establish a turning schedule for the dependent patient. Post schedule at bedside and monitor frequency. *Turning and repositioning prevent skin breakdown and improve lung expansion and prevent atelectasis.*

Assist patient with ADLs as needed *to conserve energy and avoid overexertion.*

Encourage active exercise: Provide a trapeze or other assistive device whenever possible. *Such devices simplify moving and turning for many patients and allow them to strengthen some upper body muscles.*

Inform: Teach patient the following measures *to promote participation in maintaining health status and improve ventilation*: pursed lip breathing, abdominal breathing, and relaxation techniques (deep breathing, meditation, guided imagery), taking prescribed medications (ensuring accuracy and frequency and monitoring side effects); and scheduling of activities to allow for rest periods.

Teach caregivers to assist patient with ADLs in a way that maximizes patient's potential. *This enables caregivers to participate in patient's care and encourages them to support patient's independence.*

Attend: Provide emotional support and encouragement *to improve patient's self-concept and motivate patient to perform ADLs.*

Involve patient in planning and decision making. *Having the ability to participate will encourage greater compliance with the plan for activity.*

Have patient perform self-care activities. Begin slowly and increase daily, as tolerated. *Performing self-care activities will assist patient to regain independence and enhance self-esteem.*

Schedule activities to allow for periods of rest.

Manage: Refer to case manager/social worker *to ensure that a home assessment has been done and that whatever modifications were needed to accommodate the patient's level of mobility have been made. Making adjustments in the home will allow the patient a greater degree of independence in performing ADLs, allowing better conservation of energy.*

Refer patient for evaluation of exercise potential and development of individualized exercise program. *Gradual increase in exercise will promote conditioning and ease breathing.*

SUGGESTED NIC INTERVENTIONS

Airway Management; Anxiety Reduction; Oxygen Therapy; Progressive Muscle Relaxation; Respiratory Monitoring; Ventilation Assistance

REFERENCE

Messenger, R. W. (2012, May/June). Reducing chronic obstructive pulmonary disease readmissions: The role of the durable medical equipment provider. *Professional Case Management, 17*(3), 109–114.

DEFINITION

Inadequate blood pumped by the heart to meet metabolic demands of the body

DEFINING CHARACTERISTICS

- Altered heart rate and rhythm
- Arrhythmias, palpitations, electrocardiographic changes
- Altered preload (decreased or increased CVP/PAWP, edema, fatigue, jugular vein distension, murmurs, weight gain)
- Altered afterload (cold, clammy skin; shortness of breath; oliguria; prolonged capillary refill; decreased peripheral pulses; variations in blood pressure; increased/decreased systemic vascular resistance; increased/decreased pulmonary vascular resistance; skin color changes
- Altered contractility (crackles, cough, orthopnea/paroxysmal nocturnal dyspnea, cardiac output (<4 L/minute), cardiac index (less than 2.5 L/minute), decreased ejection fraction, stroke volume index, audible S_3 or S_4 sounds
- Anxiety/restlessness

RELATED FACTORS

- Altered afterload
- Altered contractility
- Altered heart rate
- Altered heart rhythm
- Altered preload
- Altered stroke volume

ASSESSMENT FOCUS

(Refer to comprehensive assessment parameters.)

- Cardiac function
- Respiratory function
- Activity/exercise
- Fluid and electrolytes

EXPECTED OUTCOMES

The patient will

- Maintain pulse within predetermined limits.
- Maintain blood pressure within predetermined limits.
- Exhibit no arrhythmias.
- Maintain warm and dry skin.
- Exhibit no pedal edema.
- Maintain acceptable cardiac output.
- Verbalize understanding of reportable signs and symptoms.
- Understand diet, medication regimen, and prescribed activity level.

SUGGESTED NOC OUTCOMES

Cardiac Pump Effectiveness; Circulation Status; Tissue Perfusion: Peripheral; Vital Signs

INTERVENTIONS AND RATIONALES

Determine: Monitor patient at least every 4 hours for irregularities in heart rate, rhythm, dyspnea, fatigue, crackles in lungs, jugular venous distension, or chest pain. *Any or all of these may indicate impending cardiac failure or other complications. Report changes immediately.*

Perform: Administer oxygen as ordered *to increase supply to myocardium.*

Turn and reposition patient at least every 2 hours. Establish a turning schedule for the dependent patient. Post schedule at bedside and monitor frequency. *Turning and repositioning prevent skin breakdown and improve lung expansion and prevent atelectasis.*

Administer antiarrhythmic drugs, as ordered, *to reduce or eliminate rhythm disturbances. Monitor for adverse effects.*

Administer stool softeners, as prescribed, *to reduce straining during bowel movements.*

Measure and record intake and output. *Decreased urinary output without decreased fluid intake may indicate decreased renal perfusion resulting from decreased cardiac output.*

Weigh patient daily before breakfast *to detect fluid retention.*

Perform active or passive range of motion (ROM) exercises to all extremities every 2 to 4 hours. *ROM exercises foster muscle strength and tone, maintain joint mobility, and prevent contractures.*

Inspect legs and feet *for pedal edema.*

Maintain dietary restrictions, as ordered, *to prevent fluid retention, dehydration, weight gain or loss.*

Gradually increase levels of activity within prescribed limits of cardiac rate *to allow heart to adjust to increased cardiac demands.*

Inform: Educate patient and his or her family about chest pain and other reportable symptoms, prescribed diet, medications (name, dosage, frequency, and therapeutic and adverse effects), prescribed activity level, simple methods of lifting and bending, and stress-reduction techniques. *Education promotes remembering of and compliance with techniques to reduce energy consumption.*

Attend: Provide emotional support and encouragement *to help* improve patient's self-concept.

Involve patient in planning and decision making. *Having the ability to participate will encourage greater compliance with the plan of treatment.*

Have patient perform self-care activities. Begin slowly and increase daily, as tolerated. *Performing self-care activities will assist patient to regain independence and enhance self-esteem.*

Manage: Refer to case manager/social worker *to ensure that a home assessment has been done and that whatever modifications are needed to accommodate the patient's ongoing care have been made.* Refer to cardiac program for exercise when the time is appropriate.

SUGGESTED NIC INTERVENTIONS

Cardiac Precautions; Circulatory Precautions; Fluid Management; Homodynamic Regulation; Vital Signs Monitoring

REFERENCE

Albert, N. M., et al. (2012, March). Complexities of care for patients and families living with advanced cardiovascular diseases: Overview. *Journal of Cardiovascular Nursing, 27*(2), 103–113.

DEFINITION
Difficulty in performing a family caregiver role

DEFINING CHARACTERISTICS
- Difficulty performing/completing required tasks
- Preoccupation with care routine
- Apprehension about care receiver's health and caregivers' ability to provide care
- Fate of the care receiver if the caregiver becomes ill or dies, or the possible institutionalization of care receiver
- Caregiver–care receiver relationship: grief or uncertainty regarding changed relationship with care receiver
- Difficulty with watching care receiver experience the illness

RELATED FACTORS
- Caregiver health status—physical: CV disease, diabetes, fatigue, hypertension, weight change; emotional (e.g., anger, frustration, impatience, stress); socioeconomic (e.g., changes in leisure activities, withdraws from social life)
- Caregiver–care receiver relationship (e.g., difficulty, grief, or uncertainty about changes)
- Caregiving activities (e.g., apprehension, difficulty in performing or completing required tasks)
- Family processes (e.g., concerns about family members, family conflict)

ASSESSMENT FOCUS
(Refer to comprehensive assessment parameters.)
- Behavior
- Coping
- Emotional
- Home environment
- Neurocognition
- Role/relationships
- Support systems

EXPECTED OUTCOMES
The caregiver will
- Describe current stressors.
- Identify stressors that can and can't be controlled.
- Identify formal and informal sources of support.
- Show evidence of using support systems.
- Report increased ability to cope with stress.

SUGGESTED NOC OUTCOMES
Caregiver Emotional Health; Caregiver Lifestyle Disruption; Caregiver Stressors; Caregiver Well-Being; Caregiver Role Endurance; Caregiver Adaptation to Patient Institutionalization; Caregiver Home Care Readiness

INTERVENTIONS AND RATIONALES

<u>Determine:</u> Help caregivers identify current stressors *to evaluate the causes of role strain.*

<u>Perform:</u> Provide care, as indicated, *to give caregivers respite.*

<u>Inform:</u> Suggest ways for caregivers to use time more efficiently. For example, caregiver may save time by filling out insurance forms while visiting and chatting with care recipient. *Better time management may help caregiver reduce stress.*

<u>Attend:</u> Using a nonjudgmental approach, help caregiver evaluate which stressors are controllable and which aren't *to begin to develop strategies to reduce stress.*

Encourage caregiver to discuss coping skills used to overcome similar stressful situations in the past *to build confidence for managing the current situation.*

Encourage caregiver to participate in a support group. Provide information on organizations such as Alzheimer's Association, Children of Aging Parents, or the referral service of the community-acquired immunodeficiency syndrome task force *to foster mutual support and provide an opportunity for caregiver to discuss personal feelings with empathetic listeners.*

Help caregiver identify informal sources of support, such as family members, friends, church groups, and community volunteers, *to provide resources for obtaining an occasional or regularly scheduled respite.*

Help caregiver identify available formal support services, such as home health agencies, municipal or county social services, hospital social workers, physicians, clinics, and day-care centers, *to enhance coping by providing a reliable structure for support.*

If caregiver seems overly anxious or distraught, gently point out facts about care recipient's mental and physical condition. *Many times, especially when care recipient is a family member, caregiver's perspective is clouded by a long history of emotional involvement. Your input may help caregiver view the situation more objectively.*

<u>Manage:</u> If you believe that excessive emotional involvement is hindering caregiver's ability to function, consider recommending Co-Dependents Anonymous, a support group for people whose preoccupation with a relationship leads to chronic suffering and diminished effectiveness, *to provide support.*

SUGGESTED NIC INTERVENTIONS

Active Listening; Caregiver Support; Coping Enhancement; Counseling; Role Enhancement; Support Group

REFERENCE

Lohne, V., Miaskowski, C., & Rustøen, T. (2012, March/April). The relationship between hope and caregiver role strain in family caregivers of patients with advanced cancer. *Cancer Nursing, 35*(2), 99–105.

DEFINITION

Caregiver is vulnerable for felt difficulty in performing the family caregiver role

RISK FACTORS

- Not developmentally ready for caregiver role (e.g., young adult who must unexpectedly care for a middle-age parent)
- Evidence of drug or alcohol addiction in caregiver or care recipient, health impairment of caregiver, severity or unpredictable course of illness, or instability of care recipient's health
- Evidence of codependency; deviant, bizarre behavior of care recipient; dysfunctional family coping patterns that existed before the caregiving situation
- Situational factors, such as close relationship between caregiver and care recipient; discharge of family member with significant home care needs; inadequate environment or facilities for providing care; isolation, inexperience, or overwork of caregiver; lack of recreation for caregiver; presence of abuse or violence; simultaneous occurrence of other events that cause stress for family (significant personal loss, natural disaster, economic hardship, or major life events)

ASSESSMENT FOCUS

(Refer to comprehensive assessment parameters.)
- Behavior
- Coping
- Knowledge
- Neurocognition
- Role/relationships

EXPECTED OUTCOMES

The caregiver will
- Identify current stressors.
- Identify appropriate coping strategies and will state plans to incorporate strategies into daily routine.
- State intention to contact formal and informal sources of support.
- State intention to incorporate recreational activities into daily routine.
- Report satisfaction with ability to cope with stress caused by caregiving responsibilities.

SUGGESTED NOC OUTCOMES

Caregiver Emotional Health; Caregiver Home Care Readiness; Caregiver Lifestyle Disruption; Caregiver–Patient Relationship; Caregiver Physical Health; Caregiver Stressors; Caregiver Role Endurance

INTERVENTIONS AND RATIONALES

Determine: Help caregiver identify current stressors. Ask whether stress is likely to increase or decrease in the future *to evaluate the risk of caregiver role strain.*

Attend: Encourage caregiver to discuss coping skills used to overcome similar stressful situations in the past *to bolster caregiver's confidence in ability to manage current situation and explore ways to apply coping strategies before caregiver becomes overwhelmed.*

Help caregiver identify formal and informal sources of support, such as home health agencies, municipal or county social services, hospital social workers, physicians, clinics and day-care centers, family members, friends, church groups, and community volunteers, *to plan for an occasional or regularly scheduled respite.*

Encourage caregiver to discuss hobbies or diversional activities. *Incorporating enjoyable activities into the daily or weekly schedule will discipline caregiver to take needed breaks from caregiving responsibilities and thereby diminish stress.*

Encourage caregiver to participate in a support group. Provide information on organizations such as Alzheimer's Association and Children of Aging Parents *to foster mutual support and provide an outlet for expressing feelings before frustration becomes overwhelming.*

If caregiver seems overly anxious or distraught, gently point out facts about care recipient's mental and physical condition. *Many times a caregiver's perspective is clouded by a long history of emotional involvement. Your input may help caregiver view the situation more objectively.* Suggest ways for caregiver to use time efficiently. *Better time management may help caregiver reduce stress.*

Manage: If you believe that excessive emotional involvement is hindering caregiver's ability to function, consider recommending Co-Dependents Anonymous *to provide support.*

SUGGESTED NIC INTERVENTIONS

Caregiver Support; Home Maintenance Assistance; Referral; Respite Care; Role Enhancement; Support Group

REFERENCE

Conway, F., Jones, S., & Speakes-Lewis, A. (2011, April). Emotional strain in caregiving among African American grandmothers raising their grandchildren. *Journal of Women Aging, 23*(2), 113–128.

DEFINITION

Pregnancy and childbirth process and care of the newborn that does not match the environmental context, norms, and expectations

DEFINING CHARACTERISTICS

During pregnancy

- Does not access support systems; make appropriate physical preparations; report appropriate prenatal lifestyle, availability of support systems, management of unpleasant symptoms of pregnancy, realistic birth plan; failure to seek knowledge (labor and delivery, newborn care), prepare newborn care items, make prenatal visits, or respect unborn baby

During labor and delivery

- Does not access support systems; demonstrate attachment behavior to newborn; report appropriate lifestyle; respond appropriately to labor; lacks proactivity during labor and delivery

After birth

- Does not access support systems; demonstrate appropriate feeding techniques, breast care, or attachment to newborn

RELATED FACTORS

- Maternal age
- Maternal lifestyle choices, that is, tobacco smoking, substance abuse
- Maternal lack of resources
- Family unit/support system
- Cultural beliefs or expectations

ASSESSMENT FOCUS

(Refer to comprehensive assessment parameters.)

- Comfort
- Growth and development
- Nutrition
- Values/beliefs
- Fluids and electrolytes
- Physical regulation
- Respiratory function
- Tissue integrity
- Behavior
- Coping
- Emotional
- Knowledge
- Roles and relationships

EXPECTED OUTCOMES

The mother and family unit will

- Demonstrate a willingness to improve her lifestyle and adhere to medical recommendations for optimal prenatal health.
- Seek and convey confidence in knowledge about pregnancy, the labor and the delivery processes, and newborn care.
- Cooperate and follow the care directives of the health care team during labor and delivery and the postpartum period.

- Demonstrate coping and emotional strength to adapt to emergent situations during the prenatal, intrapartal, postpartal, and newborn care periods.
- Exhibit maternal interest, attachment, and bonding with the newborn.
- Perform skills for self-care and newborn care including breastfeeding skills.
- Seek to meet positive self-care needs and to meet the newborn's physical, social, nutritional, and safety needs.

SUGGESTED NOC OUTCOMES

Fetal Status: Antepartum; Fetal Status: Intrapartum; Newborn Adaptation; Breastfeeding Establishment: Infant; Breastfeeding Establishment: Maternal; Parent–Infant Attachment; Role Performance; Prenatal Health Behavior; Knowledge: Breastfeeding; Knowledge: Infant Care; Knowledge: Labor and Delivery; Maternal Status: Antepartum; Maternal Status: Intrapartum; Maternal Status: Postpartum

INTERVENTIONS AND RATIONALES

Determine. Assess baseline knowledge of prenatal self-care, labor and delivery process, and newborn care *to identify and resolve knowledge deficits.*

Assess physical and psychological states of the mother during pregnancy *in order to treat medical conditions and develop a patient-centered plan to address needs and deficits.*

Monitor physiologic vital signs and parameters at each phase of childbearing frequently *as these aid the clinicians in determining courses of action in response to evolving pathophysiologic needs.*

Monitor the emotional baseline of mother/family unit *to identify strengths needed to cope with unknown rapidly changing conditions.*

Perform: Anticipate needs and provide opportunities for mother to reach out for assistance and knowledge for her self-care and expectations of labor and delivery and newborn care. *Mother's engagement in the processes demonstrates interest and initiates autonomy.*

Provide interventions for emergent conditions according to nursing standards of practice within clinical pathway protocols. *Adherence to evidence-based standards and practice guidelines benefits the mother-neonate-family unit and provides quality, efficient team-based care.*

Inform: Teach mother self-care for common prenatal discomforts *to promote patient comfort and autonomy.*

Teach the mother about the pregnancy process and the labor and delivery. *Understanding expectations improves confidence, reduces anxiety, and aids in creating a trusting relationship.*

Demonstrate comfort techniques that aid in labor management and delivery. *As the individual is free from discomfort, she can be more accepting of instruction and assist in the labor–delivery processes.*

Include mother in planning for changes in treatment plan during labor and delivery. *This indicates respect and reduces anxiety and fear of the unknown.*

Provide accurate information to mother/family unit during crisis/emergent situations. *This aids in anxiety reduction, trust establishment, and the family unit's ability to cooperate with the treatment team for the safety of mother and fetus/newborn.*

Demonstrate techniques that match the mother's abilities to care for the newborn while newborn is undergoing therapeutic care. *Demonstrates respect and individualization of the plan of care for the mother to meet the physical and emotional needs of the newborn.*

Attend: Provide supportive environment during prenatal, intrapartum, and postpartum periods *when the mother feels comfortable and cared for, she can focus on self-care, healing, and care of newborn undergoing intensive care management.*

Provide bonding time between newborn and mother/family unit, encourage skin-to-skin cuddling, and encourage breastfeeding at delivery. *These and other actions enhance critical bond development between mother/family unit and newborn.*

Support the mother/family unit in the recovery and healing processes for the mother and the neonate following unplanned, emergent stressful events. *Allowing the mother/family unit to verbalize and explore feelings and emotions aids in the integration process of healing.*

Manage: Arrange for transportation to provider for clinic visit. *Nonadherence to prenatal and postpartum visits may be related to transportation.*

Provide antenatal and postnatal classes on self-care and care of the newborn by a certified childbirth educator. *Advanced knowledge of the childbearing process promotes empowerment and positive maternal outcomes.*

Coordinate multidisciplinary team—registered nurse, nurse midwife, physician, lactation consultant, registered dietitian, social worker. *These professionals assess and uniquely meet the needs of the mother and newborn when there have been events that interfered with the childbearing processes.*

Assist the family unit to develop the support system/network if management of medical and neonatal conditions warrants extended hospitalization. *Anticipatory guidance in seeking resources and assistance will aid the family to cope and provide autonomy in supporting the family as it supports its members in the hospital.*

SUGGESTED NIC INTERVENTIONS

Role Enhancement; Parent Education: Infant; Teaching: Infant Safety 0–3 Months; Birthing; Infant Care; Family Involvement Promotion; Coping Enhancement; Family Integration Promotion

REFERENCE

Doyle, C. S. (2012). When delivery expectations change. *AWHONN Nursing for Women's Health, 15*(6), 465–569.

DEFINITION
A pattern of preparing for, maintaining and strengthening a healthy pregnancy and childbirth process and care of newborn

DEFINING CHARACTERISTICS
During pregnancy
- Reports appropriate prenatal lifestyle, physical preparations; managing unpleasant symptoms in pregnancy
- Demonstrates respect for unborn baby
- Reports a realistic birth plan
- Prepares necessary newborn care items
- Seeks necessary knowledge (e.g., of labor and delivery, newborn care)
- Reports availability of support systems
- Has regular prenatal health visits

During labor and delivery
- Reports lifestyle that is appropriate for the stage of labor
- Responds appropriately to the onset of labor
- Is proactive in labor and delivery
- Uses relaxation techniques appropriate for the stage of labor
- Demonstrates attachment behavior to the newborn baby
- Utilizes support systems appropriately

After birth
- Demonstrates appropriate baby-feeding techniques; basic baby care techniques
- Provides safe environment for the baby
- Reports appropriate lifestyle
- Utilizes support system appropriately

ASSESSMENT FOCUS
(Refer to comprehensive assessment parameters.)
- Behavior
- Knowledge
- Roles/relationships

EXPECTED OUTCOMES
The patient/childbearing family will
- Demonstrate a willingness to maintain/modify his or her lifestyle for optimal prenatal health.
- Convey confidence and knowledge of pregnancy, the labor and delivery process, and newborn care.
- Express appropriate self-control and readily cooperate with recommendations of the health care team during labor and delivery.

- Exhibit parent–newborn attachment after delivery.
- Meet the newborn's physical, social, and nutritional needs.

SUGGESTED NOC OUTCOMES

Prenatal Health Behavior; Knowledge: Pregnancy; Knowledge: Labor & Delivery; Knowledge: Newborn Care; Parent-Infant Attachment

INTERVENTIONS AND RATIONALES

<u>Determine:</u> Assess baseline knowledge of prenatal self-care, labor and delivery process, and newborn care *to identify and resolve knowledge deficits.*

<u>Perform:</u> Provide written literature on prenatal wellness, labor and delivery expectations, and newborn care. *Providing written materials allows adequate time to synthesize and understand new information.*

<u>Inform:</u> Teach self-care for common prenatal discomforts to *promote patient autonomy.*

Teach childbearing family labor and delivery process and newborn care. *Understanding expectations improves confidence and reduces anxiety.*

<u>Attend:</u> Assist childbearing family with development of a birth plan. *This allows childbearing family to participate in managing the birth experience and promotes communication with the health care team.*

Encourage and support childbearing family throughout the course of the pregnancy *to improve self-confidence and promote patient compliance with health recommendations.*

<u>Manage:</u> Refer to certified childbirth educator for classes on prenatal care, labor and delivery (to include Cesarean birth), breastfeeding, and newborn care. *Advanced knowledge of the childbearing process promotes empowerment and positive maternal outcomes.*

SUGGESTED NIC INTERVENTIONS

Anticipatory Guidance; Childbirth Preparation; Emotional Support; Parent Education: Infant, Prenatal Care

REFERENCE

Vasquez, M. J., & Berg, O. R. (2012, January). The Baby-Friendly journey in a US public hospital. *Journal of Perinatal Nursing, 26*(1), 37–46.

DEFINITION

Risk for a pregnancy and childbirth process and care of the newborn that does not match the environmental context, norms, and expectations

RISK FACTORS

- Deficient knowledge (e.g., labor and delivery, newborn care)
- Domestic violence
- Inconsistent or lack of prenatal health visits
- Lack of appropriate role models of parenthood and/or support systems
- Lack of cognitive readiness for parenthood and/or maternal confidence
- Lack of a realistic birth plan
- Maternal powerlessness and/or psychological distress
- Suboptimal maternal nutrition
- Premature membrane rupture
- Unplanned and/or unwanted pregnancy

ASSESSMENT FOCUS

(Refer to comprehensive assessment parameters.)

- Comfort
- Nutrition
- Self-care
- Coping
- Reproduction
- Behavior
- Knowledge
- Roles/relationships
- Risk management

EXPECTED OUTCOMES

The patient will

- Demonstrate a willingness to improve her lifestyle for optimal prenatal health.
- Seek and convey confidence in knowledge about pregnancy, the labor and the delivery processes, and newborn care.
- Cooperate and follow the care directives of the health care team during labor and delivery and the postpartum period.
- Exhibit maternal interest, attachment, and bonding with the newborn.
- Performs skills for self-care and newborn care.
- Seek to meet positive self-care needs and to meet the newborn's physical, social, nutritional, and safety needs.

SUGGESTED NOC OUTCOMES

Fetal Status: Antepartum; Fetal Status: Intrapartum; Newborn Adaptation; Breastfeeding Establishment: Infant; Breastfeeding Establishment: Maternal;

Parent–Infant Attachment; Role Performance; Prenatal Health Behavior; Knowledge: Breastfeeding; Knowledge: Infant Care; Knowledge: Labor and Delivery; Maternal Status: Antepartum; Maternal Status: Intrapartum; Maternal Status: Postpartum

INTERVENTIONS AND RATIONALES

<u>Determine:</u> Assess baseline knowledge of prenatal self-care, labor and delivery process, and newborn care *to identify and resolve knowledge deficits.*

Assess physical and psychological states of the mother during pregnancy *in order to treat medical conditions and develop plan to address deficits.*

Analyze cultural beliefs contributing to mother's behavior *since understanding by the health care team can aid in determining a plan of approach and treatment that is patient centered.*

<u>Perform:</u> Convey a nonjudgmental attitude *to allow a trusting relationship to develop.*

Anticipate needs and provide opportunities for mother to reach out for assistance and knowledge for her self-care and expectations of labor and delivery and newborn care. *Mother's engagement in the processes demonstrates interest and initiates autonomy.*

Monitor intrapartal parameters according to accepted standard of practice *to maintain physiologic needs and respond to evolving pathophysiologic needs.*

Implement treatment plan prenatally or intrapartum to alleviate medical conditions *to enhance the physiologic condition of the mother.*

<u>Inform:</u> Teach mother self-care for common prenatal discomforts *to promote patient autonomy.*

Teach the mother about the pregnancy process and the labor and delivery. *Understanding expectations improves confidence, reduces anxiety, and aids in creating a trusting relationship.*

Demonstrate comfort techniques that aid in labor management and delivery. *As the individual is free from discomfort, she can be more accepting of instruction and assist in the labor–delivery processes.*

Include mother in planning for changes in treatment plan during labor and delivery. *This Indicates respect, reduces anxiety and fear of the unknown.*

Demonstrate techniques that match the mother's abilities to care for the newborn. *Demonstrates respect and individualization of the plan of care for the mother.*

<u>Attend:</u> Provide supportive environment during prenatal, intrapartum, and postpartum periods *when the mother feels comfortable and cared for, she can focus on self-care and care of newborn.*

Provide bonding time between newborn and mother, encourage skin-to-skin cuddling, and encourage breastfeeding at delivery. *These and other actions enhance critical bond development between mother and newborn.*

Provide antenatal and postnatal classes on self-care and care of the newborn by a certified childbirth educator. *Advanced knowledge of the childbearing process promotes empowerment and positive maternal outcomes.*

<u>Manage:</u> Arrange for transportation for clinic visit. *Nonadherence to prenatal and postpartum visits may be related to transportation.*

Coordinate multidisciplinary team; registered nurse, nurse midwife, physician, lactation consultant, registered dietitian, social worker. *These professionals assess and uniquely meet the needs of the mother and newborn.*

SUGGESTED NIC INTERVENTIONS

Role Enhancement; Parent Education: Infant; Teaching: Infant Safety; Birthing; Infant Care; Family Involvement Promotion; Coping Enhancement

REFERENCE

Cooke, A., Mills, T. A., & Lavender, T. (2012, January). Advanced maternal age: Delayed childbearing is rarely a conscious choice a qualitative study of women's views and experiences. *International Journal of Nursing Studies, 49*(1), 30–39.

DEFINITION

Perceived lack of ease, relief, and transcendence in physical, psychospiritual, environmental, and social dimensions

DEFINING CHARACTERISTICS

- Disturbed sleep pattern, inability to relax, and restlessness
- Insufficient resources (e.g., financial, social support)
- Lack of environmental or situational control
- Lack of privacy
- Noxious environmental stimuli
- Reports being uncomfortable, hot or cold, or hungry
- Reports distressing symptoms, anxiety, crying, irritability, and moaning
- Reports itching
- Reports lack of contentment in situation
- Treatment-related side effects (e.g., medication, radiation)

ASSESSMENT FOCUS

- Cardiac
- Muscle tone
- Pain
- Respiratory
- Sleep patterns

EXPECTED OUTCOMES

The patient will
- Maintain heart rate, rhythm, and respiration rate within expected range during rest and activity.
- Maintain muscle mass and strength.
- Report pain using pain scale.
- Report periods of restful sleep.

SUGGESTED NOC OUTCOMES

Comfort Status; Coping; Knowledge Health Promotion; Pain Control; Comfort Status: Environment, Physical, Sociocultural, and Psychospiritual

INTERVENTIONS AND RATIONALES

<u>Determine:</u> Monitor pain level using scale 1 to 10. *Using a scale will allow evaluation of the effectiveness of pain-relieving measures.*

Assess vital signs during times of discomfort, including blood pressure, heart rate and rhythm, and respirations. *Use the patient's baseline vital signs to evaluate response to pain and response to pain-relieving measures.*

Assess sleeping patterns in response to discomfort. *Interruption of sleep is common in patients experiencing discomfort.*

<u>Perform:</u> Provide a quiet and relaxing atmosphere. Encourage active exercise *to increase feeling of well-being.* Provide pain medications as ordered; evaluate response *to evaluate effectiveness of pain-relieving measures.*

<u>Inform:</u> Teach relaxation exercises and techniques *to promote reduced pain levels, sleep, and anxiety.* Teach medication administration and schedule to facilitate pain relief. Teach massage therapy to caregiver *to promote comfort.*

<u>Attend:</u> Provide support and encouragement during periods of discomfort. Include patient in plan of action *to promote self-care.*

<u>Manage:</u> Refer to pain management clinic if pain cannot be controlled through relaxation and exercise. Refer to physical therapist to accommodate patient's level of physical activity. Refer to massage therapist to promote relaxation. *All health care professionals contribute to the overall goal of maintaining comfort.*

SUGGESTED NIC INTERVENTIONS

Active Listening; Aromatherapy; Calming Technique; Massage; Environmental Management: Comfort Coping Enhancement

REFERENCE

Campbell, M. L. (2010, September). Assessing respiratory distress when the patient cannot report dyspnea. *Nursing Clinics of North America, 45*(3), 363–373.

DEFINITION

A pattern of ease, relief, and transcendence in physical, psychospiritual environmental, and/or social dimensions is sufficient for well-being and can be strengthened

DEFINING CHARACTERISTICS

- Expresses desire to enhance comfort
- Expresses desire to enhance feelings of contentment
- Expresses desire to enhance relaxation
- Expresses desire to enhance resolution of complaints

ASSESSMENT FOCUS

(Refer to comprehensive assessment parameters.)

- Behavior
- Communication
- Coping

EXPECTED OUTCOMES

The patient will

- Express positive perception of nursing assistance to perform activities that promote comfort.
- Experience physical and psychological ease.
- Develop plans to optimize level of comfort.
- Report an increase in relaxation.

SUGGESTED NOC OUTCOMES

Coping Enhancement; Client Satisfaction: Caring; Comfort Status; Environmental Management; Comfort Status: Environment, Physical, Sociocultural, and Psychospiritual

INTERVENTIONS AND RATIONALES

<u>Determine:</u> Assess patient's satisfaction with the amount of assistance the nurse is presently offering *to determine whether the patient perceives self as performing physical, psychosocial, and spiritual activities as a level that is comfortable for self-changes in status.*

Determine what enhancements to care can be made *to provide the patient a greater degree of comfort.*

Ask for feedback from the patient at least once a day *to evaluate progress.*

<u>Perform:</u> Adjust environmental factors, where possible, *to enhance the patient's feeling of a safe and comfortable environment.*

Assist patient with bathing, feeding, and toileting *to ensure that his or her needs are met.*

Turn and reposition patient every 2 hours *to promote comfort.*

Inform: Teach patient when he or she is ready about his or her disease. Present only what patient is able and willing to absorb *to prevent him or her from becoming overwhelmed.*

Avoid insisting that the patient accept information. *Readiness is an important factor in adult education.* Provide both patient and family with written information such as pamphlets and so forth.

Teach the patient and family techniques for relaxation such as guided imagery *to promote comfort and reduce anxiety.*

Attend: Provide emotional support and encouragement *to help improve ability of patient to cope with the diagnosis.*

Involve patient in planning and decision making. *Having the ability to participate will encourage greater compliance with the plan and enhance comfort.*

Encourage patient to communicate with others, asking questions and clarifying concerns based on readiness. *This will enhance the patient's learning ability.*

Manage: Maintain frequent communication with physicians and other staff *to determine what the patient is being told about his or her condition.*

Collaboration will foster consistency in what the patient is being told.

Refer patient to a mental health professional/grief counselor *if denial interferes with ability of patient to function within limits.*

SUGGESTED NIC INTERVENTIONS

Anxiety Reduction; Calming Techniques; Counseling; Health Education; Reality Orientation; Truth Telling; Environmental Management: Comfort

REFERENCE

Decker S. A., et al. (2012, August). Healingtouch for older adults with persistent pain. *Holistic Nursing Practice, 26*(4), 194–202.

DEFINITION

A pattern of exchanging information and ideas with others that is sufficient for meeting one's needs and life's goals and can be strengthened

DEFINING CHARACTERISTICS

- Expresses willingness to enhance communication ability
- Able to speak or write language clearly
- Forms words, phrases, and language with articulation
- Uses and interprets nonverbal cues appropriately
- Expresses satisfaction with ability to share information and ideas with others
- Expresses needs in an assertive way

ASSESSMENT FOCUS

(Refer to comprehensive assessment parameters.)

- Communication
- Coping
- Roles and relationships
- Values and beliefs

EXPECTED OUTCOMES

The patient will

- Express message clearly as evidenced by feedback that receiver understood message.
- Express an increased sense of confidence in communicating thoughts and feelings.
- Report enhanced ability to respond assertively to individuals.
- Report feelings of confidence in social encounters.
- Gain practice in applying enhanced communication techniques with individuals, family, and groups.
- Enhance communication by nonverbal means, such as use of electronic mail and Internet connections, pictures, and drawings.
- Use enhanced communication skills to negotiate and advocate for self.

SUGGESTED NOC OUTCOMES

Communication: Expressive; Communication: Receptive; Health-Seeking Behaviors

INTERVENTIONS AND RATIONALES

Determine: Listen for themes presented during nurse–client interactions *because themes can provide areas of focus for patient discussions with caregiver.*

Establish a clear purpose for interaction. *This provides the patient with goals and a time frame for interaction.*

<u>Perform:</u> Provide an environment that diminishes space between the patient and the nurse *to eliminate barriers to communication such as noise and lack of privacy.*

Incorporate questions that are open-ended and start with such words as "what," "how," and "could," rather than "why." *Open-minded, non threatening questioning encourages patient to discuss issues of concern and improve communication skills.*

Schedule frequent interdisciplinary treatment team meetings regarding communication skill development with patient. *Team meetings with the patient can ensure continuity of care.*

<u>Inform:</u> Educate patient and family members about the aging process. *Educating the patient and family will help them anticipate processes that will naturally occur again.*

Teach theory of assertive behavior and role-play assertive communication approaches. *Assertive training can decrease passive or aggressive communication patterns.*

Include role-playing as a teaching strategy *to model methods of enhanced verbal and nonverbal communication skills. Role-playing in a nonthreatening, safe environment can enhance communication skills.*

<u>Attend:</u> Encourage patient verbally and nonverbally to explore strategies to enhance self-advocacy communication skills with health care providers. *Self-advocacy communication can guide a patient toward autonomy, confidence, and independence.*

Provide support through active listening, appropriate periods of silence, reflection on feelings, and paraphrasing and summarizing comments. *Active listening techniques encourage patient participation in communication.*

Provide patient with clear explanations for everything that will happen to him. Ask for feedback *to ensure that the patient understands. Anxiety may impair patient's cognitive abilities.*

<u>Manage:</u> Identify appropriate social agencies and support groups for the patient and provide referrals *to ensure ongoing opportunities for the patient to increase social interaction.*

SUGGESTED NIC INTERVENTIONS

Active Listening; Anticipatory Guidance; Assertiveness Training; Behavior Modification; Social Skills; Relationship-Building Enhancement; Guided Imagery; Support Group

REFERENCE

MacCallum, A. (2012, March 22–April 11). Delivering optimal patient care through effective communication. *British Journal of Nursing, 21*(6), 383.

DEFINITION
Abrupt onset of reversible disturbances of consciousness, attention, cognition, and perception that develop over a short period of time

DEFINING CHARACTERISTICS
- Fluctuations in level of consciousness (LOC), psychomotor activity, cognition, and sleep–wake cycle
- Hallucinations
- Impaired perceptive ability
- Increased agitation or restlessness
- Misperceptions
- Lack of motivation to initiate and follow through with goal-directed behavior

RELATED FACTORS
- Delirium
- Dementia
- Drug abuse
- Fluctuations in sleep–wake cycle
- Over 60 years of age

ASSESSMENT FOCUS
(Refer to comprehensive assessment parameters.)
- Cardiac function
- Neurocognition
- Nutrition
- Respiratory function
- Risk management
- Sleep/rest

EXPECTED OUTCOMES
The patient/family will
- Experience no injury.
- Maintain a stable neurologic status.
- Start to participate in activities of daily living (ADLs).
- Report feeling increasingly calm and improved ability to cope with confused state.
- Express an understanding of the importance of informing other health care providers about episodes of acute confusion.

SUGGESTED NOC OUTCOMES
Cognition; Cognitive Orientation; Information Processing; Distorted Thought Self-Control

INTERVENTIONS AND RATIONALES
<u>Determine:</u> Assess patient's LOC and changes in behavior *to provide baseline for comparison with ongoing assessment findings.* Monitor neurologic status on a regular basis *to detect any improvement or decline in patient's neurologic function.*

<u>Perform:</u> Limit noise and environmental stimulation *to prevent additional confusion.*

Use appropriate safety measures *to protect patient from injury.* Avoid physical restraints to prevent agitating patient.

Address patient by name and tell him your name *to foster awareness of self and environment.* Also, frequently mention time, place, and date; have a clock and a calendar in sight and refer to these aids.

Give patient short, simple explanations each time you perform a procedure or task *to decrease confusion.* Speak slowly and clearly and allow time to respond *to reduce frustration.*

Schedule nursing care to include quiet times *to help avoid sensory overload.* Plan patient's routine and be consistent *to foster task completion and reduce confusion.*

Ask family members to bring labeled family photos and articles *to create a more secure environment for patient.* Keep patient's possessions in the same place. *A consistent, stable environment reduces confusion and frustration and aids completion of ADLs.*

Inform: Review home measures to use and report if patient begins to exhibit signs of confusion. Tell caregiver to provide short explanations of activities and orient the patient frequently; speak slowly and clearly and allow patient time to respond; and provide patient with a consistent routine. *Teaching empowers patient and family members to take greater responsibility for the health care needs.*

Attend: Have a staff member stay at patient's bedside, if necessary, *to protect him or her from harm.*

Enlist the aid of family member *to help calm patient.* Patiently encourage patient to perform ADLs, dividing tasks into small, critical units.

Be patient and specific in providing instructions. Allow time for patient to perform each task *These measures enhance his or her self-esteem as well as help prevent complications related to inactivity.*

Encourage family members to share stories and discuss familiar people and events with patient *to promote a sense of continuity and create a sense of security and comfort.* Support family members' attempts to interact with patient *to provide positive reinforcement.* Allow time before and after visits for family members to express feelings. *Listening to family members in an open and nonjudgmental manner promotes coping and may help you assess and monitor patient's condition.* Reassure patient and family that confusion is temporary *to help relieve anxiety.* Always include patient in discussions.

Manage: Confer with physician about diagnostic test results, patient's progress in behavior, and patient's LOC. *A collaborative approach to treatment helps ensure high-quality care and continuity of care.*

SUGGESTED NIC INTERVENTIONS

Cognitive Stimulation; Delirium Management; Hallucination Management; Orientation; Cognitive Restructuring; Delusion Management

REFERENCE

Ryu, H. H., & Kim, H. L. (2012, March). Acute confusion in dialysis patients. *Journal of Emergency Medicine, 42*(3), 311–312.

DEFINITION

Irreversible, long-standing, and/or progressive deterioration of intellect and personality characterized by decreased ability to interpret environmental stimuli; decreased capacity for intellectual thought processes; and manifested by disturbances of memory, orientation, and behavior

DEFINING CHARACTERISTICS

- Altered interpretation, response to stimuli, and/or personality
- No change in level of consciousness
- Clinical evidence of organic impairment
- Short- and long-term memory loss
- Progressive or long-standing impaired cognition or socialization

RELATED FACTORS

- Alzheimer's disease
- Cerebral vascular accident
- Head injury
- Korsakoff's psychosis
- Multi-infarct dementia

ASSESSMENT FOCUS

(Refer to comprehensive assessment parameters.)
- Neurocognition
- Role/relationships
- Self-care

EXPECTED OUTCOMES

The patient will
- Remain free of injury caused by confusion.
- Exhibit no signs of depression.
- Maintain weight.
- Have an environment structured for maximum functioning.
- Participate in selected activities to fullest extent possible.
- Receive adequate emotional support.

Family members will
- Discuss strategies to provide care and help patient cope.
- Maintain safety of patient's home environment.
- Receive information on the options available for long-term care.
- Assist patient to prepare for relocation to long-term care facility.

SUGGESTED NOC OUTCOMES

Client Satisfaction: Safety; Cognition; Cognitive Orientation; Distorted Thought Self-Control

INTERVENTIONS AND RATIONALES

Determine: Assess patient's cognitive abilities and changes in behavior *to provide baseline data.*

Weigh patient and include instructions for regular weighing as part of care plan *to monitor patient's nutritional status.*

Perform: Take steps to provide a stable physical environment and consistent daily routine for patient. *Stability and consistency enhance functioning.*

<u>Inform:</u> Teach family members or caregiver strategies to help patient cope with his condition: Place an identification bracelet on patient *to promote safety*; touch patient *to convey acceptance*; avoid unfamiliar situations when possible *to help ensure consistent environment*; provide structured rest periods *to prevent fatigue and reduce stress*; refrain from asking questions patient can't answer *to avoid frustration*; provide finger foods if patient won't sit and eat *to ensure adequate nutrition*; select activities based on patient's interests and abilities and praise him or her for participating in activities *to enhance his or her sense of self-worth*; use television and radio carefully *to avoid sensory overload*; limit choices patient has to make *to provide structure and avoid confusion*; label familiar photos *to provide a sense of security*; use symbols, rather than written signs, to identify patient's room, bathroom, and other facilities *to help patient identify surroundings*; place patient's name in large block letters on clothing and other belongings *to help him recognize his belongings and prevent them from becoming lost*.

<u>Attend:</u> Encourage family members to watch mental status assessments *to provide a more accurate view of patient's abilities.*

Evaluate patient's ability to perform self-care activities, including ability to function alone and drive a car. *Safety is a primary concern.*

Ask family members about their ability to provide care for patient *to assess the need for assistance.*

Project an attentive, nonjudgmental attitude when listening to them *to help ensure that you receive accurate information.*

<u>Manage:</u> Assist family members in contacting appropriate community services. If necessary, act as an advocate for patients within health care system *to help secure services needed for ongoing care.*

Provide family members with information concerning long-term health care facilities. If patient is to be moved to a long-term care facility, explain the decision to him in as simple and gentle terms as possible *to facilitate comprehension.*

Allow patient to express feelings regarding the move *to facilitate grieving over loss of independence.* Provide psychological support to patient and family members *to alleviate stress they may experience during relocation.*

Communicate all aspects of discharge plan to staff members at patient's new residence. *Documenting a discharge plan and communicating it to caregivers help ensure continuity of care.* Interventions should ensure patient's dignity and rights.

SUGGESTED NIC INTERVENTIONS

Cognitive Stimulation; Dementia Management; Family Involvement Promotion; Reality Orientation; Delusion Management

REFERENCE

Glassman, T. J. (2010, January/February). Alcohol measures and terms: A perfect storm for chronic confusion. *Journal of the American College of Health, 58*(4), 397–399.

DEFINITION
At risk for reversible disturbances of consciousness, attention, cognition, and perception that develop over time

RISK FACTORS
- Alcohol use
- Decreased mobility or restraints
- Dementia
- Fluctuation in sleep–wake cycle
- History of stroke
- Impaired cognition
- Infection
- Male gender
- Pharmaceutical agents (e.g., anesthesia, opioids, anticholinergics, multiple medications, psychoactive drugs)
- >60 years
- Pain
- Metabolic abnormalities (e.g., electrolyte imbalances, azotemia, dehydration)
- Sensory deprivation
- Substance abuse
- Urinary retention

ASSESSMENT FOCUS
(Refer to comprehensive assessment parameters.)
- Cardiac function
- Neurocognition
- Nutrition
- Respiratory function
- Risk management
- Sleep/rest

EXPECTED OUTCOMES
The patient will
- Remain free from injury.
- Have a stable neurologic status.
- Obtain adequate amounts of sleep.
- Maintain optimal hydration and nutrition.
- Begin to participate in activities of daily living (ADLs).
- Report feeling increasingly calm.

Family members will
- Report an improved ability to cope with the patient's confused state.
- State the causes of acute confusion.
- Express the necessity for informing health care providers about acute confusion.

SUGGESTED NOC OUTCOMES
Cognitive Orientation; Information Processing; Memory; Personal Safety Behavior

INTERVENTION AND RATIONALES
Determine: Assess patient's level of consciousness (LOC) and changes in behavior *to provide baseline for comparison with ongoing assessment findings.*

Monitor neurologic status on a regular basis *to detect improvement or decline in the patient's neurologic function.*

Perform: Use appropriate safety measures *to protect patient from injury.*
Avoid physical restraints *to prevent agitating patient.*

Address patient by name and tell him or her your name, mention time, place, and date frequently throughout day, and have a large clock and a calendar close by and refer to those aids *to foster awareness of self and environment.*

Give patient short, simple explanations each time you perform a procedure or task *to decrease confusion.* Speak slowly and clearly and allow patient ample time to respond *to reduce his or her frustration and promote task completion.*

Schedule nursing care to provide quiet times for patient *to help avoid sensory overload.* Follow consistent patient routine *to aid task completion and reduces confusion.*

Keep patient's possessions in the same place. *A consistent, stable environment reduces confusion and frustration and aids completion of ADLs.* Ask family to bring labeled family photos and other favorite articles *to create a more secure environment for patient.*

Encourage patient to perform ADLs, dividing tasks into small, critical units. Be patient and specific in providing instructions. Allow time for patient to perform each task. *These measures enhance his or her self-esteem as well as help prevent complications related to inactivity.*

Inform: Discuss episodes of acute confusion with patient and family members *to make sure they understand the cause of confusion.*

Review measures family members can take at home to help patient if he or she begins to exhibit signs of confusion and to report future episodes. Tell them to give patient short explanations of activities; remind him of time, place, and date frequently; speak slowly and clearly and allow patient ample time to respond; and provide patient with a consistent routine. *Teaching empowers patient and family to take greater responsibility for his or her health care needs.*

Attend: Have a staff member stay at patient's bedside, if necessary, *to protect patient from harm.* Enlist family member *to help calm patient.*

Encourage family to share stories and discuss familiar people and events with patient to *promote a sense of continuity, security, and comfort.*

Manage: Confer with physician about diagnostic test results, patient's progress in behavior, and patient's LOC. *A collaborative approach to treatment helps ensure high-quality care and continuity of care.*

SUGGESTED NIC INTERVENTIONS

Behavior Management: Overactivity/Inattention; Cognitive Stimulation; Delirium Management; Hallucination Management; Reality Orientation

REFERENCE

Rudolph, J. L., et al. (2011, November). Validation of a medical record-based delirium risk assessment. *Journal of the American Geriatric Society, 59*(Suppl. 2), 289–294.

DEFINITION

Decrease in normal frequency of defecation accompanied by difficult or incomplete passage of stool and/or passage of excessively hard, dry stool

DEFINING CHARACTERISTICS

- Palpable rectal or abdominal mass
- Borborygmi, hypoactive or hyperactive bowel sounds, or abdominal dullness on percussion
- Bright red blood with stools; bark-colored or black, tarry stools; hard, dry stools; or oozing liquid stools
- Change in bowel pattern; decreased frequency and volume of stool
- Changes in mental status, urinary incontinence, unexplained falls, or elevated body temperature in older adults
- Distended or tender abdomen and feeling of fullness or pressure
- General fatigue, anorexia, headache, indigestion, nausea, or vomiting
- Severe flatus; straining and possible pain during defecation

RELATED FACTORS

- *Functional*: Habitual denial or ignoring urge to defecate, irregular defecation patterns, insufficient physical activity
- *Psychological*: Depression, emotional stress, mental confusion
- *Pharmacological*: Aluminum-containing antacids, and drugs that affect bowels
- *Mechanical*: Electrolyte imbalance, hemorrhoids, prostate enlargement, rectal abscess, anal fissure, or stricture
- *Physiological*: Change in eating patterns or usual foods, dehydration, inadequate dentition or oral hygiene, insufficient fiber or fluid intake

ASSESSMENT FOCUS

(Refer to comprehensive assessment parameters.)
- Elimination
- Nutrition
- Pharmacological function
- Tissue integrity

EXPECTED OUTCOMES

The patient will
- Participate in development of bowel program.
- Report urge to defecate, as appropriate.
- Increase fluid and fiber intake.
- Report easy and complete evacuation of stools.
- Have elimination pattern within normal limits.
- Adopt personal habits that maintain normal elimination.

SUGGESTED NOC OUTCOMES

Bowel Continence; Bowel Elimination; Hydration; Nutritional Status: Food & Fluid Intake

INTERVENTIONS AND RATIONALES

<u>Determine:</u> Monitor frequency and characteristics of patient's stool daily. *Careful monitoring forms the basis of an effective treatment plan.*

Monitor and record patient's fluid intake and output. *Inadequate fluid intake contributes to dry feces and constipation.*

<u>Perform:</u> Provide privacy for elimination *to promote physiological functioning.*

Plan and implement an individualized bowel regimen *to establish a regular elimination schedule*; and exercise routine *to promote abdominal and pelvic muscle tone.*

<u>Inform:</u> Emphasize importance of responding to urge to defecate. *A timely response to the urge to defecate is necessary to maintain normal physiological functioning.*

Teach patient to locate public restrooms and to wear easily removable clothing on outings *to promote normal bowel functioning.* Teach patient to massage abdomen once per day and how to locate and gently massage along the transverse and descending colon. *In the older patient, the neural centers in the lower intestinal wall may be impaired, making it more difficult for the body to evacuate feces. Massage may help stimulate peristalsis and the urge to defecate.*

Teach patient sensible use of laxatives and enemas *to avoid laxative dependency. Overuse of laxatives and enemas may cause fluid and electrolyte loss and damage to intestinal mucosa.*

<u>Attend:</u> Encourage patient to use a bedside commode or walk to toilet facilities to encourage *normal position for evacuation.* Encourage intake of high-fiber foods *to supply bulk for normal elimination and improve muscle tone.* Unless contraindicated, encourage fluid intake of 6 to 8 glasses (1,420 to 1,900 mL) daily *to maintain normal metabolic processes.*

<u>Manage:</u> Help patient understand diet modification plan along with dietitian, if appropriate, *to encourage compliance with prescribed diet.*

SUGGESTED NIC INTERVENTIONS

Bowel Management; Bowel Training; Bowel Incontinence Care; Constipation/Impaction Management; Exercise Promotion; Fluid Management; Nutrition Management

REFERENCE

Şendir, M., et al. (2012). Postoperative constipation risk assessment in Turkish orthopedic patients. *Gastroenterology Nursing, 35*(2), 106–113.

DEFINITION
Self-diagnosis of constipation combined with abuse of laxatives, enemas, and/or suppositories to ensure a daily bowel movement

DEFINING CHARACTERISTICS
- Expectation of passage of stools at the same time each day
- Overuse of laxatives, enemas, and/or suppositories

RELATED FACTORS
- Cultural health beliefs
- Family health beliefs
- Faulty appraisal
- Impaired thought processes

ASSESSMENT FOCUS
(Refer to comprehensive assessment parameters.)
- Activity/exercise
- Coping
- Behavior
- Emotional
- Elimination
- Fluid and electrolytes
- Nutrition

EXPECTED OUTCOMES
The patient will
- Decrease use of laxatives, enemas, or suppositories.
- State understanding of normal bowel function.
- Discuss feelings about elimination pattern.
- Have a return-to-normal elimination pattern.
- Experience bowel movement every _____ day(s) without laxatives, enemas, or suppositories.
- State understanding of factors causing constipation.
- Get regular exercise.
- Describe changes in personal habits to maintain normal elimination pattern.
- State intent to use appropriate resources to help resolve emotional or psychological problems.

SUGGESTED NOC OUTCOMES
Adherence Behavior; Bowel Continence; Bowel Elimination; Health Beliefs; Health Beliefs: Perceived Threat; Knowledge: Health Behavior

INTERVENTIONS AND RATIONALES
<u>Determine:</u> Assess patient's dietary habits and encourage modification to include adequate fluids, fresh fruits and vegetables, and whole grain cereals and breads, which *supply necessary bulk for normal elimination.*

<u>Perform:</u> If not contraindicated, increase patient's fluid intake to about 3 L daily *to increase functional capacity of bowel elimination.*

Establish and implement an individualized bowel elimination regimen based on the patient's needs. *Knowledge of normal body functions will improve patient's understanding of problem.*

<u>Inform:</u> Explain normal bowel elimination habits *so patient can better understand normal and abnormal body functions.*

Instruct patient to avoid straining during elimination *to avoid tissue damage, bleeding, and pain.*

Instruct patient that abdominal massage may help relieve discomfort and promote defecation *because it triggers bowel's spastic reflex.*

Inform patient not to expect a bowel movement every day or even every other day *to avoid the use of poor health practices to stimulate elimination.*

<u>Attend:</u> Encourage patient to engage in daily exercise, such as brisk walking, *to strengthen muscle tone and stimulate circulation.*

Encourage patient to evacuate at regular times *to aid adaptation and routine physiological function.*

Urge patient to avoid taking laxatives, if possible, or to gradually decrease their use *to avoid further trauma to intestinal mucosa.* Reassure patient that normal bowel function is possible without laxatives, enemas, or suppositories *to give patient the necessary confidence for compliance.*

<u>Manage:</u> Give information about self-help groups, as appropriate, *to provide additional resources for patient and family.*

SUGGESTED NIC INTERVENTIONS

Anxiety Reduction; Bowel Training; Bowel Incontinence Care; Bowel Management; Counseling; Health Education; Nutrition Management

REFERENCE

Malaguarnera, G., et al. (2012). Probiotics in the gastrointestinal diseases of the elderly. *Journal of Nutrition Health and Aging, 16*(4), 402–410.

DEFINITION
At risk for a decrease in normal frequency of defecation accompanied by difficult or incomplete passage of stool and/or passage of excessively hard, dry stool

RISK FACTORS
- *Functional*: Habitual denial and ignoring urge to defecate, recent environmental changes, inadequate toileting, irregular defecation habits, insufficient physical activity, and abdominal muscle weakness
- *Mechanical*: Rectal abscess or ulcer, pregnancy, rectal anal stricture, postsurgical obstruction, rectal anal fissures, megacolon (Hirschsprung's disease), electrolyte imbalance, tumors, prostate enlargement, rectocele, rectal prolapse, neurologic impairment, hemorrhoids, and obesity
- *Pharmacological*: Phenothiazines, nonsteroidal anti-inflammatory agents, sedatives, aluminum-containing antacids, laxative overuse, iron salts, anticholinergics, antidepressants, anticonvulsants, antilipemic agents, calcium channel blockers, calcium carbonate, diuretics, sympathomimetics, opiates, and bismuth salts
- *Physiological*: Insufficient fiber intake, dehydration, inadequate dentition/oral hygiene, poor eating habits, insufficient fluid intake, change in usual foods/eating patterns, and decreased motility of gastrointestinal (GI) tract
- *Psychological*: Emotional stress, mental confusion, depression

ASSESSMENT FOCUS
(Refer to comprehensive assessment parameters.)
- Activity/rest
- Behavior
- Elimination
- Fluid and electrolytes
- Nutrition
- Risk management

EXPECTED OUTCOMES
The patient will
- Experience no signs or symptoms of constipation.
- Maintain bowel movement every _____ day(s).
- Consume a high-fiber or high-bulk diet, unless contraindicated.
- Maintain fluid intake of _____ mL daily (specify).
- Express understanding of the relationship between constipation and dietary intake, bulk, and activity.
- Express understanding of preventive measures, such as eating fruit and whole grain breads and cereals and engaging in mild activity, if appropriate.

SUGGESTED NOC OUTCOMES
Bowel Continence; Bowel Elimination; Self-Care: Toileting

INTERVENTIONS AND RATIONALES
<u>Determine:</u> Assess bowel sounds and check patient for abdominal distention. Monitor and record frequency and characteristics of stools *to develop an effective treatment plan for preventing constipation and fecal impaction.*

Record intake and output accurately *to ensure accurate fluid replacement therapy.*

<u>Perform:</u> Initiate bowel program. Place patient on a bedpan or commode at specific times daily, as close to usual evacuation time (if known) as possible; *to aid adaptation to routine physiological function.*

Administer a laxative, an enema, or suppositories, as prescribed, *to promote elimination of solids and gases from GI tract.* Monitor effectiveness.

<u>Inform:</u> Teach patient to gently massage along the transverse and descending colon *to stimulate the bowel's spastic reflex and aid in stools passage.*

Instruct patient, family member, or caregiver in the relationship between diet, activity and exercise, and fluid intake and constipation *to discourage departure from prescribed diet and assist in promoting elimination.*

Review care plan with patient, family member, or caregiver, emphasizing the relationship between the risk factors for constipation and preventive measures *to foster understanding.*

<u>Attend:</u> Encourage fluid intake of 2.5 L daily, unless contraindicated, *to promote fluid replacement therapy and hydration.*

<u>Manage:</u> Consult with a dietitian about how to increase fiber and bulk in patient's diet to the maximum amount prescribed by the physician *to improve intestinal muscle tone and promote comfortable elimination.*

Include a program of mild exercise in your care plan *to promote muscle tone and circulation.*

SUGGESTED NIC INTERVENTIONS
Bowel Training; Bowel Incontinence Care; Bowel Management; Constipation/Impaction Management; Exercise Promotion; Fluid Management; Fluid Monitoring; Nutrition Management

REFERENCE
Ding, M., et al. (2012). The effect of biofeedback training on patients with functional constipation. *Gastroenterological Nursing, 35*(2), 85–92.

DEFINITION
Exposure to environmental contaminants in doses sufficient to cause adverse health effects

DEFINING CHARACTERISTICS
(These are dependent on the causative agent. Agents cause a variety of individual organ responses as well as systemic responses.)
- *Pesticides*: Have dermatological, gastrointestinal (GI), neurological, pulmonary, and renal effects. Categories include insecticides, herbicides, fungicides, antimicrobials, and rodenticides
- *Chemicals*: Have dermatological, immunological, neurological, pulmonary, and renal effects. Categories include petroleum-based agents, anticholinesterases, Type I agents act on proximal tracheobronchial tract, Type II agents act on alveoli and produce systemic effects
- *Biologicals*: Have dermatological, GI, neurological, pulmonary, and renal effects
- *Radiation*: Have dermatological, GI, neurological, pulmonary, and renal effects. Categories include internal such as exposure through ingestion of radioactive material or external such as direct contact with radiological material
- *Pollution*: Have dermatological and pulmonary effects. Categories include trash, raw sewage, and industrial waste

RELATED FACTORS
- *External*: Chemical contamination of food or water, exposure to bioterrorism, radiation, and exposure to areas of contamination
- *Internal*: Extremes of age, nutritional factors, preexisting disease states, pregnancy, and previous exposure

ASSESSMENT FOCUS
(Refer to comprehensive assessment parameters.)
- Populations
- Risk management

EXPECTED OUTCOMES
The patient/community will
- Have minimized health effects associated with contamination.
- Utilize health surveillance data system to monitor for contamination incidents.
- Utilize disaster plan to evacuate and triage affected members.
- Minimize exposure to contaminants.

SUGGESTED NOC OUTCOMES
Community Disaster Readiness; Community Disaster Response; Community Health Status; Health Beliefs: Perceived Threat; Knowledge: Health Resources, Risk Control

INTERVENTIONS AND RATIONALES

Determine: Triage, stabilize, transport, and treat affected community members. *Accurate triage and early treatment provide the best chance of survival to affected persons.*

Monitor individuals for therapeutic effects, side effects, and compliance with postexposure drug therapy. *Drug therapy may extend over a long period of time and will require monitoring for compliance as well as therapeutic and side effects.*

Perform: Help individuals cope with contamination incident; use groups that have survived terrorist attacks as useful resource for victims *to aid in support; those with experience can share reactions and useful coping mechanisms.*

Help individuals deal with feelings of fear, vulnerability, and grief *to minimize risk of traumatic stress.*

Decontaminate persons, clothing, and equipment using approved procedure. *Victims may first require decontamination before entering health facility to receive care in order to prevent the spread of contamination.*

Use appropriate isolation precautions, including universal, airborne, droplet, and contact isolation. *Proper use of isolation precautions prevents cross-contamination.*

Inform: Provide accurate information on risks involved, preventive measures, and use of antibiotics and vaccines *to enhance the use of protective measures.*

Attend: Encourage individuals to talk to others about their fears. Interventions aimed at supporting an individual's coping can help the person deal with feelings of fear, helplessness, and loss of *control that are normal reactions in a crisis situation.*

Manage: Collaborate with other agencies (local health department, emergency medical services, state and federal agencies). *Communication and collaboration among agencies increase ability to handle crises efficiently and correctly.*

SUGGESTED NIC INTERVENTIONS

Bioterrorism Preparedness; Crisis Intervention; Environmental Management. Community; Infection Control; Health Education; Triage; Communicable Disease Management; Surveillance

REFERENCE

Green, P. M., & Polk, L. V. (2012). A nursing conceptual model for contamination. *International Journal of Nursing Knowledge, 23*(1), 10–17.

DEFINITION

Accentuated risk of exposure to environmental contaminants in doses sufficient to cause adverse health effects

RISK FACTORS

External

- Environmental contaminants in the home
- Exposure to heavy metals or chemicals, bioterrorism, atmospheric pollutants, disaster, radiation
- Insufficient or absent use of decontamination protocol
- Flooding, earthquakes, atmospheric pollutants, or other natural disasters
- Contamination of aquifers by septic tanks
- Industrial plant emissions, discharge of contaminants by industries
- Intentional or accidental contamination of food and water supply
- No or inappropriate use of protective clothing
- Physical factors, such as climactic conditions (temperature, wind, geographic area)
- Playing in outdoor areas where environmental contaminants are present
- Social factors, such as overcrowding, sanitation, poverty, personal and household hygiene practices, lack of access to health care

Internal

- Age (<5 years or older adult)
- Female gender
- Concomitant or previous exposures
- Developmental characteristics (gestational age during exposure)
- Nutritional factors or dietary practices
- Preexisting disease states: gender, occupation, history of smoking; presence of bacteria, viruses, toxins, vectors

ASSESSMENT FOCUS

(Refer to comprehensive assessment parameters.)

- Populations
- Risk management

EXPECTED OUTCOMES

The patient/community will

- Remain free from adverse effects of contamination.
- Utilize health surveillance data system to monitor for contamination incidents.
- Participate in mass casualty and disaster readiness drills.
- Remain free from contamination-related health effects.
- Have minimal exposure to contaminants.

SUGGESTED NOC OUTCOMES

Community Disaster Readiness; Community Disaster Response; Community Health Status; Health Beliefs: Perceived Threat; Knowledge: Health Behavior; Knowledge: Health Resources; Risk Control

INTERVENTIONS AND RATIONALES

Determine: Monitor individuals for therapeutic effects, side effects, and compliance with postexposure drug therapy. *Drug therapy may extend over a long period of time and will require monitoring for compliance as well as therapeutic and side effects.*

Perform: Conduct surveillance for environmental contamination; notify agencies authorized to protect the environment of contaminants in the area. *Early surveillance and detection are critical components of preparation.*

Assist individuals in relocating to safer environment *to decrease their risk of contamination.*

Modify environment to minimize risk. *Modification of the environment will decrease the risk of actual contamination.*

Implement decontamination of persons, clothing, and equipment by using approved procedure. Victims may first require decontamination before entering health facility *to receive care in order to prevent the spread of contamination.*

Use appropriate isolation precautions: universal, airborne, droplet, and contact isolation. *Proper use of isolation precautions prevents cross-contamination by contaminating agent.*

Inform: Provide accurate information on risks involved, preventive measures, use of antibiotics and *vaccines to reduce anxiety and increase compliance.*

Attend: Assist community members with feelings of fear and vulnerability. *Interventions aimed at supporting an individual's coping help the person deal with feelings of fear, helplessness, and loss of control that are normal reactions in a crisis situation.*

Manage: In conjunction with other health care providers, schedule mass casualty and disaster readiness drills. *Practice in handling contamination occurrences will decrease the risk of exposure during actual contamination events.*

SUGGESTED NIC INTERVENTIONS

Bioterrorism Preparedness; Communicable Disease Management; Community; Community Disaster Preparedness; Environmental Management: Community Environmental Management: Safety; Environmental Risk Protection; Health Education; Health Policy Monitoring; Health Screening; Immunization/Vaccination Management; Risk Identification; Surveillance: Safety

REFERENCE

Cristino, S., Legnani, P. P., & Leoni, E. (2012, April). Plan for the control of Legionella infections in long-term care facilities: Role of environmental monitoring. *International Journal of Hygiene and Environmental Health, 21*(3), 279–285.

DEFINITION
Usually supportive primary person (family member or close friend) provides insufficient, ineffective, or compromised support, comfort, assistance, or encouragement that may be needed by the patient to manage or master adaptive tasks related to health challenge

DEFINING CHARACTERISTICS
- Significant person attempts to assist or support the patient with unsatisfactory results
- Significant person displays protective behavior disproportionate to the patient's abilities or need for autonomy
- Client expresses concern or complains about the family's response to health problem
- Significant person reports preoccupation with personal reaction to the patient's health need

RELATED FACTORS
- Exhaustion of supportive capacity of significant people
- Inadequate/incorrect or understanding of information by a primary person
- Lack of reciprocal support
- Temporary preoccupation by a significant person

ASSESSMENT FOCUS
(Refer to comprehensive assessment parameters.)
- Behavior
- Communication
- Coping
- Emotional status

EXPECTED OUTCOMES
The family members will
- Assume responsibility for roles and activities formerly held by the patient.
- Express feelings about assuming responsibility of care for family member.

The patient and family members will
- Identify and make use of appropriate community services.
- Express satisfaction with improved ability to cope with current crisis.

SUGGESTED NOC OUTCOMES
Caregiver Emotional Health; Caregiver–Patient Relationship; Caregiver Stressors; Family Coping; Family Normalization; Family Functioning

INTERVENTIONS AND RATIONALES

<u>Determine:</u> Identify the primary caregiver in family and assess roles of other family members. Determine usual coping mechanisms employed by this patient and family. Describe patterns of communication used in problem solving. Identify what support systems exist for the family and patient outside the family. Identify strengths and weakness in the family's communication patterns. *Assessment data will assist with establishment of interventions.*

<u>Perform:</u> Direct development of short- and long-term goals by the patient and family members. *Initially, the family members will need help from the caregiver until they understand more about the process of planning.*

Identify appropriate community services for the family *to assist with* coping.

<u>Inform:</u> Educate patient and family members about the process of aging *to assist patient and family to understand how changes in the patient have affected the family.*

Teach family members ways of maximizing the use of coping strategies that seem to have worked for them in the past. Teach new coping strategies and have family member's role model them. *Practice will help the family practice the behaviors in real situations.*

<u>Attend:</u> Avoid becoming involved in a power struggle between patient and family members. *The patient may no longer be able to fill ordinary roles and the sudden shift in roles may lead to a power struggle.*

Encourage family members to express feelings about caring for an older family member. Be nonjudgmental when listening to the family; discuss the issues associated with caring for an older person. *If the nurse is judgmental, the family members may not be comfortable discussing their problem.*

Provide emotional support for primary caregiver. Some families may hesitate to accept outside help. Other families may be unwilling to make even small sacrifices to care for an older family member. If family members have not been supportive or caring for the elder member before, they are unlikely to change.

<u>Manage:</u> Refer to community agencies (e.g., adult day care, respite care, and geriatric outreach services) *that can assist the family in caring for the elder.* Communicate to the hospice nurse where the patient is at present in coping with the terminal illness.

Refer to case manager or social service *to assist with ongoing coordination of the patient's needs after hospitalization.*

Refer to a member of the clergy or a spiritual counselor when deemed appropriate. *Patients will often be more inclined to talk to a spiritual counselor.*

SUGGESTED NIC INTERVENTIONS

Support System Enhancement; Coping Enhancement; Family Involvement Promotion; Respite Care; Family Support

REFERENCE

Häggman-Laitila, A., et al. (2010, April). Effectiveness of resource-enhancing family-oriented intervention. *American Journal of Clinical Nursing, 19*(17–18), 2500–2510.

DEFINITION

Repeated projection of falsely positive self-evaluation based on a self-protective pattern that defends against underlying perceived threats to positive self-regard

DEFINING CHARACTERISTICS

- Denial of obvious problems or weaknesses
- Denial of obvious
- Difficulty establishing or maintaining relationships
- Difficulty in perception of reality testing
- Lack of follow-through or participation in treatment or therapy
- Projection of blame
- Projection of responsibility
- Rationalization of failures
- Ridicule of others
- Superior attitude toward others

RELATED FACTORS

- Conflict between self-perception and value system
- Fear of failure
- Fear of humiliation
- Fear of repercussion
- Lack of resilience
- Low level of confidence in others
- Low level of self-confidence
- Uncertainty
- Unrealistic expectation of self

ASSESSMENT FOCUS

(Refer to comprehensive assessment parameters.)

- Behavior
- Emotional
- Communication
- Coping
- Knowledge
- Roles/relationships
- Self-perception

EXPECTED OUTCOMES

The patient will
- State the reason for hospitalization.
- Verbally describe self-perception, body image, success, and failures.
- Engage in decision making about care.
- Express a responsible attitude toward own behavior.
- Demonstrate follow-through in decisions related to health care.
- Interact with others in a socially acceptable manner.

SUGGESTED NOC OUTCOMES

Acceptance: Health Status; Coping; Self-Esteem; Social Interaction Skills; Self-Direction of Care

INTERVENTIONS AND RATIONALES

<u>Determine:</u> Assess patient's understanding of current illness; relationships with family and friends; self-esteem; self-perception; support systems; spiritual support. *Specific assessment information will assist in developing an accurate plan of care for the individual.*

<u>Perform:</u> Assist patient to compile a list of this that he likes and dislikes about his present situation. *Performing this exercise can help the patient identify aspects of self and identify changes he would like to make with specific variables.*

Have patient perform as many self-care activities as possible, and make treatment-related decisions *to encourage a sense of autonomy and promote compliance.*

Provide a structured daily routine. *Structure may help provide an alternative to self-absorption.*

<u>Inform:</u> Teach patient relaxation techniques such as guided imagery, deep breathing, meditation, aromatherapy, and progressive muscle relaxation. *Purposeful relaxation efforts help reduce anxiety.*

Teach patient strategies for positive thinking. Work specifically to identify negative thoughts and rephrase them in a positive way. *Making the patient conscious of negative thoughts will help reinforce the need to think about things and people in a more positive way.*

<u>Attend:</u> Arrange for interaction between the patient and family or friends and observe the interaction patterns. *This allows the nurse to provide feedback about the effectiveness of communication.*

Allow time for patient to talk about his or her frustration. *Speaking to a sensitive listener may help to reduce some frustration and may lead to new ideas about how to help the patient resolve his or her issues.*

Provide positive feedback to patient when he or she assumes responsibility for his or her own behavior *in order to reinforce positive coping behaviors.*

<u>Manage:</u> Encourage the patient to meet with someone who is coping successfully with a similar problem. *This may assist the patient to work toward a positive outcome.*

Encourage the patient to consider participating in a support group. *Participation in such a group may help the patient cope more effectively, as well as establish new relationships.*

Refer to case manager/social worker to ensure that follow-up is provided.

SUGGESTED NIC INTERVENTIONS

Calming Techniques; Coping Enhancement; Emotional Support; Self-Awareness Enhancement; Self-Responsibility Facilitation; Self-Modification Assistance

REFERENCE

Bahtı, T. (2010). Coping issues among people living with advanced cancer. *Seminars in Oncology Nursing, 26*(3), 175–182.

DEFINITION

Behavior of significant person (family members or other primary person) that disables his or her capabilities and the patient's capabilities to effectively address tasks essential to either person's adaptation to the health challenge

DEFINING CHARACTERISTICS

- Intolerance
- Agitation, depression, aggression, hostility
- Taking on illness signs of patient
- Rejection
- Psychosomaticism
- Neglectful relationships with other family members
- Neglectful care of patient in regard to basic human needs
- Distortion of reality regarding patient
- Impaired restructuring of a meaningful life

RELATED FACTORS

- Arbitrary handling of family's resistance to treatment
- Dissonant coping styles among significant people
- Significant person with chronically unexpressed feelings (e.g., guilt, anxiety, hostility, despair)

ASSESSMENT FOCUS

(Refer to comprehensive assessment parameters.)
- Communication
- Coping
- Knowledge
- Values and beliefs

EXPECTED OUTCOMES

To the extent possible, family members will participate in aspects of patient's care without evidence of increased conflict.

The patient will
- Express confidence in his or her ability to make decisions despite pressure from family members.
- Contact appropriate sources of support outside the family.
- Take steps to ensure that care needs are met despite family's shortcomings.
- Express greater understanding of emotional limitations of family members.

SUGGESTED NOC OUTCOMES

Caregiver Emotional Health; Caregiver–Patient Relationship; Caregiving Endurance Potential; Family Coping; Family Support During Treatment

INTERVENTIONS AND RATIONALES

Determine: Assess effects of patient's disease on ability of family to cope *to identify strengths and weaknesses in patient's patterns of coping.*

Describe role relationships in the family. Evaluate changes that occur in family relationships during the course of the patient's hospitalization. *This information will be helpful in making a plan.*

Have patient identify support systems outside the family *to encourage responsibility for knowing what support systems are helpful.*

Perform: Engage family in assisting with physical aspects of patient care. *Family members should have an opportunity to overcome dysfunctional behavior.*

Develop short- and long-term goals with both patient and family. *Problems associated with coping may will require long-term planning to resolve.*

Inform: Teach patient strategies to discuss, *to confront in a positive way that will help cope with the present situation.* Role-play coping strategies with the patient *to reinforce new adaptive behaviors.*

Educate family members about resources in the community *that can assist them with the patient after hospitalization.*

Teach *patient decision-making skills and assist* him or her to practice with simple decisions. *Beginning with simple decisions will begin helping the patient lay out options before deciding.*

Attend: Maintain objectivity when dealing with family conflicts. Do not become embroiled in the dynamics of a dysfunctional family *in order to maintain objectivity and effectiveness.*

Focus on being a patient advocate. Reaffirm patient's right to make decisions without interference from family members. Encourage patient to seek help family cannot provide by participating in support group. *Help patient select a support group that best meets personal needs. Participation in a support group may improve the patient's ability to cope as well as provide meaningful relationships.*

Listen attentively to patient's expression of pain over unresolved conflicts with family members. The patient may have to grieve over the fact that he or she does not have an "ideal" family, capable of meeting his emotional needs. *Therapeutic listening helps patient to understand himself and his family better and to understand how conflicts from the past affect his behavior.*

Manage: Refer patient to a home health agency, homemaker service, meals-on-wheels, or other appropriate community services for assistance and follow-up. *Use of various community services may help make up the family's shortcomings in coping.*

SUGGESTED NIC INTERVENTIONS
Anger Control Assistance; Caregiver Support; Family Involvement Promotion; Family Mobilization; Family Support; Family Integrity Promotion; Case Management

REFERENCE

Davidson, J. E., et al. (2010, April–June). Facilitated sensemaking: A feasibility study for the provision of a family support program in the intensive care unit. *Critical Care Nursing, 33*(2), 177–189.

DEFINITION

Inability to form a valid appraisal of the stressors, inadequate choices of practiced responses, and/or inability to use available resources

DEFINING CHARACTERISTICS

- Change in communication patterns
- Decreased use of social support
- Destructive behavior toward self or others
- Difficulty asking for help
- Fatigue
- High illness rate
- Inability to meet basic needs and role expectations
- Statements indicating inability to cope
- Substance abuse

RELATED FACTORS

- High degree of threat
- Inability to conserve adaptive energies
- Inadequate resources available
- Maturational or situational crisis

ASSESSMENT FOCUS

(Refer to comprehensive assessment parameters.)

- Behavior
- Communication
- Coping

EXPECTED OUTCOMES

The patient will

- Verbalize increased ability to cope.
- Expand support network to meet social and emotional needs.
- Locate and use appropriate resources for help in problem solving.
- Report increased ability to meet demands of daily living.
- Make changes to environment to ensure enhanced coping or move into long-term care facility, as needed.

SUGGESTED NOC OUTCOMES

Coping; Decision Making; Impulse Self-Control; Information Processing; Social Interaction Skills; Social Support

INTERVENTIONS AND RATIONALES

Determine: Monitor physiological responses to increased activity level, including respirations, heart rate and rhythm, and blood pressure. *Vital signs are likely to change as the patient deals with the frustration from poor coping strategies.* Assess understanding of the current health problem and desire *to participate in treatment.*

Perform: Listen to the patient. Respond in a matter-of-fact, nonjudgmental manner. *Judgmental responses will impede the development of a trusting relationship.* Practice guided imagery and deep breathing with the patient *to help the patient relax.*

Inform: Provide patient with information about relaxation techniques. *These techniques take practice. Information will help the patient understand the benefit.*

Teach patient about her disease process and explain treatments *to allay fear and allow the patient to regain sense of control.*

Teach positive coping strategies and have patient role-play them and give praise for successful modeling. *This will help to reinforce coping behaviors.*

Attend: Assist patient to develop short- and long-term goals *to encourage better coping and a roadmap to measure progress.* Provide emotional support and encouragement *to help improve patient's negative self-concept and motivate the patient to perform activities of daily living.* Involve patient in planning and decision making. *Having the ability to participate will encourage greater compliance with treatment plan.* Encourage patient to engage in social activities with people of all age groups. *Participation once a week will help relieve the patient's sense of isolation.*

Manage: Refer patient for professional psychological counseling. *Formal counseling helps ease the nurse's frustration, increases objectivity, and fosters collaborative approach to patient's care.*

Before discharge, refer patient to case manager who can help patient become involved in informal community programs, such as volunteer, foster grandparents, or religious groups, *to provide peer and social contact and decrease the patient's loneliness and isolation.* Refer patient to a support group. *In the context of a group, the patient may develop a more positive view in the present situation.*

SUGGESTED NIC INTERVENTIONS

Coping Enhancement; Decision-Making Support; Emotional Support; Environmental Management; Impulse Control Training; Support System Enhancement

REFERENCE

Bossi, L., & Porter, S. (2011, November). Calming and coping strategies for the school nurse's new year: Using mind-body concepts. *NASN School Nurse*, 26(6), 368–372.

DEFINITION

Pattern of community activities for adaptation and problem-solving that is unsatisfactory for meeting the demands or needs of the community

DEFINING CHARACTERISTICS

- Deficits in participation
- Excessive conflicts
- Expressed powerlessness and vulnerability
- Failure of community to meet its own expectations
- High illness rate
- Increased social problems (abuse, divorce, and unemployment)
- Perception of stressors as excessive

RELATED FACTORS

- Deficits in community social support services
- Deficits in community social resources
- Natural disasters
- Man-made disasters
- Inadequate resources for problem solving
- Ineffective community systems (e.g., lack of disaster planning system)

ASSESSMENT FOCUS

(Refer to comprehensive assessment parameters.)

- Communication
- Coping
- Health care system
- Risk management
- Values and beliefs

EXPECTED OUTCOMES

Community members will

- Express awareness of seriousness of high school adolescent pregnancy rate in their community.
- Express need for plan to reduce prevalence of teen pregnancy.
- Develop and implement plan to reduce teen pregnancy
- Evaluate success of plan in meeting goals and objectives and will continue to revise it, as necessary.
- Report reduction in rate of teen pregnancy.

SUGGESTED NOC OUTCOMES

Community Competence; Community Health Status

INTERVENTIONS AND RATIONALES

<u>Determine:</u> Assess the following: community demographics; number of teen pregnancies in the community in the past 2 years; attitudes toward teen mothers and their infants; availability of programs in the schools

that help teen mothers continue their education; teens' knowledge about sex and sexuality; religious attitudes in the community toward sex and sexuality; influence of religious groups on educators. *Assessment information will be useful in establishing appropriate interventions.*

<u>Perform:</u> Collect statistical data from schools *to analyze teen pregnancy rates as a basis for evaluating a pregnancy prevention program.* Plan a teen pregnancy program that can be used in schools. Include information on risks, problems, and complications of teen pregnancy. Contact local corporations *for financial assistance in supporting educational programs.*

Establish clubs for adolescent girls in the community. *These can be used as a method for educating as well as helping girls establish healthy relationships.*

Establish therapeutic relationships with pregnant adolescents to *build support during this difficult period.*

<u>Inform:</u> Provide education on birth-control measures (including abstinence from sex) and have this information available at school.

Encourage an information campaign *to educate adolescents, parents, and community members about problems related to teen pregnancy.*

Teach parent to observe behavioral cues from child. For example, the child may become fussy when he is ready for a nap or may pull his ear if he has an earache *to indicate that he has pain.* Explain the range of options for responding to these cues in positive ways. *Parents may be unfamiliar with cues from child behavior.*

Teach parents to give physical care when the need exists. *The parents may need instruction on the importance and proper way of providing care.* Teach relaxation techniques that can be done by the parents such as guided imagery, progressive muscle relaxation, and meditation. *These measures restore psychological and physical equilibrium by decreasing autonomic response to anxiety.*

Encourage local youth groups and religious and social organizations to feature guest speakers on pregnancy prevention at their meetings. *Speakers with expertise in the area of teen pregnancy are better able to provide information that may help teens make better choices in sexual behavior.*

<u>Attend:</u> Encourage community members to establish school-based clinics that allow teen's access to reproductive-system models, pregnancy tests, and nonprescription birth-control measures *to support teens who choose to protect themselves from unwanted pregnancy.*

<u>Manage:</u> Develop a referral list for teens that includes resources such as hospitals with human sexuality courses, charities that provide prenatal care and childbirth services, women's clinics, and Planned Parenthood *to compensate for restricted access to information in the schools.*

SUGGESTED NIC INTERVENTIONS

Community Health Development; Health Education; Health Screening; Program Development; Health Policy Monitoring

REFERENCE

Daley, A. M. (2012, June). Rethinking school-based health centers as complex adaptive systems: Maximizing opportunities for the prevention of teen pregnancy and sexually transmitted infections. *Advances in Nursing Science*, *35*(2), E37–E46.

DEFINITION

A pattern of cognitive and behavioral efforts to manage demands that is sufficient for well-being and can be strengthened

DEFINING CHARACTERISTICS

- Defines stressors as manageable
- Acknowledges power; aware of possible environmental changes
- Seeks knowledge of new strategies
- Seeks social support
- Uses a broad range of problem-oriented and emotion-oriented strategies
- Uses spiritual resources

ASSESSMENT FOCUS

(Refer to comprehensive assessment parameters.)
- Behavior
- Communication
- Coping
- Roles/relationships
- Self-perception

EXPECTED OUTCOMES

The patient will
- Identify major issues that require ongoing enhancement of coping strategies.
- Express feelings associated with coping strategies.
- Demonstrate readiness to develop enhanced strategies.
- Identify support persons and activities that will assist in goal attainment.

SUGGESTED NOC OUTCOMES

Coping; Quality of Life; Personal Autonomy

INTERVENTIONS AND RATIONALES

<u>Determine:</u> Assess patient's usual coping mechanisms, roles and responsibilities, social support, spiritual resources, and use of alcohol and tobacco *in order to decide on a focus for interventions.*

<u>Perform:</u> Establish a trusting relationship with patient by spending time with the patient each shift, *which will encourage the patient to be more honest and open.*

Begin discussions at patient's level of comfort. *If patient wants to express anger or other emotion, listen carefully. Until the patient has had an opportunity to talk, you will not be able to move him to a place where the issue can be discussed logically.*

<u>Inform:</u> Provide information on informed consent *because parents will be making decisions for the child's care.*

Teach additional skills that enhance coping strategies. Help the patient develop a program by using relaxation strategies (i.e., meditation, guided imagery, yoga, exercise); *these strategies will help to reduce anxiety and allow the patient to concentrate.*

Teach problem-solving skills. Have patient role-play *to demonstrate how to set up options and choose from among them.*

Attend: Encourage patient to continue adhering to his plan for enhanced coping strategies. *Compliance with the plan will produce results for the patient. It will also help patient measure success.*

Encourage patient to continue involvement in a wide range of activities. *More activities will involve more choices.*

Encourage patient to look for volunteer opportunities in the *community* as a way of keeping the patient involved with others.

Offer to meet with patient regularly, if desired, *to help patient continue developing enhanced coping skills.*

Manage: Refer patients to support groups and offer ideas about educational opportunities in the community.

SUGGESTED NIC INTERVENTIONS

Active Listening; Coping Enhancement; Guided Imagery; Massage; Meditation Facilitation

REFERENCE

Whittemore, R., Jaser, S. S., Jeon, S., Liberti, L., Delamater, A., Murphy, K., Faulkner, M. S., & Grey, M. (2012, September). An Internet coping skills training program for youth with Type I Diabetes: Six month outcomes. *Nursing Research* 61(6): 395–404.

DEFINITION

Pattern of community activities for adaptation and problem solving that is sufficient for meeting the demands or needs of the community but can be improved for management of current and future problems/stressors

DEFINING CHARACTERISTICS

- Active planning by community to handle predicted stressors
- Active problem solving by community when faced with issues
- Agreement that community carries responsibility for stress management
- Positive communication among community members and between community members and larger organizations
- Programs available for recreation and relaxation
- Resources sufficient for managing stressors

ASSESSMENT FOCUS

(Refer to comprehensive assessment parameters.)
- Communication
- Coping
- Populations
- Risk management

EXPECTED OUTCOMES

Community members will
- Express understanding of problems associated with failure to immunize population and will recognize the needs to reduce the number of adults and children who are not immunized.
- Initiate a plan to increase the number of immunizations in population and provide adequate protection from communicable diseases.
- Work to reduce spread of communicable diseases and increase the number of immunizations.
- Evaluate established plans for ensuring that all children become immunized and will make changes to plans as needed.

SUGGESTED NOC OUTCOMES

Community Competence; Community Health Status: Immunity; Community Risk Control: Communicable Disease

INTERVENTIONS AND RATIONALES

<u>Determine:</u> Assess community member's level of understanding of the importance of immunization. If level of compliance is low, survey community needs to determine why. Determine ease of access in the community for members to comply with immunization requirements/needs. Identify new members of the community, such as immigrants or refugees. *This assessment will assist in identifying appropriate intervention.*

<u>Perform:</u> Collect statistical data from community health sources, such as the health department and schools *to continue to identify children who have not been immunized.* Recruit local agencies with an adequate number of professionals able to deliver the immunization services.

Contact parents personally or by handwritten note about children who have not been immunized. *Make it clear to the parents that your purpose is to protect the children.*

<u>Inform:</u> Provide extensive educational opportunities in the community about communicable diseases and the importance of immunization. *Educate persons in the community in their first language to ensure adequate understanding.*

<u>Attend:</u> Encourage community members to implement a program to disseminate information about problems associated with inadequate immunization *to educate residents and promote the community's established immunization program.*

Encourage health departments, clinics, and practitioners' offices to provide information on the recommended childhood immunization schedule to the public *to foster understanding about the importance of educating the public.*

Conduct a follow-up survey on immunization rates *to measure the effectiveness of educational initiatives.*

<u>Manage:</u> Supply a list of referrals for the parents of children who are not immunized. Include information on low-cost health insurance, city health centers, and well-baby clinics to encourage compliance. *Helping the parents by giving referrals will empower them to meet their child's health care needs.*

SUGGESTED NIC INTERVENTIONS

Communicable Disease Management; Community Health Development; Health Education; Health Policy Monitoring; Immunization/Vaccination Management

REFERENCE

Eisenman, D. P., et al. (2012, August). The public health disaster trust scale: Validation of a brief measure. *Journal of Public Health Management, 18*(4), 11–18.

DEFINITION

A pattern of management of adaptive tasks by primary person involved with the client's health challenge that is sufficient for health and growth, in regard to self and in relation to the client, and can be strengthened

DEFINING CHARACTERISTICS

- Individual expresses interest in making contact with others who have experienced a similar situation
- Significant person attempts to describe growth impact of crisis
- Significant person moves in direction of enriching lifestyle
- Significant person moves in direction of health promotion
- Significant person expresses interest in making contact with others who have experienced a similar situation

ASSESSMENT FOCUS

(Refer to comprehensive assessment parameters.)
- Behavior
- Coping
- Emotional status
- Roles/responsibilities

EXPECTED OUTCOMES

Family members will
- Discuss the impact of patient's illness and feelings about it with health care professional.
- Participate in treatment plan.
- Establish a visiting routine beneficial to the patient.
- Demonstrate the care needed to maintain patient's health status.
- Identify and use available support systems.

SUGGESTED NOC OUTCOMES

Caregiver–Patient Relationship; Caregiver Well-Being; Family Coping; Family Normalization; Health-Promoting Behavior

INTERVENTIONS AND RATIONALES

Determine: Assess normal pattern of communication among family members; understanding and knowledge of family members about patient's condition; family's past response to crises; patient's perception of health problem. Assess patient and family's spiritual needs, including religious beliefs and affiliation. *Assessment of these factors will assist in selecting appropriate interventions.*

Perform: Schedule time to meet with family and patient *in order to listen to ways in which they plan to enhance their coping skills in the present situation.*

Provide comfort measures such as bathing, massage, regulation of environmental temperature, and mouth care, according to the patient's needs and preferences. *Comfort can promote ability to cooperate with the plan.*

Establish a visiting schedule that will not tax patient's or family's resources. Use patient's daily routine to aid in planning (e.g., no visiting during treatments or during periods of uninterrupted rest). *Establishing a routine will allow the patient to have consistency and a measure of control.*

Inform: Teach self-healing techniques to patient and family such as meditation, guided imagery, yoga, and prayer. *These strategies promote anxiety reduction.*

Teach patient how to incorporate the use of self-healing techniques in carrying out usual daily activities *in order to encourage ongoing use of the strategies.*

Demonstrate procedures and encourage participation in patient's care in a way that maximizes patient's comfort. *Both patient and family need to work together to implement the plan with patient's comfort in mind.*

Provide patient with concise information about condition. Be aware of what family members already know. *Honesty is important when conveying information.*

Attend: Reinforce family's efforts to care for patient. Let family know they are doing well *to ease adaptation to new caregiver roles.*

Ensure privacy for patient and family visits *to foster open communication.*

Encourage family to support patient's independence. Encourage patient's cooperation as you continue with healing techniques, such as therapeutic touch. *There is a need to allow for as much independence on the part of the patient as possible. At times the family will try to promote dependency to the detriment of the patient.*

Provide emotional support to family by being available to answer questions. *Availability will communicate to the family that you are concerned for them and the patient.*

Manage: Refer family to community resources and support groups available *to assist in managing patient's illness and providing emotional and financial assistance to caregivers.*

Refer to a member of the clergy or a spiritual counselor, according to the patient's preference, *to show respect for the patient's beliefs and provide spiritual care.*

SUGGESTED NIC INTERVENTIONS

Coping Enhancement; Family Process Management

REFERENCE

Carson, V. B., & Yambor, S. J. (2012, May). Managing patients with bipolar disorder at home: A family affair and a psychiatric challenge in home healthcare. *Home Healthcare Nurse, 30*(5), 280–291.

DEFINITION
Vague uneasy feeling of discomfort or dread generated by perceptions of a real or imagined threat to one's existence

DEFINING CHARACTERISTICS
- Reports concerns of overworking the caregiver
- Reports deep sadness, fear of developing terminal illness, fears of loss of mental faculties
- Reports fears of death, process of death, pain, premature death, prolonged dying, suffering
- Reports feeling powerless over dying
- Worry about the impact of one's death on significant others
- Negative death images or unpleasant thoughts about events related to death or dying

RELATED FACTORS
- Anticipating the impact of death on others
- Anticipating suffering
- Experiencing the dying process
- Uncertainty about life after death
- Uncertainty about the existence of a higher power

ASSESSMENT FOCUS
(Refer to comprehensive assessment parameters.)
- Behavior
- Communication
- Emotional status

EXPECTED OUTCOMES
The patient will
- Identify time alone and time needed with others.
- Communicate important thoughts and feelings to family members.
- Obtain the level of spiritual support desired.
- Use available support systems.
- Perform self-care activities to tolerance level.
- Express feelings of comfort and peacefulness.

SUGGESTED NOC OUTCOMES
Acceptance: Health Status; Anxiety Level; Depression Level; Dignified Life Closure; Fear Self-Control; Hope

INTERVENTIONS AND RATIONALES
Determine: Assess how much support the patient desires. *Patients may want a higher degree of independence in dealing with death than the caregiver wants to allow.*

Assess patient's spiritual needs. *Often as death approaches, individuals begin thinking more about the needs of the spirit.*

Determine which comfort measures the family believes will enhance feelings of well-being. *Dying patients have the right to decide how much physical, emotional, and spiritual care they wish to have.*

<u>Perform:</u> Administer medication to relieve pain and provide comfort as required. Medicating at an appropriate level does much to relieve pain and often *helps the dying person maintain greater feeling of self-control.*

Turn and reposition patient at least every 2 hours. Establish a turning schedule for the dependent patient. Post schedule at bedside and monitor frequency. *Turning and repositioning may prevent skin breakdown, improve lung expansion, and prevent atelectasis.*

Provide simple physical gestures of support such as holding hands with the patient and encouraging family members to do the same. *Patient may want to experience less touching when he or she begins to let go.*

Provide comfort measures including bath, massage, regulation of environmental temperature, and mouth care *according to patient's preferences. These measures promote relaxation and feelings of well-being.*

<u>Inform:</u> Teach family members ways of discerning unobtrusively what the patient's desires for comfort and peace are at this time *because some patients prefer not to be bothered unless they specifically request comfort measures. Being sensitive to patient needs promotes individualized care.*

Teach caregivers to assist patient with self-care activities in a way that maximizes patient's rights to choose. *This enables caregivers to participate in patient's care while supporting patient's independence.*

<u>Attend:</u> Help family identify, discuss, and resolve issues related to patient's dying. Provide emotional support and encouragement to help. Clear communication promotes family integrity.

Demonstrate to patient willingness to discuss the spiritual aspects of death and dying *to foster an open discussion.* Keep conversation focused on patient's spiritual values and the role they play coping with dying. *Meeting the patient's spiritual needs conveys respect for the importance of all aspects of care.*

If patient is confused, provide reassurance by telling him or her who is in the room. *This information may help to reduce anxiety.*

<u>Manage:</u> Refer to hospice for end-of-life care if this has not already been done. Communicate to the hospice nurse where the patient is at present in coping with the terminal illness. Continuity of care is crucial during times of stress.

Refer to a member of the clergy or a spiritual counselor, according to the patient's preference, *to show respect for the patient's beliefs and provide spiritual care.*

SUGGESTED NIC INTERVENTIONS

Active Listening; Anticipatory Guidance; Family Involvement Promotion; Pain Management; Spiritual Support; Touch

REFERENCE

Lehto, R. H. (2012, February). The challenge of existential issues in acute care: Nursing considerations for a patient with a new diagnosis of lung cancer. *Clinical Journal of Oncology Nursing, 16*(1), E6–E8.

DEFINITION

A pattern of choosing courses of action that is sufficient for meeting short- and long-term health-related goals and can be strengthened

DEFINING CHARACTERISTICS

- Expresses desire to enhance decision making
- Expresses desire to enhance congruency of decisions with personal values and goals
- Expresses desire to enhance congruency between decisions and sociocultural goals and values
- Expresses desire to enhance risk–benefit analysis of decisions
- Expresses desire to enhance the understanding of choices
- Expresses desire to enhance use of reliable evidence for decisions

ASSESSMENT FOCUS

(Refer to comprehensive assessment parameters.)

- Coping
- Communication
- Knowledge
- Values and beliefs

EXPECTED OUTCOMES

The patient will

- Express the desire to make effective decisions.
- Verbalize decision-making goals and concerns.
- Discuss measures used to evaluate decisions.
- Make decisions that promote maximal physical, mental, social, and psychological well-being.
- Involve family, friends, and clergy in health care decision making when appropriate.

SUGGESTED NOC OUTCOMES

Decision Making; Participation in Healthcare Decisions; Self-Care: IADLs; Coping

INTERVENTIONS AND RATIONALES

<u>Determine:</u> Assess usual coping strategies employed by the patient when making decisions; determine how the patient goes about making difficult decisions; have the patient describe several challenging decisions he or she made in the past year. *Assessment information will help identify appropriate interventions.*

Evaluate support systems available to the patient when it is necessary to make decisions. *Patients often need support of families or other support systems when they are faced with major decisions.*

<u>Perform:</u> Provide assistance with activities of daily living as required. *As the patient receives assistance, it is important to allow him or her to be as independent as possible.*

Make changes in the environment *to reduce unnecessary stimulation and promote a sense of calm.*

<u>Inform:</u> Teach patient simple decision-making techniques and role-play the same. *Return demonstration from the patient will give him or her confidence that he or she can choose wisely among options.*

Educate family about the importance of allowing the patient to think and act for him or herself *in order to give the patient a sense of control over the present situation.*

<u>Attend:</u> Provide emotional support and encouragement *to help improve patient's confidence in his or her ability to make logical decisions.*

Provide patient with all necessary support during hospitalization *to prepare him and his family to continue the process of having the patient make decisions about his own care.*

Involve patient in planning and decision making. *Having the ability to participate will encourage greater compliance with the treatment plan.*

<u>Manage:</u> If patient continues to have difficulty, refer to case manager/social worker/mental health professional *for continued follow-up.*

Provide appropriate assistance to the family members when they are trying to provide; it might be helpful in working with the patient.

SUGGESTED NIC INTERVENTIONS

Decision-Making Support; Health System Guidance; Self Responsibility Facilitation; Self-Efficacy Enhancement

REFERENCE

Knopf Kerstin et al. As If the Cancer Wasn't Enough: A Case Study of Depression in Terminal Illness, Journal of Hospice and Palliative Nursing: 14(5): 319-329, July 2012.

DEFINITION

Uncertainty about course of action to be taken when choice among competing actions involves risk, loss, or challenge to values and beliefs

DEFINING CHARACTERISTICS

- Delayed decision making
- Focusing on self
- Lack of experience or interference with decision making
- Questioning personal values or beliefs while attempting to make a decision
- Vacillation between alternative choices
- Verbal statements describing undesirable consequences of alternative actions being considered
- Verbal expression of distress and uncertainty

RELATED FACTORS

- Divergent sources of information
- Interference with decision making
- Lack of experience with decision making
- Lack of relevant information
- Moral obligations require actions
- Moral obligations require no action
- Unclear personal beliefs or values

ASSESSMENT FOCUS

(Refer to comprehensive assessment parameters.)
- Communication
- Roles and relationships
- Values and beliefs

EXPECTED OUTCOMES

The patient will
- State feelings about the current situation.
- Discuss benefits and drawbacks of treatment options.
- Make minor decisions related to daily activities.
- Accept assistance from family, friends, clergy, and other support persons.
- Report feeling comfortable about ability to make an appropriate, rational choice.

SUGGESTED NOC OUTCOMES

Decision Making; Information Processing; Participation in Health Care Decisions

INTERVENTIONS AND RATIONALES

Determine: Assess major challenges patient will face in making decisions about care, as well as factors that influence patient's present decision-making skills. *This information will be useful in establishing appropriate interventions.*

<u>Perform:</u> Arrange patient's environment *to promote relaxation and comfort while the patient is trying to gain control of decision making.*

Assist with self-care activities while patient needs help *to ensure that activities of daily living are met.*

Offer massage *to reduce tension and assist patient to relax.*

Help patient make decisions about daily activities *to enhance her feelings of control.*

Help patient identify available options and possible consequences *to assist with rational, logical decision making.*

<u>Inform:</u> Teach techniques for progressive muscle relaxation *to decrease physical and psychological signs of tension.*

<u>Attend:</u> Encourage visits with family, friends, and clergy; provide privacy during visits *to foster emotional support.*

Encourage patient to express concerns about frustrations in making decisions. Take the time to assist the patient *to explore or sort out aspects of decision making that cause him or her difficulty.*

<u>Manage:</u> Offer written information, a reading list, or a referral to a support group *to ensure that patient will have reference material when it is needed.*

Refer to home health nurse *for a follow-up visit in the home.*

Refer to a nutritionist *for information on good nutrition and fluid management.*

SUGGESTED NIC INTERVENTIONS

Active Listening; Assertiveness Training; Decision-Making Support; Learning Facilitation; Mutual Goal-Setting

REFERENCE

Allen, J. D. & Berry, D. L. (2011, August). Multi-media support for informed/ shared decision-making before and after a cancer diagnosis. *Seminars in Oncology Nursing, 27*(3), 192–202.

DEFINITION

Conscious or unconscious attempt to disavow the knowledge or meaning of an event to reduce anxiety/fear, but leading to the detriment of health

DEFINING CHARACTERISTICS

- Delay in seeking or refusal of medical attention to detriment of health
- Displacement of fear about condition's impact
- Displacement of sources of symptoms to other organs
- Failure to perceive personal relevance or danger of symptoms
- Inability to admit impact of disease on life pattern
- Inappropriate affect
- Minimization of symptoms
- Refusal to admit fear of death or invalidism
- Uses self-treatment

RELATED FACTORS

- Anxiety
- Fear of death and loss of autonomy
- Threat of inadequacy in dealing with strong emotions
- Lack of control of the situation
- Overwhelming stress
- Threat of unpleasant reality
- Lack of competency in using effective coping mechanisms

ASSESSMENT FOCUS

(Refer to comprehensive assessment parameters.)
- Behavior
- Communication
- Coping
- Values and beliefs

EXPECTED OUTCOMES

The patient will
- Describe knowledge and perception of present health problem.
- Describe life pattern and report any changes.
- Express knowledge of stages of grieving.
- Demonstrate behavior associated with the grief process.
- Indicate, either verbally or through behavior, an increased awareness of reality.

SUGGESTED NOC OUTCOMES

Acceptance: Health Status; Anxiety Level; Coping; Fear Self-Control; Health Beliefs: Perceived Threat; Symptom Control

INTERVENTIONS AND RATIONALES

Determine: Assess patient's understanding and perception of present health state, including awareness of diagnosis, and perception of relevance on life pattern and description of symptoms.

Evaluate coping status and mental status, including mood, affect, memory, and judgment. *Assessment of these factors will help identify appropriate interventions.*

Perform: Schedule a specific amount of uninterrupted non-care-related time each day with the patient *to allow patient to express feelings and concerns.*

Assist patient with activities of living as needed *to conserve energy and avoid overexertion.* Assist with grooming (e.g., shaving for men, hair and makeup for women). Offer massage *to enhance comfort and promote relaxation.*

Encourage active exercise (e.g., provide a trapeze or other assistive device if needed). *Exercise will promote positive attitude.*

Inform: Discuss stages of anticipatory *grieving to increase understanding of what is happening and increase patient's ability to cope.*

Teach patient about diagnosis and treatment as he or she demonstrates readiness to learn. Provide brochures and simple written materials *to help with the learning process.*

Attend: Provide emotional support and encouragement *to help improve patient's self-concept and motivate the patient to be more involved in planning care*

Involve patient in planning and decision making. *Having the ability to participate will encourage greater compliance with the plan for treatment.*

Have patient perform self-care activities. Begin slowly and increase daily, as tolerated. *Performing self-care activities will assist patient to regain independence and enhance self-esteem.*

Schedule treatments apart from visiting *to allow for periods of rest.*

Maintain frequent discussions with physicians and staff *to be certain what patient has been told by other care providers.*

Manage: Refer to case manager/social worker *for follow-up care.*

Refer to clergy person *for spiritual care* if patient expresses interest.

SUGGESTED NIC INTERVENTIONS

Anxiety Reduction, Behavior Modification; Calming; Counseling; Decision-Making Support; Truth Telling

REFERENCE

Harvath, T. A. (2010, January). Hope versus denial. *Journal of Gerontology Nursing, 36*(1), 3–4.

DEFINITION
Disruption in tooth development and eruption patterns or structural integrity of individual teeth

DEFINING CHARACTERISTICS
- Caries; extractions; evidence of periodontal disease
- Evulsion
- Malocclusion; plaque; toothache
- Loose teeth; premature loss of primary teeth
- Erosion of enamel or discoloration

RELATED FACTORS
- Barriers to self-care
- Bruxism
- Chronic use of coffee, tea, red wine, or tobacco
- Chronic vomiting
- Ineffective oral hygiene
- Nutritional deficits
- Sensitivity to cold or heat
- Deficient knowledge regarding dental health

ASSESSMENT FOCUS
(Refer to comprehensive assessment parameters.)
- Knowledge
- Nutrition
- Roles/responsibilities
- Values and beliefs

EXPECTED OUTCOMES
The individual will
- Brush teeth with minimal supervision.
- Demonstrate good brushing technique.
- Not show evidence of dental caries, periodontal disease, or malocclusion.
- Reduce quantity of cariogenic foods in his or her diet.
- Show evidence of good daily oral hygiene.

SUGGESTED NOC OUTCOME
Oral Hygiene; Self-Care: Oral Hygiene

INTERVENTIONS AND RATIONALES
<u>Determine:</u> Assess dental history; primary and secondary tooth development; frequency of visits to dentist; frequency of brushing; condition of the teeth; nutritional status; medications; socioeconomic status. *Assessment of these factors will help to identify appropriate interventions.*
<u>Perform:</u> Provide tooth brush, toothpaste, and dental floss *to ensure that supplies are available.*

Schedule times for brushing and have patient begin keeping a record. *Keeping a record will promote compliance.*

Inform: Teach child principles of good oral hygiene by using teaching methods appropriate to his age-group *to foster compliance.*

Teach the child and his or her parents or caregiver about the relationship between diet and dental health. Show the child pictures that promote good dental health and pictures of foods that lead to dental decay. If the child can read, teach him or her to read labels; teach him or her to avoid products with excessive sucrose. *Sucrose is a simple sugar that promotes dental decay.*

Demonstrate good brushing technique. Stress the importance of having teeth feel clean rather than the need to follow a specific procedure *to reinforce good dental hygiene habits.*

Attend: Encourage parents to create a pleasant mealtime environment with nutritious foods made to look appealing to a child *so that the child will learn to recognize nutritious foods.*

Give positive reinforcement for good choices. Be supportive to the parents as they try to help the child modify diet to include more nutritional foods. *It is not easy to teach children to make right food choices, and parents benefit from encouragement to keep reinforcing good healthy choices.*

Encourage ample fluid intake to keep gums well hydrated. *Adequate fluids promote healthy gums*

Manage: Refer to dentist *for assessment of dental health.*

Schedule a follow-up appointment with parents *to ensure they have taken child to the dentist.*

Where it is indicated, refer to a nutritionist *for help in modifying diet.*

SUGGESTED NIC INTERVENTIONS

Oral Health Maintenance; Oral Health Promotion; Teaching: Individual

REFERENCE

Your child's growing smile. (2012, January). *Journal of the American Dental Association, 143*(1), 88.

DEFINITION

At risk for delay of 25% or more in one or more of the areas of social or self-regulatory behavior, or in cognitive, language, gross or fine motor skills

RISK FACTORS

- Prenatal (e.g., endocrine or genetic disorder, economically disadvantaged, illiteracy, inadequate nutrition or prenatal care, infections, maternal age <15 or >35, substance abuse, unplanned or unwanted pregnancy)
- Individual (e.g., adopted child, behavior disorders, brain damage, chronic illness, congenital disorders, foster child, hearing impairment, inadequate nutrition, genetic disorders, lead poisoning, substance abuse, vision impairment, prematurity, seizures, technology dependent, treatment-related side effects)
- Environmental (e.g., economically disadvantaged, violence)
- Caregiver (e.g., abuse, learning disabilities, mental illness)

ASSESSMENT FOCUS

(Refer to comprehensive assessment parameters.)

- Coping
- Communication
- Emotional
- Roles/relationship
- Values/beliefs

EXPECTED OUTCOMES

The child will

- Continue to grow and gain weight in accordance with growth chart of age and sex.
- Consume _____ calories and _____ mL of fluids representing _____ servings (specify for each food group).
- Participate in activities and be provided with a supervised, unconfined environment that includes age-appropriate toys and fosters interaction with child's development.

The parents will

- Express understanding of measures to reduce child's risk for delayed development.
- Identify risk factors that may interfere with child's development.

SUGGESTED NOC OUTCOMES

Family Functioning; Growth; Parenting Performance; Risk Control; Child Development: 1 Month through Adolescence; Decision Making; Knowledge: Parenting

INTERVENTION AND RATIONALES

<u>Determine:</u> Assess family's developmental stage; family roles; family rules; socioeconomic status; family health history; history of substance abuse; history of sexual abuse of spouse or children; problem-solving

and decision-making skills; religious affiliation; ethnicity. *Assessment information will aid in developing a workable plan of care.*

<u>Perform:</u> Weigh and measure child. Review growth chart *to establish current height and weight values.*

Establish a meal program *to meet the child's nutritional needs.*

Create an environment in which family members can express themselves openly and honestly. Establish rules for communication during meetings with the family. *Having rules allows everyone to participate and keep the discussion on the designated topic.*

<u>Inform:</u> Teach parents about nutritional requirements needed for child of specific weight and age. Discuss various meal choices available to the child. *Providing instruction in writing simplifies the parents' role in selecting healthy foods.*

Educate parents about child's need for quality interaction with family members and others. Inform parents about age-appropriate activities and toys as well as potential playmates for a child of specific age. Emphasize importance of providing an unconfined, supervised environment in which the child can *play to encourage play that encourages the child to move freely.*

Educate parents about risk factors that may lead to delayed development, such as lack of supportive interactions or age-appropriate activities. *The ability to recognize risk factors will promote getting help for the parents and child sooner.*

Teach coping skills to parents *to enable them to deal effectively with the child's needs.*

<u>Attend:</u> Encourage parents to listen to the child and communicate in a loving, supportive way *in order to allow the child to maintain a positive attitude.*

Encourage parents to identify preventive measures they may initiate at home to ensure continuity of care. *Consistency in providing care will help the child understand that the plan carries over to all aspects of his or her life.*

<u>Manage:</u> Provide parents with a copy of child's teaching plan. *This helps to reinforce what the child is learning.*

Refer to case manager/social worker *to ensure that a home assessment is done.*

Refer to nutritionist *for follow-up with food issues.*

SUGGESTED NIC INTERVENTIONS

Family Process Maintenance; Coping Enhancement; Family Integrity Promotion; Normalization Promotion; Risk Identification; Developmental Enhancement

REFERENCE

Doyle, L. W., Davis, P. G., Schmidt, B., & Anderson, P. J. (2012, February). Cognitive outcome at 24 months is more predictive than at 18 months for IQ at 8–9 years in extremely low birth weight children. *Early Human Development, 88*(2), 95–98.

DEFINITION

Passage of loose, unformed stools

DEFINING CHARACTERISTICS

- Abdominal pain and cramping
- At least three loose, liquid stools per day
- Hyperactive bowel sounds
- Urgency

RELATED FACTORS

- *Psychological*: Anxiety, high stress levels
- *Physiological*: Malabsorption, infectious processes, irritation, parasites, inflammation
- *Situational*: Adverse effects of medications, alcohol abuse, toxins, laxative abuse, contaminants, radiation, tube feedings, travel

ASSESSMENT FOCUS

(Refer to comprehensive assessment parameters.)

- Coping
- Emotional
- Elimination
- Fluid and electrolytes
- Nutrition

EXPECTED OUTCOMES

The patient will

- Have less or no diarrheal episodes.
- Resume usual bowel pattern.
- Maintain weight and fluid and electrolyte balance.
- Keep skin clean and free from irritation or ulcerations.
- Explain causative factors and preventive measures.
- Discuss relationship of stress and anxiety to episodes of diarrhea.
- State plans to use stress-reduction techniques (specify).
- Demonstrate ability to use at least one stress-reduction technique.

SUGGESTED NOC OUTCOMES

Bowel Continence; Hydration; Symptom Control; Bowel Elimination

INTERVENTIONS AND RATIONALES

Determine: Monitor and record frequency and characteristics of stools *to monitor treatment effectiveness.*

Identify stressors and help the patient solve problems *to provide more realistic approach to care.*

Monitor perianal skin for irritation and ulceration; treat according to established protocol *to promote comfort, skin integrity, and freedom from infection.*

Perform: Administer antidiarrheal medications, as ordered, *to improve body function, promote comfort, and balance body fluids, salts, and acid–base levels.* Monitor and report effectiveness of medication.

Provide replacement fluids and electrolytes as prescribed. Maintain accurate records *to ensure balanced fluid intake and output.*

Inform: Teach patient to use relaxation techniques *to reduce muscle tension and nervousness;* recognize and reduce intake of diarrhea-producing foods or substances (such as dairy products and fruit) to reduce residual waste matter and decrease intestinal irritation.

Instruct patient to record diarrheal episodes and report them to staff to *promote comfort and maintain effective patient–staff communication.*

Attend: Encourage patient to ventilate stresses and anxiety; *release of pent-up emotions can temporarily relieve emotional distress.*

Encourage and assist patient to practice relaxation techniques *to reduce tension and promote self-knowledge and growth.*

Spend at least 10 minutes with patient twice daily to discuss stress-reducing techniques; *this can help patient pinpoint specific fears.*

Manage: Consult with dietician *to determine foods that may be related to diarrheal episodes.*

SUGGESTED NIC INTERVENTIONS

Diarrhea Management; Nutrition Management; Skin Surveillance; Anxiety Reduction

REFERENCE

Salfi, S. F. & Holt, K. (2012, May). The role of probiotics in diarrheal management. *Holistic Nursing Practice, 26*(3), 142–149.

DEFINITION
At risk for deterioration of body systems as the result of prescribed or unavoidable musculoskeletal inactivity

RISK FACTORS
- Altered level of consciousness
- Mechanical immobilization
- Paralysis
- Prescribed immobilization
- Severe pain

ASSESSMENT FOCUS
(Refer to comprehensive assessment parameters.)
- Activity/exercise
- Cardiac function
- Coping
- Elimination; nutrition
- Fluid and electrolytes
- Neurocognition
- Respiratory function
- Risk management
- Tissue integrity

EXPECTED OUTCOMES
The patient will
- Have no evidence of altered mental, sensory, or motor ability.
- Have no evidence of thrombus formation or venous stasis.
- Have no evidence of decreased chest movement, cough stimulus, depth of ventilation, pooling of secretions, or signs of infection.
- Maintain normal bowel elimination patterns.
- Maintain adequate dietary intake, hydration, and weight.
- Have no evidence of urine retention, infection, or renal calculi.
- Maintain muscle strength and tone and joint range of motion (ROM).
- Have no evidence of contractures or skin breakdown.
- Maintain normal neurologic, cardiovascular, respiratory, gastrointestinal, nutritional, genitourinary, musculoskeletal, and integumentary functioning during period of inactivity.

SUGGESTED NOC OUTCOMES
Coordinated Movement; Endurance; Immobility Consequences: Physiological; Immobility Consequences: Psycho-Cognitive; Mobility; Risk Control; Comfort Status

INTERVENTIONS AND RATIONALES
<u>Determine:</u> Inspect skin every shift and follow facility policy for prevention of pressure ulcers *to prevent or mitigate skin breakdown.*

Administer anticoagulant therapy, if ordered; monitor for signs and symptoms of bleeding. *Anticoagulant therapy may cause hemorrhage.*

Monitor vital signs every 4 hours: Monitor breath sounds and respiratory rate, rhythm, and depth *to rule out respiratory complications.* Monitor arterial blood gas levels or pulse oximetry *to assess oxygenation, ventilation, and metabolic status.*

Monitor urine characteristics and patient's subjective complaints typical of urinary tract of infections (UTIs), such as burning, frequency, and urgency. Obtain urine cultures, as ordered. *These measures aid early detection of UTI.*

Identify functional level *to provide baseline for future assessment,* and encourage appropriate participation in care *to prevent complications of immobility and increase patient's feelings of self-esteem.*

<u>Perform:</u> Avoid positions that put prolonged pressure on body parts and compress blood vessels; reposition patient at least every 2 hours within prescribed limits. *These measures enhance circulation and help prevent tissue or skin breakdown.*

Use pressure-reducing or pressure-equalizing equipment, as indicated or ordered (flotation pad, air pressure mattress, sheepskin pads, or special bed). *This helps prevent skin breakdown by relieving pressure.*

Apply antiembolism stockings; remove for 1 hours every 8 hours. *Stockings promote venous return to heart, prevent venous stasis, and decrease or prevent swelling of lower extremities.*

Suction airway, as needed and ordered, *to clear airway and stimulate cough reflex.* Note secretion characteristics.

Provide small, frequent meals of favorite foods *to increase dietary intake.* Increase fiber content *to enhance bowel elimination.* Increase protein and vitamin C *to promote wound healing*; limit calcium *to reduce risk of renal and bladder calculi.*

Perform active or passive ROM exercises at least once per shift. Teach and monitor appropriate isotonic and isometric exercises. *These measures prevent joint contractures, muscle atrophy, and other complications of prolonged inactivity.*

Provide or help with daily hygiene; keep skin dry and lubricated *to prevent cracking and possible infection.*

<u>Inform:</u> Teach and monitor deep breathing, coughing, and use of incentive spirometer to *help clear airways, expand lungs, and prevent respiratory complications.* Maintain regimen every 2 hours.

Instruct patient to avoid straining during bowel movements *that may be hazardous to patients with cardiovascular disorders and increased intracranial pressure.* Teach to administer stool softeners, suppositories, or laxatives, as ordered, and monitor effectiveness.

<u>Attend:</u> Encourage fluid intake of 2.5 to 3.5 L daily, unless contraindicated, *to maintain urine output and aid bowel elimination.* Encourage patient and family to verbalize frustrations *to help patient and family cope with treatment.*

SUGGESTED NIC INTERVENTIONS

Activity Therapy; Body Mechanics Promotion; Cognitive Stimulation; Energy Management; Exercise Promotion; Exercise Therapy: Ambulation and Joint Mobility; Fluid Management; Nutrition Management

REFERENCE

Clarke, K., & Levine, T. (2011, August). Clinical recognition and management of amyotrophic lateral sclerosis: The nurse's role. *Journal of Neuroscience Nursing, 43*(4), 205–214.

DEFINITION

Decreased stimulation from (or interest or engagement in) recreational or leisure activities

DEFINING CHARACTERISTICS

- Usual hobbies cannot be undertaken in the current setting.
- Reports feelings of boredom or wishing for something to do.

RELATED FACTORS

- Environmental lack of diversional activity

ASSESSMENT FOCUS

(Refer to comprehensive assessment parameters.)

- Cardiac function
- Emotional status
- Neurocognition
- Physical status
- Respiratory function

EXPECTED OUTCOMES

The patient will

- Express interest in using leisure time meaningfully.
- Express interest and participate in activities that can be provided (e.g., watch selected television program, listen to radio or music daily).
- Report satisfaction with use of leisure time.
- Modify environment to provide maximum stimulation (e.g., hanging posters or cards and moving bed next to a window).

SUGGESTED NOC OUTCOMES

Leisure Participation; Motivation; Social Involvement; Personal Well-Being

INTERVENTIONS AND RATIONALES

<u>Determine:</u> Assess leisure activity preferences. Identify the type of music patient prefers; seek help from family and hospital resources *to provide selected music daily that relieves boredom and stimulates interest.*

<u>Perform:</u> Provide supplies and set time to indulge in hobby. Obtain radio, television, or crochet hook and yarn (if desired). Allow patient to (if TV or radio) select programs. Communicate patient's desires to coworkers (e.g., Turn on television set at _____ [time] to _____ [channel]. Give crochet hook and yarn to patient daily at _____ [time]). *Specifying time for activity indicates its value.* Avoid scheduling activities during leisure time, *which is integral to quality of life.*

Ask volunteers (friends, family, or hospital volunteer) to read newspapers, books, or magazines to patient at specific times. *Personal contact helps alleviate boredom.*

Engage patient in conversation while carrying out routine care. Discuss patient's favorite topics as much as possible. *Conversation conveys caring and recognition of patient's worth.*

Provide talking books or I-Pod if available. *These provide low-effort sources of enjoyment for bedridden patient.*

Obtain an adapter for television to provide captions *for hearing-impaired patient.*

Provide plants for the patient to tend to. *Caring for live plants may stimulate interest.*

Change scenery when possible; for example, take the patient outside in a wheelchair *to help reduce boredom.*

<u>Attend:</u> Encourage discussion of previously enjoyed hobbies, interests, or skills to direct planning of new activities. Suggest performing an activity helpful to others or otherwise productive *to promote interest.*

Encourage patient's family or caregiver to bring personal articles (posters, cards, and pictures) *to help make environment more stimulating (the patient may respond better to objects with personal meaning).*

<u>Manage:</u> Make referral to recreational, occupational, or physical therapist for consultation on adaptive equipment to carry out desired activity; arrange for therapy sessions. *Adaptive equipment allows patient to continue enjoying activities or may stimulate interest in new activities.*

SUGGESTED NIC INTERVENTIONS

Activity Therapy; Animal-Assisted Therapy; Art Therapy; Recreation Therapy

REFERENCE

Mische, L. L., et al. (2012, May). Patient perceptions of an art making experience in an outpatient blood and marrow transplant clinic. *European Journal of Cancer Care, 21*(3), 403–411.

DEFINITION
At risk for eye discomfort or damage to the cornea and conjunctiva due to reduced quantity of tears to moisten the eye

RISK FACTORS
- Aging
- Autoimmune diseases (rheumatoid arthritis, diabetes mellitus, thyroid disease, gout, osteoporosis, etc.)
- Contact lenses
- Environmental factors (e.g., air-conditioning, excessive wind, sunlight exposure, air pollution, low humidity)
- Female gender
- History of allergy
- Hormones
- Lifestyle (e.g., smoking, caffeine use, prolonged reading)
- Mechanical ventilation therapy
- Neurological lesions with sensory or motor reflex loss (e.g., lagophthalmos, lack of spontaneous blink reflex due to decreased consciousness and other medical conditions)
- Ocular surface damage
- Place of living
- Treatment-related side effects (e.g., pharmacological agents such as angiotensin-converting enzyme inhibitors, antidepressants, tranquilizers, analgesics, sedatives, neuromuscular blockage agents, surgical operations)
- Vitamin A deficiency

ASSESSMENT FOCUS
(Refer to comprehensive assessment parameters.)
- Risk management
- Pharmacological function
- Tissue integrity
- Knowledge

EXPECTED OUTCOMES
The patient will
- State personal risk factors for dry eye
- Take steps to minimize risk factors
- Understand the need for collaboration with health care team if signs/symptoms occur/persist

SUGGESTED NOC OUTCOMES
Risk Control; Risk Detection; Tissue Integrity: Skin/Mucous Membranes; Knowledge: Health Behavior

INTERVENTIONS AND RATIONALES
<u>Determine:</u> Identify use of systemic medications that may decrease tear production and lifestyle behaviors that may potentiate dry eye

conditions. *Assessment data may influence interventions.* Assess for history of medical conditions *to determine underlying risks for dry eye syndrome.*

<u>Perform:</u> Modify physical environment to increase humidity, minimize excessive air movement, and control dust *which can decrease tear production.* Administer artificial tears as indicated *to relieve symptoms.* Perform protective measures such as preservative free artificial tears or polyethylene eye cover for critically ill patients *to prevent eye damage due to dry eye syndrome*

<u>Inform:</u> Teach about simple environmental modifications *to reduce evaporation of tears.* Encourage patient to take frequent breaks from visually demanding activities *to help minimize risk factors.* Suggest diet rich in Omega-3 fatty acid or dietary supplement. *Diet low in Omega-3 fatty acids can increase risk of dry eye syndrome.* Instruct patient on the use of sunglasses *to limit exposure to light.* Instruct patient to try over-the-counter artificial tears *for temporary relief of dry eye.*

<u>Attend:</u> Encourage adherence to lifestyle modifications *which will improve quality of life and decrease the risk of eye damage.*

<u>Manage:</u> Refer to eye specialist if symptoms persist *for further evaluation and continued care.* Collaborate with primary care provider regarding possible changes in medications *that may be contributing to dry eye condition.* Encourage annual eye exam *to monitor for any changes.* Offer written treatment guidelines as needed *to reinforce learning.*

SUGGESTED NIC INTERVENTIONS

Risk Management; Risk Identification; Behavior Management; Eye Care

REFERENCE

Abetz, L., Rajagopalan, K., Mertzanis, P., Begley, C., Barnes, R., & Chalmers, R. (2011). Development and validation of the impact of dry eye on everyday life (IDEEL) questionnaire, a patient-reported outcomes (PRO) measure for assessment of the burden of dry eye on patients. *Health and Quality of Life Outcomes, 9,* 111.

DEFINITION

At risk for change in serum electrolyte levels that may compromise health

RISK FACTORS

- Deficient or excess fluid volume
- Treatment-related side effects (e.g., medications, drains)
- Diarrhea
- Vomiting
- Renal dysfunction
- Endocrine dysfunction
- Impaired regulatory mechanisms (e.g., diabetes insipidus, syndrome of inappropriate antidiuretic hormone [SIADH])

ASSESSMENT FOCUS

(Refer to comprehensive assessment parameters.)
- Fluid and electrolytes
- Physical regulation

EXPECTED OUTCOMES

The patient will
- Maintain electrolyte levels within the normal limits.
- Maintain adequate fluid balance consistent with underlying disease restrictions.
- Identify health situations that increase risk for electrolyte imbalance and verbalize interventions to promote balance.
- Verbalize signs and symptoms that require immediate intervention by health care provider.
- Remain safe from injury associated with electrolyte imbalance.

SUGGESTED NOC OUTCOMES

Electrolyte & Acid–Base Balance, Fluid Balance

INTERVENTIONS AND RATIONALES

Determine: Assess patient's fluid status. *Patients who demonstrate fluid volume alterations are likely to have electrolyte alterations as well.*

Monitor patient for physical signs of electrolyte imbalance. *Many cardiac, neurological, and musculoskeletal symptoms are indicative of specific electrolyte abnormalities.*

Perform: Collect and evaluate serum electrolyte results as ordered *to allow for prompt diagnosis and treatment of any abnormalities.*

Treat underlying medical condition. *Correction of the underlying cause of electrolyte imbalance is the first step in correcting electrolyte imbalance.*

Inform: Educate patient and family regarding risks for electrolyte disturbances associated with their particular medical condition and possible interventions if symptoms occur. *Early identification and intervention may prevent life-threatening complications of electrolyte imbalance.*

<u>Attend:</u> Provide support and encouragement to patient and family in their efforts to participate in the management of the condition. *Positive feedback will increase self-confidence and feeling of partnership in care.*
<u>Manage:</u> Coordinate care with other members of the health care team to provide safe environment. *Electrolyte imbalances can cause poor coordination, weakness, and altered gait.*

SUGGESTED NIC INTERVENTIONS

Electrolyte Management, Electrolyte Monitoring, Fluid–Electrolyte Management; Laboratory Data Interpretation

REFERENCE

Hinkle, C. (2011, December). Electrolyte disorders in the cardiac patient. *Critical Care Nursing Clinics of North America, 23*(4), 635–643.

DEFINITION

Disruption of the flow of energy surrounding a person's being that results in disharmony of body, mind, and/or spirit

DEFINING CHARACTERISTICS

Perceptions of changes in patterns of energy flow, such as changes in:
- Sounds (tones, words)
- Perception of movement (wave spike, tingling, dense, flowing)
- Temperature
- Sight (image, color)
- Disruption of field (deficit, hole, spike, bulge, obstruction, congestion, diminished flow in energy field)

RELATED FACTORS

Factors secondary to the slowing or blocking of energy flows may be as follows:
- Maturational (age-related developmental crisis and/or developmental [mental] difficulties)
- Pathophysiologic (illness, injury, and pregnancy)
- Situational (anxiety, fear, grieving, and pain)
- Treatment-related (chemotherapy, immobility, labor and delivery, perioperative experience)

ASSESSMENT FOCUS

(Refer to comprehensive assessment parameters.)
- Behavior
- Coping
- Emotional status
- Sensation/perception

EXPECTED OUTCOMES

The patient will
- Feel increasingly relaxed by slower and deeper breathing, skin flushing in treated area, audible sighing, or verbal reports of feeling more relaxed.
- Visualize images that relax him.
- Report feeling less tension or pain.
- Use self-healing techniques such as meditation, guided imagery, yoga, and prayer.

SUGGESTED NOC OUTCOMES

Comfort Level; Health Beliefs; Personal Health Status; Personal Well-Being; Spiritual Health

INTERVENTIONS AND RATIONALES

Determine: Assess how much support patient desires. Evaluate the presence of a disorder that is life threatening or requires surgery. Monitor levels of pain and disorders that may affect the senses. Assess patient's spiritual needs, including religious beliefs and affiliation. *Assessment of these areas will help to identify appropriate interventions.*

<u>Perform:</u> Implement measures to promote therapeutic healing. Place your hands 4 to 6 in. above the patient's body. Pass hands over the entire skin surface to become intoned to the patient's energy fields, which is the flow of energy that surrounds the human being. Identify areas where there is energy disturbance considering cues such as cold, heat, tingling, and electric sensation. *This technique helps you become attuned to patient's energy field, the flow of energy that surrounds a person's being; it is a therapy that requires advanced study.*

Administer medication as ordered *to relieve pain.*

Turn and reposition patient at least every 2 hours. Establish a turning schedule for the dependent patient. Post schedule at bedside and monitor frequency. *Turning and repositioning prevent skin breakdown, improve lung expansion, and prevent atelectasis.*

Provide comfort measures such as bathing, massage, regulation of environmental temperature, and mouth care, according to the patient's preferences. *Comfort measures done for and with the patient reduce anxiety and promote feelings of well-being.*

<u>Inform:</u> Teach self-healing techniques to both the patient and family (e.g., meditation, guided imagery, yoga, and prayer). Teach patient how to incorporate the use of self-healing techniques in carrying out usual daily activities. *It will take repeated use of strategies to induce a spirit of well-being.*

Teach caregivers to assist patient with self-care activities in a way that maximizes his or her comfort. *Caregivers may need assistance with techniques. Lack of skill can cause the patient unnecessary pain.*

<u>Attend:</u> Encourage patient's cooperation as you continue with healing techniques, such as therapeutic touch. Listen for evidence of effectiveness of treatment by patient's statements about reduction in tension or pain. *One treatment rarely restores a full sense of well-being.*

<u>Manage:</u> Refer to mental health specialist or other community agencies as needed. *It is important for patient to have ongoing support.*

Refer to a member of the clergy or a spiritual counselor, according to the patient's preference, *to show respect for the patient's beliefs and provide spiritual care.*

SUGGESTED NIC INTERVENTIONS

Therapeutic Touch; Discharge Planning; Anxiety Reduction; Pain Management; Aroma Therapy; Relaxation Therapy

REFERENCE

Fouladbakhshs, J. (2012, March). Complementary and alternative modalities to relieve osteoarthritis symptoms. *American Journal of Nursing, 112*(3, Suppl. 1), S44–S51.

DEFINITION

Consistent lack of orientation to person, place, time, or circumstances over more than 3 to 6 months necessitating a protective environment

DEFINING CHARACTERISTICS

- Chronic confusion
- Consistent disorientation
- Inability to reason, concentrate, or follow simple directions
- Loss of occupation or social function
- Slow response to questions

RELATED FACTORS

- Dementia
- Depression
- Huntington's disease

ASSESSMENT FOCUS

(Refer to comprehensive assessment parameters.)

- Behavior
- Communication
- Knowledge
- Sensory perception

EXPECTED OUTCOMES

The patient will

- Acknowledge and respond to efforts by others to establish communication.
- Identify physical changes without making disparaging comments.
- Remain oriented to the environment to the fullest possible extent.
- Remain free from injuries.

The caregiver will

- Describe measures for helping the patient cope with disorientation.
- Demonstrate reorientation techniques.
- Describe ways to make sure that the home is safe for the patient.
- Identify and contact appropriate support services for the patient.

SUGGESTED NOC OUTCOMES

Cognitive Orientation; Concentration; Fall-Prevention Behavior; Memory; Safe Home Environment

INTERVENTIONS AND RATIONALES

<u>Determine:</u> Assess cultural status, functional ability and coordination, interaction with others in social settings, and presence of vision or hearing deficits. *Assessment of these factors will help in identifying appropriate interventions.*

<u>Perform:</u> Orient patient to reality, as needed: call patient by name; tell patient your name; provide day, date, year, and place; place a photograph or patient's name on the door; keep all items in the same place. *Consistency and continuity will reduce confusion and decrease frustration.*

Place patient in a room near the nurse's station *to provide immediate assistance from staff, if needed.*

Clear patient's room of any hazardous materials, and accompany patient who wanders *to prevent injury.*

Work with patient and caregivers to establish goals for coping with disorientation. *Practice with coping skills can prevent fear.*

When speaking to the patient, face him and maintain eye contact *to foster trust and communication.*

Promote independence while performing activities of living (ADLs) measures patient is unable to perform *to reduce feelings of dependence.*

Inform: Provide written information to caregivers on reorientation techniques. Demonstrate reorientation techniques to caregiver *to prepare caregiver to cope with the patient when he or she returns home.*

Teach caregivers to assist patient with self-care activities in a way that maximizes patient's potential *to encourage patient's independence.*

Attend: Be attentive to the patient when you are with him. Be aware that patient may be sensitive to your unspoken feelings about him *in order to inspire confidence in the caregiver.*

Help patient and caregivers cope with feelings associated with the disease. *Understanding promotes affective coping.*

Have patient perform ADLs. Begin slowly and increase daily, as tolerated *to assist patient to regain independence and enhance self-esteem.* Provide reassurance and praise for completing simple tasks. Focus on patient's strengths.

Involve caregiver and patient in planning and decision making *as a cooperative effort supports patient's needs.*

Encourage patient to engage in social activities with people of all age groups once a week *to help relieve the patient's sense of isolation.*

Manage: Refer patient to case manager/social worker to ensure that patient receives longer term assistance *to ensure continued care.*

Refer caregiver to a support group. *Caregivers need continuous support from others to cope with the need to provide constant supervision to the patient.*

SUGGESTED NIC INTERVENTIONS

Anxiety Reduction; Behavior Management; Dementia Management; Emotional Support; Mood Management; Reality Orientation; Socialization Enhancement

REFERENCE

Umegaki, H., et al. (2012, June 4). Cognitive impairments and functional declines in older adults at high risk for care needs. *Geriatric and Gerontology International.*

DEFINITION

Progressive functional deterioration of a physical and cognitive nature. The individual's ability to live with multisystem diseases, cope with ensuing problems, and manage his or her care are remarkably diminished

DEFINING CHARACTERISTICS

- Cognitive decline, as evidenced by problems with responding appropriately to environmental stimuli and decreased perception
- Consumption of limited to no food at most meals (i.e., consumes <75% of normal replacements); weight loss
- Decreased participation in activities of living that were once enjoyed
- Decreased social skills or social withdrawal
- Difficulty performing simple self-care tasks
- Frequent exacerbations of chronic health problems, such as pneumonia or urinary tract problems
- Neglect of home environment or financial responsibilities

RELATED FACTOR

- Depression

ASSESSMENT FOCUS

(Refer to comprehensive assessment parameters.)
- Knowledge
- Coping
- Emotional
- Nutrition
- Sleep patterns
- Values and beliefs

EXPECTED OUTCOMES

The patient will
- Express understanding of causes of failure to thrive.
- Express realization that he or she is depressed.
- Consume sufficient amounts of food and nutrients.
- Sleep for ___ hours without interruption.
- Gain weight.
- Verbalize feelings of safety.
- Follow up with psychiatric evaluation/social service assistance.

SUGGESTED NOC OUTCOMES

Nutritional Status; Physical Aging; Psychosocial Adjustment: Life Change; Will to Live

INTERVENTIONS AND RATIONALES

Determine: Assess daily food intake; meal preparation; sleep patterns; mobility status; education, activity, and exercise; religious affiliation;

involvement in social activities; and access to transportation. *Assessment factors will help identify appropriate interventions.*

Monitor fluids and electrolytes. *Imbalance can be life-threatening.*

Perform: Record daily weights at the same time each day *to provide consistent information.*

Report abnormal electrolyte levels *to ensure that therapy will reverse and levels will not deteriorate.*

Monitor fluid intake and output every 8 hours to ensure that fluids are balanced. *Imbalance can lead to heart failure or dehydration.*

Record amount of food consumed and supplements given to patient *to ensure that the patient is getting sufficient nutrition.*

Plan activities and exercise consistent with patient's capabilities. *It is important that the patient be able to enjoy activity. Overexertion can lead to cardiac problems.*

Arrange for social interaction with other patients. Arrange for the nurse to spend several short periods of uninterrupted time with the patient each day *to instill trust and a sense of caring.*

Teach caregiver how to make meals that may be appetizing to the patient. Encourage caregiver to record food consumed by patient. *Appetizing foods may help motivate the patient to eat when he or she claims not to be hungry.*

Attend: Create a pleasant mealtime environment for patient. Provide unlimited access to nourishing foods and nutritional supplements. Attempt to accommodate ethnic food preferences. *This will encourage patient when he or she is hungry rather than when food is put in front of him or her.*

Encourage family members and caregivers to establish a plan for addressing patient's failure to thrive *in order to take responsibility for meeting the patient's needs to the extent they are able.*

Encourage patient to participate in active exercise during the day to the extent he or she is able. *Exercise is essential to a feeling of well-being.*

Manage: Refer patient and family to appropriate agencies in the community such as meal programs, senior support/activities groups, and so forth. *This kind of follow-up will ensure that the plan has a chance of succeeding.*

Refer patient and family to social services *for appropriate resources.*

Refer to clergy person *for spiritual help* if patient wishes.

SUGGESTED NIC INTERVENTIONS

Coping Enhancement; Home Maintenance Assistance; Nutritional Monitoring; Spiritual Support

REFERENCE

Wallis, A., Mortimer, A., & Planner, A. (2011, June). Failure to thrive: An unexpected finding after Whipple's resection. *Gastroenterology, 140*(7), e1–e2.

DEFINITION
Increasing susceptibility to falling that may cause physical harm

RISK FACTORS
Adult/Environment/Medications/Physiological
- Age >65 years
- Lives alone
- Environmental hazards (e.g., cluttered environment; poor lighting, dimly lit room)
- Presence of lower limb prosthesis; use of assistive devices for walking
- History of falls
- Use of alcohol, diuretics, and tranquilizers
- Presence of anemia, diarrhea, acute illness, incontinence, impaired mobility
- Verbalizes faintness when extending or turning neck
- Difficulties with hearing or vision
- Incontinence

Child
- Age <2 years
- Environmental hazards (e.g., bed located near window, lack of gate on stairs)
- Lack of parental supervision
- Unattended infant on elevated surface (e.g., bed/changing table)

ASSESSMENT FOCUS
(Refer to comprehensive assessment parameters.)
- Activity/exercise
- Cardiac function
- Knowledge
- Neurocognition
- Sensation/perception

EXPECTED OUTCOMES
Patient and family will
- Identify factors that increase potential for falling.
- Assist in identifying and applying safety measures to prevent injury.
- Make necessary changes in the physical environment to ensure safety for the patient.
- Develop long-term strategies to promote safety and prevent falls.
- Optimize patient's ability to carry out activities of living within sensor motor limitations.

SUGGESTED NOC OUTCOMES
Balance; Cognition; Risk Control; Knowledge: Fall Prevention; Safe Home Environment; Fall Prevention Behavior, Falls Occurrence

INTERVENTIONS AND RATIONALES
Determine: For adults, assess severity of sensory or motor deficits; environmental hazards, and inadequate lighting; medication use; improper use of assistive devices.

For children, assess sensory or motor deficits, recent illnesses, unsteady balance, running at speeds beyond capability, and inadequate supervision. *Assessment factors will help identify appropriate interventions.*

<u>Perform:</u> For older adults, make necessary changes in environment (i.e., remove throw rugs). Orient patient to environment. Post a notice that the patient is at risk for falling. Place side rails up and bed position down when the patient is in bed. Place personal items within the patient's reach. *These measures prevent injury to patient.*

For children, make necessary changes in environment (i.e., apply window guards); keep toys and other objects from lying around on the floor; use a gate when necessary to keep the child in a confined area; provide adequate supervision *to prevent injury to the patient.*

<u>Inform:</u> Provide family with a list of all the things they need to do to prevent the patient from falling. Go over each item and explain the reason for each cautionary measure. *Written instructions will reinforce the need for prevention.*

Teach patient with an unstable gait how to use assistive devices properly. *Improper use of assistive devices can put the patient at greater risk of falling.*

Teach patient and family about the use of safe lighting. Advise patients to wear sunglasses to reduce glare. *Proper lighting is always considered as a preventive measure.*

Teach patient about medications that have been prescribed for him or her. *Overmedication in older adults is one of the major risk factors in falls. Understanding on the part of the patient and family can reduce the incidence of falls in the home.*

<u>Attend:</u> Ask frequently during hospitalization whether patient and family have questions about the modifications needed to prevent falls. Listen carefully to statement or ideas the patient and/or family may present about potential for falls in their individual home settings. *Greater awareness on the part of both patient and family can markedly reduce the risk of falls.*

Encourage adult patient to express feelings about the fear of falling. *Being able to express the fear will raise the nurse's awareness of what the patient considers problem areas.*

<u>Manage:</u> Arrange for social service/case manager to make a home visit *to help prepare the family for the patient's return to a safe environment.*

Refer patient and family to community resources *that may offer assistance to the patient when needed.*

Refer to home health nurse *for a follow-up visit in the home.*

SUGGESTED NIC INTERVENTIONS

Environmental Management: Safety; Exercise Therapy: Balance; Fall Prevention; Medication Management; Teaching

REFERENCE

Lindus, L. (2012, January 18). Preventing falls in older people. *Nursing Standard,* 26(20), 59.

DEFINITION

Psychosocial, spiritual, and physiological functions of the family unit are chronically disorganized, which leads to conflict, denial of problems, resistance to change, ineffective problem solving, and a series of self-perpetuating crises

DEFINING CHARACTERISTICS

- Behavioral (e.g., Agitation, alcohol or substance abuse, blaming, criticizing, broken promises, chaos, contradictory or paradoxical communication, power struggles, dependency, harsh self-judgment and self-blame, immaturity, inability to express or accept wide range of feelings, ineffective problem-solving skills, isolation, verbal abuse of spouse or parent)
- Feelings (e.g., abandonment, anger, suppressed rage, anxiety, tension, distress, being "different" from other people, being unloved, confusing love and pity, confusion, decreased self-esteem or worthlessness, depression, dissatisfaction, emotional isolation or loneliness, fear, frustration, powerlessness, rejection, shame/embarrassment, unhappiness, vulnerability)
- Roles and relationships (e.g., deterioration in family relationships or disturbed family dynamics, inconsistent parenting or low perception of parental support, altered role function or disruption of family roles, chronic family problems, ineffective spouse communication or marital problems, intimacy dysfunction, pattern of rejection, reduced ability to relate to each other for mutual growth and maturation, triangulating family relationships, unable to meet security needs of its members)

RELATED FACTORS

- Inadequate coping skills; lack of problem-solving skills
- Addictive personality
- Biochemical influences
- Family history of substance abuse or resistance to treatment
- Genetic predisposition to substance abuse

ASSESSMENT FOCUS

(Refer to comprehensive assessment parameters.)
- Behavior
- Emotional
- Coping
- Values and beliefs
- Communication
- Knowledge
- Self-perception

EXPECTED OUTCOMES

Family members will

- Acknowledge there is a problem with alcoholism within the family.
- Sign contracts stating they will not engage in abusive behavior.
- Communicate their needs, using "I" statements.
- Discuss problems in an open, safe environment.
- Acknowledge their strengths and progress in resolving problems.
- State plans to continue to seek counseling and attend appropriate support group meetings.

SUGGESTED NOC OUTCOMES

Family Coping; Family Functioning; Family Normalization; Role Performance; Substance Addiction Consequences; Risk Control: Alcohol Abuse and Drug Use

INTERVENTIONS AND RATIONALES

<u>Determine:</u> Assess drinking pattern; use of other substances; patterns of withdrawal; ability of alcoholic member to function in occupational and familial roles; ability of family members to function in their roles; family health history; affiliation with a religious group and religious practices. *Assessment factors will assist in identifying appropriate interventions.*

<u>Perform:</u> Create an environment in which family members feel free to express themselves honestly about the present situation *to decrease their anxiety and help family members develop confidence in their ability to resolve problems.*

Inform alcoholic family member that he will have to acknowledge his alcoholism before progress can be made in rebuilding family relations *to establish abstinence as a basis for treatment.*

<u>Inform:</u> Teach family members to communicate their needs assertively. Have them practice using "I" statements to express feelings *to help them get in touch with their feelings.*

Inform patient and family about the symptoms and effects of addictive behaviors on both the patient and the family *to help them understand the role they play in both the disease and the recovery process.*

Do interactive planning and role-playing with the patient and family to help them gain the skills needed to effect necessary changes in communication patterns in the family. *Role-playing helps create a realistic view of the behaviors that reinforce behaviors in themselves and the patient.*

<u>Attend:</u> Encourage family members to acknowledge that alcoholism is a problem within the family *in order to break through family denial.*

Ask alcoholic family member to sign a contract stating he will abstain from alcohol *to help him take responsibility for his own behavior.*

Help family members evaluate the consequences of abusive and violent behavior. Inform them that any suspected abuse will be reported. Ask family members to sign contracts so they will not continue to abuse one another *to make them take responsibility for their behavior. Being able to identify strengths provides the confidence the family needs to continue working toward a positive outcome for both patient and family.*

Assist family members to identify their strengths and talk about progress they have made in resolving problems associated with alcoholism or living with a family member who has alcoholism.

Provide additional emotional support to the head of the family about altered role and additional responsibility *to build self-esteem.*

Manage: Refer family for continued family therapy *so they can continue the process of restructuring their lives.*

Refer patient and family to AA, Al-Anon, or other appropriate support group *to establish the importance of abstinence.*

SUGGESTED NIC INTERVENTIONS

Coping Enhancement; Family Process Maintenance; Family Support; Substance Use Prevention; Substance Use Treatment

REFERENCE

Lange, B., & Greif, S. (2011, December). An emic view of caring for self: Grandmothers who care for children of mothers with substance use disorders. *Contemporary Nurse, 40*(1), 15–26.

DEFINITION
Change in family relationship or functioning

DEFINING CHARACTERISTICS
Changes in:
- Assigned tasks
- Availability for affective responses and/or emotional support
- Communication patterns
- Effectiveness in completing assigned tasks
- Expressions of conflict within family and/or community resources
- Expressions of isolation from community resources
- Intimacy
- Participation in problem solving and/or decision making
- Stress-reduction behaviors

RELATED FACTORS
- Developmental crises or transition
- Family role shift
- Interaction with community
- Modification in family finances
- Modification in family social status
- Situational transition or crises

ASSESSMENT FOCUS
(Refer to comprehensive assessment parameters.)
- Communication
- Coping
- Emotional
- Roles/relationship

EXPECTED OUTCOMES
Family members will
- Not experience physical, verbal, emotional, or sexual abuse.
- Communicate clearly, honestly, consistently, and directly.
- Establish clearly defined roles and equitable responsibilities.
- Express understanding of rules and expectations.
- Report the methods of problem solving and resolving conflicts have improved.
- Report a decrease in the number and intensity of family crises.
- Seek ongoing treatment.

SUGGESTED NOC OUTCOMES
Family Coping; Family Functioning; Family Normalization; Social Interaction Skills; Substance Addiction Consequences

INTERVENTION AND RATIONALES

<u>Determine:</u> Assess family's developmental stage, roles, rules, socioeconomic status, health history, history of substance abuse; history of sexual abuse of spouse or children, problem-solving and decision-making skills, and patterns of communication. *Assessment information will provide development of appropriate interventions.*

<u>Perform:</u> Meet with family members to establish levels of authority and responsibility in the family. *Understanding the family dynamics provides information about the kinds of support the family needs to work with the patient's issues.*

Create an environment in which family members can express themselves openly and honestly *to build trust and self-esteem.*

Establish rules for communication during meetings with the family to *assist family members to take responsibility for their own behavior.*

<u>Inform:</u> Teach family members basic communication skills *to enable them to discuss issues in a positive way.* Have them role-play with one another numerous times *to demonstrate what has been learned.*

Involve the family in exercises *to reduce stress and deal with anger.*

<u>Attend:</u> Hold adults accountable for their alcohol or substance abuse and have them sign a "Use contract" *to decrease denial, increase trust, and promote positive change.*

Involve patient in planning and decision making. *Having the ability to participate will encourage greater compliance with the plan.*

Assist family to set limits on abusive behaviors and have them sign "Abuse contracts" *to foster feelings of safety and trust.*

<u>Manage:</u> Refer to case manager/social worker *to ensure that a home assessment is done.*

Refer to support groups that deal with substance abuse, domestic violence, or sexual abuse depending on the needs of the patient and/or family *to enhance interpersonal skills and strengthen the family unit.*

Provide all appropriate phone numbers so that the family members can initiate whatever follow-up is needed.

SUGGESTED NIC INTERVENTIONS

Coping Enhancement; Family Integrity Promotion; Family Process Maintenance; Family Support; Normalization Promotion; Substance Use Prevention; Substance Use Treatment

REFERENCE

Jannone, L. (2011, December). Community services for victims of interpersonal violence.*Nursing Clinics of North America, 46*(4), 471–476.

DEFINITION
A pattern of family functioning that is sufficient to support the well-being of family members and can be strengthened

DEFINING CHARACTERISTICS
- Activities support the growth of family members
- Activities support the safety of family members
- Balance exists between autonomy and cohesiveness
- Boundaries of family members are maintained
- Energy level of family supports activities of living
- Family adapts to change
- Relationships are generally positive
- Respect for family members is positive

ASSESSMENT FOCUS
(Refer to comprehensive assessment parameters.)
- Roles/relationship
- Communication
- Coping
- Values/beliefs

EXPECTED OUTCOMES
Family members will
- Identify family goals and structured directions.
- Express enjoyment and satisfaction with their roles in the family.
- Express a willingness to enhance roles in family dynamics.
- Participate regularly in traditional family activities.
- Maintain open and positive communication.
- Maintain a safe home environment.
- Seek regular health screenings and immunizations.
- Identify and acknowledge family risk factors.
- Make plans to deal with life changes and events.

SUGGESTED NOC OUTCOMES
Family Coping; Family Functioning; Family Health Status; Family Integrity; Family Normalization; Family Social Climate

INTERVENTIONS AND RATIONALES
<u>Determine:</u> Assess family composition, roles within the family, communication patterns, family developmental stages, developmental tasks, health patterns, coping mechanisms, socioeconomics, educational levels, ethnicity, and cultural and religious beliefs. *Assessment information helps identify appropriate interventions.*

<u>Perform:</u> Establish an environment in which family members can openly share their issues and concerns in *comfort to reduce anxiety and develop their ability to resolve problems.*

<u>Inform:</u> Explain importance of setting goals as a method of establishing boundaries that will be respected by all family members. *Family functioning with structural direction will enhance the potential to meet physical, social, and psychological needs.*

Show family how to develop a Genogram to identify genetic risk factors. *Information from the Genogram will highlight things that can modify a family's health patterns, lead to early identification of genetically related diseases, and may delay onset of disease.*

Teach value of daily exercise, well-balanced diet, and use of proven holistic strategies *to improve health.*

Provide family with information on recommended health screenings and immunization schedules. *It is essential to keep immunizations given according to schedule to prevent loss of immunity.*

<u>Attend:</u> *Encourage family members to identify individual and* family goals and a structured direction toward sound health habits for the entire family. *Developing a structured plan will assist in having everyone work together toward goals set by the family for themselves.*

Involve family in planning and decision making. *Having the ability to participate encourages greater compliance with the plan.*

Encourage family to spend time together enjoying traditional activities that everyone likes doing *to promote a healthy lifestyle and encourage strong family unity.*

<u>Manage:</u> Refer, where requested, for follow-up for a family member who needs exercise, weight management, diet assistance, health screenings, and so forth. *Providing referrals will help to provide continuity of care for the patient.*

SUGGESTED NIC INTERVENTIONS

Family Support; Family Integrity Promotion; Family Maintenance

REFERENCE

Abraham, M., et al. (2012, January/February). Implementing patient-family centered care: Part 1 understanding the challenge. *Pediatric Nursing, 38*(1), 33–38.

DEFINITION

An overwhelming sustained sense of exhaustion and decreased capacity for physical and mental work at usual level

DEFINING CHARACTERISTICS

- Decreased libido or performance
- Disinterest in surroundings
- Drowsiness
- Failure of sleep to restore energy
- Lack of energy
- Guilt for not meeting responsibilities
- Inability to maintain usual routines
- Impaired concentration
- Increased need for rest
- Increased physical complaints
- Lethargy or listlessness
- Perceived need for more energy for routine tasks
- Verbalization of overwhelming lack of energy

RELATED FACTORS

- Psychological (e.g., anxiety, depression, stress)
- Physiological (e.g., anemia, disease states, malnutrition, pregnancy, poor physical condition)
- Environmental (e.g., humidity, lights, noise, temperature)
- Situational (e.g., negative life events, occupation)

ASSESSMENT FOCUS

(Refer to comprehensive assessment parameters.)

- Activity/exercise
- Cardiovascular function
- Coping
- Neurocognition
- Nutrition
- Reproduction
- Respiratory function
- Risk management
- Sleep/rest

EXPECTED OUTCOMES

The patient will

- Identify and employ measures to prevent or modify fatigue.
- Explain relationship of fatigue to disease process and activity level.
- Verbally express increased energy.
- Articulate plan to resolve fatigue problems.

SUGGESTED NOC OUTCOMES

Fatigue Level; Activity Tolerance; Endurance; Energy Conservation; Nutritional Status: Energy; Psychomotor Energy; Personal Well-Being

INTERVENTIONS AND RATIONALES

<u>Determine:</u> Assess usual patterns of sleep and activity *to establish a baseline.*

<u>Perform:</u> Conserve energy through rest, planning, and setting priorities *to prevent or alleviate fatigue.* Alternate activities with periods of rest. Avoid scheduling two energy-draining procedures on the same day. Encourage activities that can be completed in short periods. *These measures help to avoid overexertion and increase stamina.*

Reduce demands placed on patient (e.g., ask one family member to call at specified times and relay messages to friends and other family members) *to reduce physical and emotional stress.*

Structure environment (e.g., set up daily schedule on the basis of patient needs and desires) *to encourage compliance with treatment regimen.*

Postpone eating when patient is fatigued, *to avoid aggravating condition.* Provide small, frequent feedings *to conserve patient's energy and encourage increased dietary intake.*

Establish a regular sleeping pattern. Getting 8 to 10 hours of sleep nightly helps reduce fatigue.

<u>Inform:</u> Discuss effect of fatigue on daily living and personal goals. Explore with patient relationship between fatigue and disease process *to help increase patient compliance with schedule for activity and rest.*

<u>Attend:</u> Encourage patient to eat foods rich in iron and minerals, unless contraindicated *to help avoid anemia and demineralization.*

<u>Manage:</u> Encourage patient to explore feelings and emotions with a supportive counselor, clergy, or other professional *to help cope with illness and avoid aggravating fatigue.*

SUGGESTED NIC INTERVENTIONS

Activity Therapy; Coping Enhancement; Energy Management; Exercise Promotion; Sleep Enhancement; Autogenic Training; Progressive Muscle Relaxation

REFERENCE

Fitch, M. I., et al. (2011, January). The fatigue pictogram: Psychometric evaluation of a new clinical tool. *Canadian Oncology Nursing Journal, 21*(4), 205–217.

DEFINITION

Response to a perceived threat that is consciously recognized as a danger

DEFINING CHARACTERISTICS

- Behaviors involving aggression, avoidance, impulsiveness, increased alertness, and narrowed focus of the source of fear
- Cognitive effects such as decreased self-assurance, productivity, and ability to problem solve
- Feelings of alarm, apprehension, increased tension, panic, and terror
- Physiological changes including increased heart rate, respiration rate, perspiration, and/or blood pressure; anorexia, nausea, vomiting, diarrhea, muscle tightness, fatigue, and shortness of breath and pallor

RELATED FACTORS

- Language barrier
- Learned response
- Phobic stimulus
- Sensory impairment
- Separation from support system
- Unfamiliarity with environmental experience

ASSESSMENT FOCUS

(Refer to comprehensive assessment parameters.)
- Behavior
- Coping
- Physical regulation
- Risk management
- Sleep/rest

EXPECTED OUTCOMES

The patient will
- Identify source of fear.
- Communicate feelings about separation from support systems.
- Communicate feelings of comfort or satisfaction.
- Use situational supports to reduce fear.
- Integrate into daily behavior at least one fear-reducing coping mechanism, such as asking questions about treatment progress or making decisions about care.

SUGGESTED NOC OUTCOMES

Anxiety Control; Comfort Level; Coping; Fear Level; Fear Control; Pain Level

INTERVENTIONS AND RATIONALES

<u>Determine:</u> Ask patient to identify source of fear; assess patient's understanding of situation. *Perceptions may be erroneously based.*

<u>Perform:</u> Help patient maintain daily contact with family: Arrange for telephone calls; help write letters; promptly convey messages to patient from family and vice versa; encourage patient to have pictures of loved ones; provide privacy for visits; take patient to day room or other quiet area. *These measures help patient reestablish and maintain social relationships.*

Involve patient in planning care and setting goals to renew confidence and give a sense of control in a crisis situation. If patient has no visitors, spend an extra 15 minutes each shift in casual conversation; encourage other staff members to stop for brief visits. *These measures help patient cope with separation.*

Administer antianxiety medications, as ordered, and monitor effectiveness. *Drug therapy may be needed to manage high anxiety levels or panic disorders.*

<u>Inform:</u> Instruct patient in relaxation techniques such as imagery and progressive muscle relaxation *to reduce symptoms of sympathetic stimulation.*

Answer questions and help patient understand care *to reduce anxiety and correct misconceptions.*

<u>Attend:</u> When feasible and where policies permit, relax visiting restrictions *to reduce patient's sense of isolation.*

Allow a close family member or friend to participate in care *to provide an additional source of support.*

Support family and friends in their efforts to understand patient's fear and to respond accordingly *to help them understand that patient's emotions are appropriate in context of situation.*

<u>Manage:</u> Refer patient to community or professional mental health resources *to provide assistance.*

SUGGESTED NIC INTERVENTIONS

Active Listening; Anxiety Reduction; Cognitive Restructuring; Counseling; Coping Enhancement; Decision-Making Support; Security Enhancement; Presence; Support Group; Relaxation Therapy

REFERENCE

McGinty, H. L., Goldenberg, J. L., & Jacobsen, P. B. (2012, February). Relationship of threat appraisal with coping appraisal to fear of cancer recurrence in breast cancer survivors. *Psychooncology, 21*(2), 203–210.

DEFINITION

Impaired ability of an infant to suck or coordinate the suck/swallow response resulting in inadequate oral nutrition for metabolic needs

DEFINING CHARACTERISTICS

- Inability to coordinate sucking, swallowing, and breathing
- Inability to initiate or sustain effective suck

RELATED FACTORS

- Anatomic abnormality
- Neurological delay or impairment
- Oral hypersensitivity
- Prematurity
- Prolonged NPO status

ASSESSMENT FOCUS

(Refer to comprehensive assessment parameters.)

- Fluid and electrolytes
- Growth and development
- Nutrition
- Roles/relationships

EXPECTED OUTCOMES

The neonate will

- Not lose more than 10% of birth weight within first week of life.
- Gain 4 to 7 oz (113.5 to 198.5 g) after first week of life.
- Remain hydrated.
- Receive adequate supplemental nutrition until able to suckle sufficiently.
- Establish effective suck-and-swallow reflexes that allow for adequate intake of nutrients.

The parents will

- Identify factors that interfere with neonate establishing effective feeding pattern.
- Express increased confidence in their ability to perform appropriate feeding techniques.

SUGGESTED NOC OUTCOMES

Breast-Feeding Establishment: Infant; Breast-Feeding Maintenance; Nutritional Status: Food & Fluid Intake; Swallowing Status; Newborn Adaptation; Knowledge: Breastfeeding

INTERVENTIONS AND RATIONALES

<u>Determine:</u> Weigh neonate at the same time each day on the same scale *to detect excessive weight loss early.*

Continuously assess neonate's sucking pattern *to monitor for ineffective patterns.*

Assess parents' knowledge of feeding techniques *to help identify and clear up misconceptions.*

Assess parents' level of anxiety about the neonate's feeding difficulty. *Anxiety may interfere with the parents' ability to learn new techniques.*

Monitor neonate for poor skin turgor, dry mucous membranes, decreased or concentrated urine, and sunken fontanels and eyeballs *to detect possible dehydration and allow for immediate intervention.*

Record the number of stools and amount of urine voided each shift. *An altered bowel elimination pattern may indicate decreased food intake; decreased amounts of concentrated urine may indicate dehydration.*

Assess the need for gavage feeding. *The neonate may temporarily require alternative means of obtaining adequate fluids and calories.*

If neonate requires intravenous nourishment, assess the insertion site, amount infused, and infusion rate every hour *to monitor fluid intake and identify possible complications, such as infiltration and phlebitis.*

<u>Perform:</u> Remain with the parents and neonate during the feeding *to identify problem areas and direct interventions.*

For bottle-feeding, record the amount ingested at each feeding; for breastfeeding, record the number of minutes the neonate nurses at each breast and the amount of any supplement ingested *to monitor for inadequate caloric and fluid intake.*

Provide an alternative nipple, such as a preemie nipple. *A preemie nipple has a larger hole and softer texture, which makes it easier for the neonate to obtain formula.*

For breastfeeding, ensure that the neonate's tongue is properly positioned under the mother's nipple *to promote adequate sucking.*

Alternate oral and gavage feeding *to conserve the neonate's energy.*

<u>Inform:</u> Teach parents to place the neonate in the upright position during feeding *to prevent aspiration.*

Teach parents to unwrap and position a sleepy neonate before feeding *to ensure that the neonate is awake and alert enough to suckle sufficiently.*

<u>Attend:</u> Provide positive reinforcement for the parents' efforts *to improve their feeding technique to decrease anxiety and enhance feelings of success.*

<u>Manage:</u> Assess neonate for neurologic deficits or other pathophysiologic causes of ineffective sucking *to identify the need for referral for more extensive evaluation.*

SUGGESTED NIC INTERVENTIONS

Attachment Promotion; Breastfeeding Assistance; Lactation Counseling; Nonnutritive Sucking; Teaching: Infant Nutrition; Parent Education: Infant

REFERENCE

Gale, C., et al. (2012, March). Effect of breastfeeding compared with formula feeding on infant body composition: A systematic review and meta-analysis. *American Journal of Clinical Nutrition, 95*(3), 656–669.

DEFINITION

A pattern of equilibrium between fluid volume and chemical composition of body fluids that is sufficient for meeting physical needs and can be strengthened

DEFINING CHARACTERISTICS

- Verbalization of willingness to enhance fluid balance
- Stable weight
- Moist mucous membranes
- Food and fluid intake adequate for daily needs
- Straw-colored urine with specific gravity within normal limits
- Good tissue turgor
- No excessive thirst
- Urine output appropriate for intake
- No evidence of edema or dehydration

ASSESSMENT FOCUS

(Refer to comprehensive assessment parameters.)
- Activity/exercise
- Cardiac function
- Elimination
- Fluid and electrolytes
- Neurocognition
- Respiratory function

EXPECTED OUTCOMES

The patient will
- Have stable vital signs within normal ranges; electrocardiograph shows no abnormality in rhythm.
- Have normal skin temperature, moistness, turgor, and color.
- Have moist and intact mucous membranes.
- Have stable weight.
- Have adequate fluid volume intake and thirst satiety.
- Produce adequate urine volume (approximately equal to fluid intake) of light to straw-colored urine.
- Maintain a urine specific gravity between 1.015 and 1.025.
- Have normal values for plasma and serum for electrolytes, osmolarity, glucose, blood urea nitrogen, hematocrit (HCT), and hemoglobin (Hb).
- Be alert and respond to demands of living; react appropriately to reflex needs (i.e., thirst); have normal muscle reflexes, strength, and tone.
- Express understanding of factors that contribute to normal fluid and electrolyte balance.
- Adhere to prescribed therapies to manage such coexisting disease processes.

SUGGESTED NOC OUTCOMES

Fluid Balance; Hydration; Nutritional Status: Food & Fluid Intake; Tissue Integrity: Skin & Mucous Membranes; Vital Signs; Knowledge: Health Promotion

INTERVENTIONS AND RATIONALES

<u>Determine:</u> Assess usual fluid intake and desire to improve fluid status *to establish a baseline.*

<u>Inform:</u> Teach patient to read and interpret labels on beverage and food containers. For example, humans require 0.5 g (500 mg) of sodium per day; typical intake is 3500 mg daily. *Reducing the amount of sodium reduces the amount of fluid volume in the vascular system.*

Encourage adequate water intake (1,200 to 2,000 mL) during exercise or high environmental temperatures; *unmeasured fluid losses through diaphoresis and lung evaporation can be significant.*

Teach signs and symptoms of dehydration (dry mouth and mucous membranes), light-headedness (blood pressure and vital sign changes), scant urine output (glycosuria and polyuria), and overhydration (cough, increased weight gain, dependent edema, and jugular vein distention). *Teaching prevents severe complications.*

<u>Attend:</u> Encourage patient to select healthy beverages such as water and limit beverages such as soda or sports drinks that have high sugar content *(which increase the osmolar content of the body, causing greater thirst and increased load on the renal system and diuresis)* and caffeine *(which causes diuresis and may cause an increased fluid loss),* alcoholic beverages during hot weather *because these can cause fluid and electrolyte disturbances through excess diuresis.*

SUGGESTED NIC INTERVENTIONS

Electrolyte Management; Fluid/Electrolyte Management; Fluid Management; Fluid Monitoring

REFERENCE

Matura, L. A., et al. (2012, June). Predictors of health-related quality of life in patients with idiopathic pulmonary arterial hypertension. *Journal of Hospice and Palliative Nursing, 14*(4), 283–292.

DEFINITION

Decreased intravascular, interstitial, or intracellular fluid; water loss alone without change in sodium

DEFINING CHARACTERISTICS

- Changes in mental status
- Decreased pulse volume and pressure, urine output, and venous filling
- Dry skin and mucous membranes
- Increased body temperature, HCT, pulse rate, and urine concentration
- Low blood pressure
- Poor turgor of skin or tongue
- Sudden weight loss
- Thirst
- Weakness

RELATED FACTORS

- Active fluid volume loss
- Failure of regulatory mechanisms

ASSESSMENT FOCUS

(Refer to comprehensive assessment parameters.)
- Fluid and electrolytes
- Physical regulation

EXPECTED OUTCOMES

The patient will
- Maintain stable vital signs.
- Have normal skin color.
- Have electrolyte levels within normal range.
- Maintain an adequate fluid volume.
- Maintain an adequate urine volume.
- Have normal skin turgor and moist mucous membranes.
- Have a urine specific gravity between 1.005 and 1.010.
- Have normal fluid and blood volume.
- Express understanding of factors that caused fluid volume deficit

SUGGESTED NOC OUTCOMES

Electrolyte & Acid/Base Balance; Fluid Balance; Hydration; Nutritional Status: Food & Fluid Intake

INTERVENTIONS AND RATIONALES

Determine: Monitor and record vital signs every 2 hours or as often as necessary until stable. Then monitor and record vital signs every 4 hours. *Tachycardia, dyspnea, or hypotension may indicate fluid volume deficit or electrolyte imbalance.*

Measure intake and output every 1 to 4 hours. Record and report significant changes. Include urine, stools, vomitus, wound drainage, nasogastric drainage, chest tube drainage, and any other output. *Low urine output and high specific gravity indicate hypovolemia.*

Weigh patient daily at same time to give more accurate and consistent data. *Weight is a good indicator of fluid status.*

Assess skin turgor and oral mucous membranes every 8 hours *to check for dehydration.* Give meticulous mouth care every 4 hours *to avoid dehydrating mucous membranes.*

Test urine specific gravity every 8 hours. *Elevated specific gravity may indicate dehydration.*

Measure abdominal girth every shift *to monitor for ascites and third-space shift. Report changes.*

Perform: Cover patient lightly. Avoid overheating *to prevent vasodilation, blood pooling in extremities, and reduced circulating blood volume.*

Administer fluids, blood or blood products, or plasma expanders *to replace fluids and whole blood loss and facilitate fluid movement into intravascular space.* Monitor and record effectiveness and any adverse effects.

Don't allow patient to sit or stand up quickly as long as circulation is compromised *to avoid orthostatic hypotension and possible syncope.*

Administer and monitor medications *to prevent further fluid loss.*

Inform: Explain reasons for fluid loss, and teach patient how to monitor fluid volume; for example, by recording daily weight and measuring intake and output. *This encourages patient involvement in personal care.*

SUGGESTED NIC INTERVENTIONS

Acid–Base Management; Acid-Base Monitoring; Electrolyte Monitoring; Fluid Management; Hypovolemia Management; Electrolyte Management; Fluid Monitoring

REFERENCE

Rowat, A., et al. (2011, September). A pilot study to assess if urine specific gravity and urine colour charts are useful indicators of dehydration in acute stroke patients. *Journal of Advanced Nursing, 67*(9), 1976–1983.

DEFINITION
Increased isotonic fluid retention

DEFINING CHARACTERISTICS
- Altered mental status or respiratory pattern
- Anasarca
- Azotemia
- Changes in blood pressure, pulmonary artery pressure, urine specific gravity, and electrolyte levels
- Crackles
- Decreased Hb and HCT levels
- Dyspnea
- Edema
- Increased central venous pressure (CVP)
- Intake greater than output
- Jugular vein distention
- Oliguria
- Orthopnea
- Pleural effusion
- Positive hepatojugular reflex
- Pulmonary congestion
- Rapid weight gain
- Restlessness and anxiety
- S_3 heart sound

RELATED FACTORS
- Compromised regulatory mechanism
- Excess fluid intake
- Excess sodium intake

ASSESSMENT FOCUS
(Refer to comprehensive assessment parameters.)
- Cardiac function
- Elimination
- Fluid and electrolytes
- Neurocognition
- Nutrition
- Respiratory function

EXPECTED OUTCOMES
The patient will
- State ability to breathe comfortably.
- Maintain fluid intake at ___ mL/day.
- Return to baseline weight.
- Maintain vital signs within normal limits (specify).
- Exhibit urine specific gravity of 1.005 to 1.010.
- Have normal skin turgor.
- Show electrolyte level within normal range (specify).
- Avoid complications of excess fluid.

SUGGESTED NOC OUTCOMES
Electrolyte & Acid/Base Balance; Fluid Balance; Fluid Overload Severity; Kidney Function; Nutritional Status: Food & Fluid Intake

INTERVENTIONS AND RATIONALES

Determine: Monitor and record vital signs at least every 4 hours. *Changes may indicate fluid or electrolyte imbalances.* Measure and record intake and output. *Intake greater than output may indicate fluid retention and possible overload.*

Weigh patient at same time each day *to obtain consistent readings.* Test urine specific gravity every 8 hours and record results. Monitor laboratory values and report significant changes to physician. *High specific gravity indicates fluid retention. Fluid overload may alter electrolyte levels.*

Assess patient daily for edema, including ascites and dependent or sacral edema. *Fluid overload or decreased osmotic pressure may result in edema, especially in dependent areas.*

Perform: Help patient into a position that aids breathing, such as Fowler's or semi-Fowler's, *to increase chest expansion and improve ventilation.*

Administer oxygen, as ordered, *to enhance arterial blood oxygenation.* Restrict fluids to ____ mL/shift. *Excessive fluids will worsen patient's condition.*

Administer diuretics, as ordered, *to promote fluid excretion.* Record effects. Maintain patient on sodium-restricted diet, as ordered, *to reduce excess fluid and prevent reaccumulation.*

Reposition patient every 2 hours, inspect skin for redness with each turn, and institute measures as needed *to prevent skin breakdown.*

Apply antiembolism stockings or intermittent pneumatic compression stockings *to increase venous return.* Remove for 1 hours every 8 hours or according to facility policy.

Inform: Educate patient regarding maintenance of daily weight record, daily measuring and recording of intake and output, diuretic therapy, and dietary restrictions, especially sodium. *These measures encourage patient and caregivers to participate more fully.*

Attend: Encourage patient to cough and deep breathe every 2 to 4 hours *to prevent pulmonary complications.*

SUGGESTED NIC INTERVENTIONS

Acid–Base Management; Acid–Base Monitoring; Electrolyte Management; Fluid Management; Fluid Monitoring; Nutrition Management; Electrolyte Monitoring; Hypervolemia Management

REFERENCE

Wu, S. J., et al. (2011, March). Hydration status of nursing home residents in Taiwan: A cross-sectional study. *Journal of Advanced Nursing, 67*(3), 583–590.

DEFINITION

At risk for experiencing decreased intravascular, intracellular, and/or interstitial fluid. This refers to a risk for dehydration, water loss alone without change in sodium

RISK FACTORS

- Conditions that influence fluid needs (e.g., hypermetabolic state)
- Excessive loss of fluid from normal routes (e.g., diarrhea)
- Extremes of age or weight
- Factors that affect intake or absorption of, or access to, fluids (e.g., immobility)
- Knowledge deficit related to fluid volume
- Loss of fluid through abnormal routes (e.g., drainage tube)
- Medications that cause fluid loss

ASSESSMENT FOCUS

(Refer to comprehensive assessment parameters.)
- Fluid and electrolytes
- Physical regulation

EXPECTED OUTCOMES

The patient will
- Maintain stable vital signs.
- Have normal skin color.
- Maintain urine output of at least ___ mL /hr.
- Maintain electrolyte values within normal range.
- Maintain intake at _____ mL/24 hr.
- Have an intake equal to or exceeding output.
- Express understanding of need to maintain adequate fluid intake.
- Demonstrate skill in weighing himself or herself accurately and recording weight.
- Measure and record own intake and output.
- Return to normal, appropriate diet.

SUGGESTED NOC OUTCOMES

Electrolyte & Acid–Base Balance; Fluid Balance; Hydration; Nutritional Status: Food & Fluid Intake; Risk Detection; Urinary Elimination

INTERVENTIONS AND RATIONALES

Determine: Monitor and record vital signs every 4 hours. *Fever, tachycardia, dyspnea, or hypotension may indicate hypovolemia.*

Determine patient's fluid preferences *to enhance intake.*

Maintain accurate record of intake and output *to aid estimation of patient's fluid balance.* Measure urine output every hour. Record and report output of less than ____ mL/hr. *Decreased urine output may indicate reduced fluid volume.* Measure and record drainage from all tubes and catheters *to take such losses into account when replacing fluid.*

When copious drainage appears on dressings, weigh dressings every 8 hours and record with other output sources. *Excessive wound drainage causes significant fluid imbalances* (1 kg dressing equals about 1 L of fluid).

Test urine specific gravity each shift. Monitor laboratory values and report abnormal findings to physician. *Increased urine specific gravity may indicate dehydration. Elevated HCT and Hb levels also indicate dehydration.*

Monitor serum electrolyte levels and report abnormalities. *Fluid loss may cause significant electrolyte imbalance.*

Obtain and record patient's weight at same time every day to help ensure accurate data. *Daily weighing helps estimate body fluid status.*

Monitor skin turgor each shift to check for dehydration; report any decrease in turgor. *Poor skin turgor is a sign of dehydration.*

Examine oral mucous membranes each shift. *Dry mucous membranes are a sign of dehydration.*

<u>Perform:</u> Cover wounds to minimize fluid loss and prevent skin excoriation.

Keep oral fluids at bedside within patient's reach and encourage patient to drink. *This gives patient some control over fluid intake and supplements parenteral fluid intake.*

Force oral fluids when possible and indicated *to enhance replacement of lost fluids. (Bowel sounds should be present and patient awake before giving oral fluids.)*

Administer parenteral fluids, as prescribed, to replace fluid losses. Maintain parenteral fluids or blood transfusions at prescribed rate *to prevent further fluid loss or overload.*

Progress patient to appropriate diet, as prescribed, *to help achieve fluid and electrolyte balance.*

<u>Inform:</u> Instruct patient in maintaining appropriate fluid intake, including recording daily weight, measuring intake and output, and recognizing signs of dehydration. *This encourages patient and caregiver participation and enhances patient's sense of control.*

SUGGESTED NIC INTERVENTIONS

Acid–Base Management; Acid–Base Monitoring; Fluid Management; Fluid Monitoring; Hypovolemia Management; Surveillance; Intravenous (IV) Therapy

REFERENCE

Magder, S. (2010, August). Fluid status and fluid responsiveness. *Current Opinion in Critical Care, 16*(4), 289–296.

DEFINITION

At risk for a decrease, increase, or rapid shift from one to the other of intravascular, interstitial, and/or intracellular fluid. This refers to body fluid loss, gain, or both

RISK FACTORS

- Receiving apheresis
- Abdominal surgery
- Traumatic injury
- Burns
- Intestinal obstruction
- Sepsis
- Pancreatitis
- Ascites

ASSESSMENT FOCUS

(Refer to comprehensive assessment parameters.)
- Cardiac function
- Fluid and electrolytes
- Physical regulation

EXPECTED OUTCOMES

The patient will
- Remain hemodynamically stable.
- Not experience electrolyte imbalance.
- Maintain adequate urine output.
- Identify risk factors contributing to possible imbalanced fluid volume.

SUGGESTED NOC OUTCOMES

Fluid Balance; Hydration; Vital Signs; Electrolyte & Acid/Base Balance

INTERVENTIONS AND RATIONALES

<u>Determine:</u> Assess for conditions that may contribute to imbalanced fluid volume. *Prompt treatment of the underlying cause may prevent serious complications of fluid imbalance.*

Monitor vital signs and other assessment parameters frequently. *Changes in heart rate and rhythm, blood pressure, and breath sounds may indicate altered fluid status.*

Monitor intake and output *to evaluate need for fluid replacement.*

<u>Perform:</u> Collect and evaluate urine output frequently. Measure urine specific gravity as indicated. Decreased *urine volume and elevated specific gravity indicate hypovolemia.*

Collect and evaluate serum electrolyte levels. *Fluid alterations may affect electrolyte levels.*

Administer intravenous fluids as indicated. *Proactive fluid management may prevent serious imbalances.*

Inform: Educate patient and family regarding fluid restrictions or need for increased fluids, depending on underlying condition. *Knowledge will enhance feeling of participation and sense of control.*

Attend: Provide encouragement and support for cooperation with prescribed treatment regimen. *Positive reinforcement will promote compliance.*

Manage: Coordinate care with other members of health care team *to effectively manage underlying medical condition and prevent any alteration in fluid balance.*

SUGGESTED NIC INTERVENTIONS

Fluid Management; Fluid Monitoring; Intravenous (IV) Therapy; Electrolyte Management; Electrolyte Monitoring

REFERENCE

Collins, M., & Claros, E. (2011, August). Recognizing the face of dehydration. *Nursing, 41*(8), 26–31, quiz 31–32.

DEFINITION

Excess or deficit in oxygenation and/or carbon dioxide elimination at the alveolar-capillary membrane

DEFINING CHARACTERISTICS

- Abnormal pH and arterial blood gases levels
- Abnormal respiratory rate, rhythm, and depth
- Confusion
- Cyanosis
- Diaphoresis
- Dyspnea
- Headache upon awakening
- Hypoxia and hypoxemia
- Increased or decreased carbon dioxide levels
- Irritability/restlessness
- Nasal flaring
- Pale, dusky skin
- Tachycardia

RELATED FACTORS

- Alveolar-capillary membrane changes
- Ventilation–perfusion changes

ASSESSMENT FOCUS

(Refer to comprehensive assessment parameters.)

- Activity/exercise
- Cardiac function
- Neurocognition
- Respiratory function

EXPECTED OUTCOMES

The patient will

- Maintain respiratory rate within 5 breaths of baseline.
- Carry out activities of living (ADLs) without weakness or fatigue.
- Maintain normal Hb and HCT levels.
- Express feelings of comfort in maintaining air exchange.
- Cough effectively and expectorate sputum.
- Be free from adventitious breath sounds.
- Perform relaxation techniques every 4 hours.
- Use correct bronchial hygiene.

SUGGESTED NOC OUTCOMES

Respiratory Status: Airway Patency; Respiratory Status. Ventilation; Respiratory Status: Gas Exchange; Vital Signs; Tissue Perfusion: Pulmonary

INTERVENTIONS AND RATIONALES

Determine: Monitor respiratory status; rate and depth of breaths; chest expansion; accessory muscle use; cough and amount and color of sputum; and auscultation of breath sounds every 4 hours *to detect early signs of respiratory failure.*

Monitor vital signs, arterial blood gases, and Hb levels *to detect changes in gas exchange.*

Report signs of fluid overload or dehydration immediately. *This can lead to changes in acid–base balance and affect respiratory status.*

<u>Perform:</u> Elevate head 30 to facilitate lung expansion and prevent atelectasis. Assist with ADLs as needed *to decrease tissue oxygen.*

Perform bronchial hygiene as ordered (e.g., coughing, percussing, postural drainage, and suctioning) *to promote drainage and keep airways clear.* Administer bronchodilators, antibiotics, and steroids, as ordered.

Record intake and output every *8 hours to monitor fluid balance.*

Auscultate lungs every 4 hours and report abnormalities *to detect decreased or adventitious breath sounds.*

Orient patient to the environment, that is, use of call bell, side rails, and bed positioning controls. Place side rails up and bed position down when the patient is in bed. Place personal items within the patient's reach. Assist patient when he or she is getting out of bed in case of dizziness. *These measures prevent risk of falling.* Move patient slowly *to avoid hypostatic hypotension.* Post a notice where it can be seen that the patient is at risk for falling.

<u>Inform:</u> Teach and demonstrate correct breathing and coughing techniques such as diaphragmatic or abdominal breathing and have patient return demonstration *to ensure patient understands proper technique and promote effective coughing and deep breathing.*

Teach patient correct way of using inhalers. Remind patient about mouth care after each dose. *Failure to clean the mouth after inhaling can cause candidiasis in the throat.*

Review all medications with patient and family and list side effects for each *to ensure that the patient recognizes side effects and reports them to the physician.*

Encourage relaxation techniques *to reduce oxygen demand.*

<u>Attend:</u> Encourage patient to express feelings. Attentive listening helps build a trusting relationship.

Encourage family members to stay with the patient, especially during times of anxiety *to promote relaxation which reduces oxygen demand.*

<u>Manage:</u> Request for a case manager to make a home visit to help prepare family for the patient's return to a safe environment.

Refer patient to community resources and offer written information *that can be referred to when needed.*

SUGGESTED NIC INTERVENTIONS

Airway Management; Airway Suctioning; Anxiety Reduction; Energy Management; Exercise Promotion; Fluid Management; Cough Enhancement

REFERENCE

Messenger, R. W. (2012, May–June). Reducing chronic obstructive pulmonary disease readmissions: The role of the durable medical equipment provider. *Professional Care Management, 17*(3), 109–114.

DEFINITION

Increased, decreased, ineffective, or lack of peristaltic activity within the gastrointestinal (GI) system

DEFINING CHARACTERISTICS

- Nausea
- Vomiting
- Abdominal distension
- Change in bowel sounds (e.g., absent, hypoactive, hyperactive)
- Increased bile-colored and/or gastric residual
- Abdominal pain
- Absence of flatus
- Hard, dry stool
- Difficulty passing stool
- Diarrhea
- Abdominal cramping
- Accelerated gastric emptying

RELATED FACTORS

- Anxiety
- Surgery
- Immobility
- Pharmacological agents (e.g., narcotics, laxatives, antibiotics, anesthesia)
- Aging
- Malnutrition
- Food intolerance (e.g., lactose, gluten)
- Ingestion of contaminants (e.g., food, water)
- Enteral feedings
- Inactive lifestyle

ASSESSMENT FOCUS

(Refer to comprehensive assessment parameters.)

- Elimination
- Fluid and electrolytes
- Physical regulation

EXPECTED OUTCOMES

The patient will

- Verbalize strategies to promote healthy bowel function.
- Acknowledge the importance of seeking medical help for persistent alteration in GI motility.
- Not experience any fluid and electrolyte imbalance as a result of altered motility.

- Understand the need for early ambulation following abdominal surgery.

SUGGESTED NOC OUTCOMES

Bowel Elimination; Electrolyte & Acid/Base Balance; Gastrointestinal Function

INTERVENTIONS AND RATIONALES

<u>Determine:</u> Assess abdomen including auscultation in all four quadrants noting character and frequency *to determine increased or decreased motility.*

Assess current manifestations of altered GI motility *to help identify the cause of the alteration and guide development of nursing interventions.*

Monitor intake and output *to identify need for restoration of fluid balance.*

<u>Perform:</u> Collect and evaluate laboratory electrolyte specimens. *Some altered motility states may require electrolyte replacement therapy.*

Insert nasogastric tube as prescribed for patients with absent bowel sounds *to relieve the pressures caused by accumulation of air and fluid.*

<u>Inform:</u> Educate patients regarding importance of maintaining diet high in natural fiber and adequate fluid intake. *Fiber increases stool bulk and softens the stool. Fluid will promote normal bowel elimination pattern.*

<u>Attend:</u> Encourage activities such as walking as tolerated for patients with decreased GI motility. *Increased activity will stimulate peristalsis and facilitate elimination.*

<u>Manage:</u> Coordinate with dietitian and other health care professionals as needed *to meet the unique needs of each individual patient.*

SUGGESTED NIC INTERVENTIONS

Fluid/Electrolyte Management; Gastrointestinal Intubation; Tube Care: Gastrointestinal

REFERENCE

Li, B., Wang, J. R., & Ma, Y. L. (2012, January–February). Bowel sounds and monitoring gastrointestinal motility in critically ill patients. *Clinical Nurse Specialist, 26*(1), 29–34.

DEFINITION

At risk for increased, decreased, ineffective, or lack of peristaltic activity within the gastrointestinal (GI) system

RISK FACTORS

- Abdominal surgery
- Diabetes
- Prematurity
- Decreased GI circulation
- Pharmaceutical agents (e.g., narcotics, antibiotics, proton pump inhibitors, and laxatives)
- Gastroesophageal reflux disease (GERD)
- Unsanitary food preparation
- Anxiety
- Lifestyle
- Immobility
- Food intolerance (e.g., gluten, lactose)

ASSESSMENT FOCUS

(Refer to comprehensive assessment parameters.)
- Nutrition
- Elimination
- Fluid and electrolytes
- Physical regulation

EXPECTED OUTCOMES

The patient will
- Maintain adequate fluid and electrolyte balance.
- Identify diet selections and lifestyle changes that would promote healthy GI function.
- Not experience altered GI motility related to prescribed medications.
- Recognize chronic conditions that may contribute to altered GI motility, for example, diabetes, GERD.

SUGGESTED NOC OUTCOMES

Electrolyte & Acid/Base Balance; Fluid Balance; Bowel Elimination

INTERVENTIONS AND RATIONALES

<u>Determine:</u> Assess patient for signs of fluid or electrolyte imbalance related to increased or decreased GI motility. *Fluid and electrolyte alterations can result from either increased or decreased GI motility.*

Assess patient for positive risk factors for altered GI motility. *This will allow for timely interventions to prevent complications associated with GI dysfunction.*

<u>Perform:</u> Assist patients taking prescribed medications that affect motility with strategies to avoid GI complications. *Awareness of preventive measures will decrease GI complications.*

Encourage early ambulation for postoperative patients receiving opioids for pain control. *Early ambulation will reduce the risk of narcotic-related constipation.*

Inform: Educate patient regarding the risk factors related to altered GI motility, including certain food choices, fluid intake, medications, and activity. *Promotion of healthy lifestyle choices will contribute to positive patient outcomes.*

Attend: Provide encouragement and support for behaviors that enhance GI health. *Positive reinforcement results in improved confidence in self-management of health behaviors.*

Manage: Coordinate care with other disciplines as needed *to reinforce positive behaviors or to assist with complex situations.*

SUGGESTED NIC INTERVENTIONS

Diarrhea Management; Electrolyte Monitoring; Fluid Management; Nutrition Management; Electrolyte Management; Acid–Base Management; Acid–Base Monitoring

REFERENCE

Smout, A., & Fox, M. (2012, March 24). Weak and absent peristalsis. *Neurogastroenterology Motility,* (Suppl. 1), 40–47.

DEFINITION

At risk for decrease in gastrointestinal (GI) circulation that may compromise health

RISK FACTORS

- Abdominal aortic aneurysm or compartment syndrome
- Anemia
- Diabetes mellitus
- GI disease (e.g., duodenal or gastric ulcer, ischemic colitis, ischemic pancreatitis, gastroesophageal varices, GI hemorrhage)
- Treatment side effects (e.g., cardiopulmonary bypass, medication, anesthesia, gastric surgery)
- Abnormal partial thromboplastin time or prothrombin time
- Age >60 or female gender
- Coagulopathy, hemodynamic instability, renal failure, or liver dysfunction
- Smoking, stroke, or trauma
- Vascular disease (e.g., peripheral vascular disease, aortoiliac occlusive disease)

ASSESSMENT FOCUS

- Cardiac function
- Elimination
- Fluid and electrolytes

EXPECTED OUTCOMES

The patient will

- Acknowledge the need to report any sudden increase in abdominal pain.
- Not experience any organ injury related to decrease in GI perfusion.
- Understand the rationale and need for frequent abdominal assessment.
- Verbalize strategies to decrease identified individual risk factors.

SUGGESTED NOC OUTCOMES

Tissue Perfusion: Abdominal Organs, Fluid Balance, Gastrointestinal Function; Vital Signs

INTERVENTIONS AND RATIONALES

<u>Determine:</u> Assess bowel sounds for motility. *Impaired motility can cause functional, nonmechanical obstruction, for example, ileus.*

Assess abdomen for distention *that can compromise blood flow and result in ischemia.*

<u>Perform:</u> Monitor vital signs closely and provide early intervention for those at risk *to ensure adequate GI perfusion.*

<u>Inform:</u> Educate patients at risk to promptly report any abdominal pain. *Abdominal pain is a sensitive, nonspecific indicator of GI dysfunction.*

<u>Attend:</u> Encourage at-risk patients to ask questions and share concerns *to promote understanding and decrease anxiety.*

Manage: Coordinate care and promote early intervention for evidence of decreased GI perfusion. *Early intervention will result in improved patient outcomes.*

SUGGESTED NIC INTERVENTIONS

Risk Identification; Circulatory Care: Arterial Insufficiency; Vital Signs Monitoring

REFERENCE

Mensink, P. B., Moons, L. M., & Kuipers, E. J. (2011, May). Chronic gastrointestinal ischaemia: Shifting paradigms. *Gut, 60*(5), 722–737.

DEFINITION

A normal complex process that includes emotional, physical, spiritual, social, and intellectual responses and behaviors by which individuals, families, and communities incorporate an actual, anticipated, or perceived loss into their daily lives

DEFINING CHARACTERISTICS

- Anger, blame, detachment, despair, disorganization, pain, panic behavior, personal growth, psychological distress
- Change in eating, sleep and dream patterns, activity level, or libido
- Maintaining connection to the deceased
- Experiencing relief
- Making meaning of the loss

RELATED FACTORS

- Anticipatory loss of significant object or other
- Death of a significant other
- Loss of significant object (e.g., possession, job, status)

ASSESSMENT FOCUS

(Refer to comprehensive assessment parameters.)

- Behavior
- Communication
- Emotional
- Growth and development
- Risk management
- Roles/relationships
- Values/beliefs

EXPECTED OUTCOMES

The patient will

- Express and accept feelings about anticipated death.
- Progress through stages of grieving process in his or her own way.
- Practice religious rituals and use other coping mechanisms appropriate to end of life.
- Have participation of family members or significant other in providing supportive care and comfort to patient.

SUGGESTED NOC OUTCOMES

Coping; Family Coping; Grief Resolution; Psychosocial Adjustment: Life Change; Dignified Life Closure; Comfortable Death

INTERVENTIONS AND RATIONALES

Determine: Assess stage of grieving *to establish a baseline.*

Perform: Demonstrate acceptance of patient's response to his or her anticipated death, whatever that response may be: crying, sadness, anger, fear, or denial. Each patient responds to dying in his or her own way. *Helping patient express feelings freely will enhance ability to cope.*

Help patient progress through psychological stages associated with anticipated death, including shock and denial, anger, bargaining, depression, and acceptance, *to help you anticipate the dying patient's psychological needs.* Keep in mind, however, that not all dying patients go through each stage.

Provide time for patient to express his or her feelings about death or terminal illness. *Active listening helps the patient lessen feelings of loneliness and isolation.* Refrain from approaching patient with a busy, hurried attitude, *which can block communication.*

Establish a relationship that encourages patient to express concerns about death. *Basic nursing care combined with genuine interest in the patient fosters trust and understanding.*

Guide patient in life review. Encourage patient to write or tape-record his or her life history as a lasting gift to family members. *Life review allows patient to survey events from his or her past and give them meaningful interpretation.*

Inform: Inform patient about hospice services that emphasize symptomatic relief and caring, with the aim of improving patient and family comfort until death occurs, instead of prolonging life for its own sake. *Hospice care is an appropriate alternative for a patient with an incurable illness.*

Attend: Encourage family members to become involved in the care of the dying patient. Communicate with patient and family members honestly and compassionately. Giving family members a role in patient care helps relieve anxiety and lessen feelings of regret and guilt. *Honest communication is important because family members need an opportunity to acknowledge their loss and say farewell.*

Support patient's spiritual coping behaviors. For example, arrange for patient to have objects that provide spiritual comfort (such as a copy of Bible, prayer shawl, pictures, statues, or rosary beads) at the bedside. *Even patients for whom religious practice hasn't been a dominant part of life may turn to religion when confronted by death or serious illness.*

Manage: Involve an interdisciplinary team (including a psychologist, nurse, the patient, a nutritionist, physician, physical therapist, and chaplain) in providing care for a dying patient. *Each team member offers unique expertise for meeting the dying patient's needs.*

Provide referrals for home health care assistance if the patient will be cared for at home *to support the patient's decision to remain at home.*

SUGGESTED NIC INTERVENTIONS

Anticipatory Guidance; Coping Enhancement; Family Support; Grief Work Facilitation; Dying Care

REFERENCE

Harner, H. M. (2010, June 25). Grief interrupted: The experience of loss among incarcerated women. *Qualitative Health Research, 21*(4), 454–464.

DEFINITION
A disorder that occurs after the death of a significant other, in which the experience of distress accompanying bereavement fails to follow normative expectations and manifests in functional impairment

DEFINING CHARACTERISTICS
- Decreased functioning in life roles
- Decreased sense of well-being
- Depression
- Fatigue
- Grief avoidance
- Longing for the deceased
- Low levels of intimacy
- Persistent emotional distress
- Preoccupation with thoughts of the deceased
- Rumination
- Searching for the deceased
- Verbalization of anxiety; distress about the deceased; detachment from others; self-blame, disbelief, mistrust, failure to accept the death; feeling dazed, empty, in shock, or stunned; persistent painful memories

RELATED FACTORS
- Death of a significant other
- Emotional instability
- Lack of social support
- Sudden death of significant other

ASSESSMENT FOCUS
(Refer to comprehensive assessment parameters.)

- Coping
- Emotional
- Nutrition
- Roles/relationships
- Sleep/rest
- Values/beliefs

EXPECTED OUTCOMES
The patient will
- Express appropriate feelings of loss, guilt, fear, anger, or sadness.
- Identify the loss and describe what it means to him.
- Appropriately move through stages of grief.
- Maintain healthy patterns of sleep, activity, and eating.
- Verbalize understanding that grief is normal.
- Use healthy coping mechanisms and social support systems.
- Seek fulfillment through preferred spiritual practices.
- Begin planning for future.

SUGGESTED NOC OUTCOMES

Grief Resolution; Psychosocial Adjustment: Life Change

INTERVENTIONS AND RATIONALES

<u>Determine:</u> Identify previous losses and assess for depression. Older patients may experience losses frequently and without adequate recovery time before the next loss. *Multiple losses contribute to depression.*

<u>Perform:</u> Help patient identify an area of hope in his or her life. *Focusing on a life purpose may decrease anger and feelings of frustration.*

Help patient focus realistically on changes the loss has brought about. *This will assist patient in forming plans for the future and improving social relationships.*

Help patient formulate goals for the future *to place loss in perspective and move on to new situations and relationships.*

<u>Attend:</u> Encourage patient to express grief and feelings of anger, guilt, and sadness. *Inability to express these feelings may result in maladaptive behaviors.*

Encourage journaling to express grief and loss. *Writing and exploring feelings is an active process, which may assist in grieving.*

Encourage patient and family to engage in reminiscing *to give purpose and meaning to the loss and assist in maintenance of self-esteem.*

<u>Manage:</u> Contact patient's preferred spiritual leader, if patient desires, *to provide relief from spiritual distress.*

Refer patient to community support systems to help him deal with his bereavement and grief process.

SUGGESTED NIC INTERVENTIONS

Coping Enhancement; Counseling; Emotional Support; Family Therapy; Grief Facilitation Work; Reminiscence Therapy

REFERENCE

Holtslander, L. F., & McMillan, S. C. (2011, January). Depressive symptoms, grief, and complicated grief among family caregivers of patients with advanced cancer three months into bereavement. *Oncology Nursing Forum, 38*(1), 60–65.

DEFINITION

At risk for a disorder that occurs after the death of a significant other, in which the experience of distress accompanying bereavement fails to follow normative expectations and manifests in functional impairment

RISK FACTORS

- Death of a significant other
- Emotional instability
- Lack of social support

ASSESSMENT FOCUS

(Refer to comprehensive assessment parameters.)

- Coping
- Emotional status
- Nutrition status
- Roles/relationships
- Sleep/rest
- Values/beliefs

EXPECTED OUTCOMES

The patient will

- Express appropriate feelings of loss, guilt, fear, anger, or sadness.
- Identify loss and describe meaning of loss.
- Appropriately move through stages of grieving.
- Maintain healthy patterns of sleep, activity, and eating.
- List personal strengths.
- Use healthy coping mechanisms and social support systems.
- Seek fulfillment through preferred spiritual practices.
- Begin planning for future.

SUGGESTED NOC OUTCOMES

Grief Resolution; Psychosocial Adjustment: Life Change; Comfort Status: Psychospiritual; Hope

INTERVENTIONS AND RATIONALES

<u>Determine:</u> Identify areas of hope in patient's life *to help decrease anger and feelings of frustration.*

Identify previous losses and assess for depression *to establish a baseline.*

<u>Perform:</u> Perform interventions to promote sleep such as giving snack, pillows, backrub, or shower *to enhance rest.*

<u>Inform:</u> Teach patient relaxation techniques such as guided imagery, meditation, or progressive muscle relaxation *to promote feelings of comfort.*

<u>Attend:</u> Encourage patient to express grief and feelings of anger, guilt, and sadness. *Inability to express these feelings may result in maladaptive behaviors.*

Encourage patient to express feelings in a way he is most comfortable with, for example, crying, talking, writing, and/or drawing. *Dysfunctional grieving may result from an inability to express feelings freely.*

Encourage patient to keep a journal to express feelings of grief and loss. The act of writing about feelings may aid in grieving process. *Help patient form goals for the future to place the loss in perspective and to move on to new situations and relationships.*

Manage: Refer patient to community support systems to assist with grieving process. Contact patient's preferred spiritual leader if patient desires. *This may provide relief from spiritual distress.*

SUGGESTED NIC INTERVENTIONS

Coping Enhancement; Counseling; Emotional Support; Family Therapy; Grief Facilitation Work; Hope Inspiration

REFERENCE

Paun, O., & Farran, C. J. (2011, November). Chronic grief management for dementia caregivers in transition: Intervention development and implementation. *Journal of Gerontology Nursing, 37*(12), 28–35.

DEFINITION

At risk for growth above the 97th percentile or below the 3rd percentile for age, crossing two percentile channels

RISK FACTORS

- Caregiver (e.g., abuse, learning difficulties, mental illness, severe learning disability)
- Environmental (e.g., deprivation, lead poisoning, economically disadvantaged, natural disasters, teratogen, violence)
- Prenatal influences (e.g., maternal infection or malnutrition, congenital disorders, multiple gestation, substance abuse, teratogen exposure

ASSESSMENT FOCUS

(*Refer to comprehensive assessment parameters.*)
- Nutrition
- Activity
- Sleep
- Coping

EXPECTED OUTCOMES

The child will
- Grow and gain weight as expected on the basis of growth-chart norms for age and gender.
- Consume _____ calories and ___mL of fluids representing ___ servings (specify for each food group).
- Achieve _____ hours of uninterrupted sleep daily.
- Maintain age-appropriate activity level.

Parents will
- Identify risk factors that may lead to disproportionate growth.
- State understanding of preventive measures to reduce risk of disproportionate growth.

SUGGESTED NOC OUTCOMES

Appetite; Body Image; Child Development: 1 month through Adolescence; Risk Control; Weight: Body Mass; Knowledge: Parenting

INTERVENTIONS AND RATIONALES

<u>Determine:</u> Monitor weight and height weekly *to evaluate progress.*

Monitor temperature, activity levels, sleep patterns, and changes in nutritional status. Monitor prescribed and over-the-counter medications taken. Determine exposure to tobacco smoke and/or other environmental contaminants. *These assessment parameters will assist in developing appropriate interventions.*

<u>Perform:</u> Weigh and measure the child weekly *to evaluate progress.* Review growth-chart curve *to compare with growth history.*

Establish meal program *that meets the child's nutritional needs.*

Establish routine sleep schedule for the child. Help child keep a chart *to encourage increased levels of self-care.*

List age-appropriate activities and exercises for the child *to stimulate bone and muscle development and promote cardiovascular health.*

Administer prescribed drugs and treatments as ordered. Ensure that the child and parents understand the intended action and side effects that may *occur to ensure that therapy can continue without interruption.*

Provide an environment that is conducive to promote changes the child must make. *Environment can be a powerful motivator.*

Inform: Educate child and parents on nutritional requirements for child's age and gender. Discuss meals available to the child at home *to promote growth.*

Teach child and parents about risk factors associated with disproportionate growth, such as poor nutrition, lack of regular sleep, environmental hazards, or lack of age-appropriate activities. Help to identify preventive measures to be taken in the home *to promote continuity of care.*

Attend: Encourage healthy, loving interactions between child and other family members. Demonstrate healthy and positive interactions with the child. *Disproportionate growth may be associated with emotional deprivation.*

Encourage child and parents to express feelings about present state of child's health. Listen attentively with understanding about the self-esteem associated with what is considered by peers to be other than normal. *Parents will need help in supporting the child through difficulties coping with normal peers.*

Manage: If a medical or psychiatric illness places child at risk for disproportionate growth, make sure child gets adequate follow-up medical care and ensure that the care is appropriate and professional. *This will ensure the child's right to receive remedial and educational care in accordance with his disability, as guaranteed by federal law.*

If financial hardship interferes with the family's ability to provide for child with disproportionate growth, offer a referral to a social worker *to improve the family's access to community resources.*

SUGGESTED NIC INTERVENTIONS

Active Listening; Behavior Modification; Coping Enhancement; Counseling; Nutritional Management; Patient Contracting; Weight Management; Developmental Enhancement: Child and Adolescent; Financial Resource Assistance

REFERENCE

Baptiste-Roberts, K., Nicholson, W. K., Wany, N. Y., & Brancati, F. L. (2012, January). Gestational diabetes and subsequent growth patterns of offspring: The National Collaborative Perinatal project. *Maternal Child Health Journal, 16*(10), 125–132.

DEFINITION
Deviations from age-group norms

DEFINING CHARACTERISTICS
- Altered physical growth
- Delay or difficulty in performing motor, social, or expressive skills typical of age group
- Flat affect
- Listlessness and decreased response
- Inability to perform self-care activities or maintain self-control at age-appropriate level

RELATED FACTORS
- Effects of physical disability
- Environmental deficiencies
- Inadequate caretaking
- Inconsistent responsiveness
- Indifference
- Multiple caretakers
- Prescribed dependence
- Separation from significant others
- Stimulation deficiencies

ASSESSMENT FOCUS
(Refer to comprehensive assessment parameters.)
- Activity
- Cardiac function
- Communication
- Family roles and responsibilities
- Nutrition
- Sleep

EXPECTED OUTCOMES
The child will
- Demonstrate skills appropriate for age.
- Participate in developmental stimulation program to increase skill levels.

The parents will
- Express understanding of norms for growth and development.
- Use community resources to promote child's development.
- Provide play activities to promote child's development.

SUGGESTED NOC OUTCOMES
Child Development: 1 month through Adolescence; Growth; Physical Maturation: Female; Physical Maturation: Male

INTERVENTIONS AND RATIONALES
Determine: Monitor weight and height weekly. Monitor nutritional intake, activity level, and sleep patterns. *Documentation of these factors will help measure progress over time.*

Assess cardiac functioning and respiratory status *to ensure that child is healthy enough to participate in activities.*

Assess child's motor skills, communication patterns, social skills, and cognitive abilities *to evaluate where skill development may be needed.*

Assess *support systems available to child and parents. Where there are gaps, other sources of support may need to be put in place.*

<u>Perform:</u> Establish a meal program *to promote nutritional needs.* Weigh and measure child weekly and review growth-chart curve *to monitor progress.*

Establish a routine sleep schedule for child *to ensure that the child is healthy enough to participate in an activity.*

List age-appropriate activities and exercises *to stimulate bone and muscle development and promote cardiovascular health.* Provide appropriate play activities, such as building blocks, dolls, crayons, or games *to promote development.*

Administer prescribed drugs and treatments as ordered. Ensure parents and child understand intended action and possible side effects *to ensure therapy will continue as planned.*

Provide an environment that is conducive *to promote changes the child must make. Environment can be a powerful motivator.*

<u>Inform:</u> Provide parents with information about the causes of delayed growth and development. Provide written information *to help them know what they can expect as a result of treatment.*

Discuss age appropriate nutritional requirements with parents and child and teach additional risk factors associated with delayed growth (e.g., lack of regular sleep, environmental hazards). Teach appropriate activities and encourage frequent play with child. *These measures promote continuity of care.*

<u>Attend:</u> Five child positive reinforcement for demonstrating appropriate skills and behavior and encourage parents to do the same *to encourage the child to continue developing skills.*

Encourage child and parents to express feelings about present state of child's health. Listen attentively with understanding about the self-esteem associated with what is considered by peers to be other than normal. Parents need to be encouraged first to accept the child as he is and then encourage the child to develop new skills *Development can occur only when parents and staff are both realistic about the child's present stage of development.*

<u>Manage:</u> Provide parents with referrals to appropriate community resources, including sources for financial assistance, child care, and suppliers of adaptive equipment, *to ensure the child's right to receive remedial and educational support in accordance with the disability, as guaranteed by federal law.*

SUGGESTED NIC INTERVENTIONS

Developmental Enhancement: Child and Adolescent; Health Screening; Nutrition Management; Risk Identification; Self-Responsibility Facilitation

REFERENCES

Johnson, J. L., Lashley, J., Stonek, A. V., & Bonjour, A. (2012). Children with developmental disabilities at a pediatric hospital: Staff education to prevent and manage challenging behaviors. *Journal of Pediatric Nursing, 27*(6), 742–749.

Kempton, D. (2012, January). Asthma, ICSs and growth. Are temporary growth delays worth the tradeoff in children with asthma? *Advance for NPs/PAs, 3*(1), 35–36.

DEFINITION

Absence of sufficient professional, governmental, social, and financial/economic resources to provide for the community's health

DEFINING CHARACTERISTICS

- Incidence of risks relating to hospitalization, physiological states, psychological states, or health problems experienced by aggregates or populations
- No program available to enhance wellness, prevent, reduce, or eliminate one or more health problems for an aggregate or population

RELATED FACTORS

- Vulnerable populations
- Characteristics of populations (age, gender, ethnic/racial, education and income levels)
- Migrant and ethnically concentrated groups of individuals
- Rurality and geographic and environmental features
- Urbanicity and density/crowding of population

ASSESSMENT FOCUS

(*Refer to comprehensive assessment parameters.*)
- Values/beliefs
- Populations
- Roles/relationships
- Health care system

EXPECTED OUTCOMES

The community will
- Conduct a formal comprehensive survey assessing the parameters of the community that impact its health.
- Develop a plan to secure professional, governmental, social, and financial/economic resources that sustain a community's health.
- Develop processes that enable individuals, organizations, and agencies to work together to accomplish the community's health goals.
- Implement systems that meet the community's health needs.

SUGGESTED NOC OUTCOMES

Health-Promoting Behavior; Health-Seeking Behavior; Knowledge: Health Behavior; Knowledge: Health Resources; Community Health Status

INTERVENTIONS AND RATIONALES

<u>Determine:</u> Select a qualified leader/coordinator to establish and direct community resources to assess the health care needs of the residents. *A leader is necessary to coordinate the efforts of individuals working to improve the structures supporting community health.*

Communicate widely and through multiple media outlets the need for participation in surveys and assessments to determine deficiencies in community health. *Understanding proposed actions and expectations reduces anxiety and suspicion; it increases cooperation among the community and residents.*

Assess the community demographics. *An understanding of who has health needs to be addressed provides efficiency and effectiveness in delivering care.*

Evaluate the prevalence of health problems and risk behaviors. *An understanding of what the medical conditions and nursing needs are is helpful to align professional services for the continuum of care.*

Establish the scope of need and the reality of resources available to meet the needs. *Integrating the knowledge gained about the community deficit enables the community leaders to identify scope of need, scope of work and means to accomplish it.*

<u>Perform:</u> Create opportunities for community resources to begin services to the community residents in need. *Volunteers and concerned individuals can provide local services to meet the needs of "their neighbors" and promote goodwill.*

Foster relationships at all levels (local, regional, and national) that secure resources to enable policy, funding, and actions plans to evolve for solutions to deficiencies in the community health. *In communities of any size, working together for common goals creates synergy and moves the agendas forward.*

Plan for resident (community) centered, safe, equitable, effective, efficient, quality, and timely delivery of health care. *These aims from the Institute of Medicine provide guidance in the outcomes desired for the community health care delivery.*

<u>Inform:</u> Teach the community members about their roles in self-care, disease management, and community care. *This facilitates autonomy to improve health and promote community centered care.*

Educate students within the school systems about their responsibilities, self-care, health maintenance, and health protection. *Positive health habits, positive self-esteem, disease avoidance, pregnancy avoidance, and successful completion of high school coupled with plans for a vocation or higher education reduces the current and future burden on the community's health.*

<u>Attend:</u> Support and encourage the community as it moves forward. *Barriers and challenges to initiatives may develop and can be surmounted with professional guidance.*

Encourage groups, agencies, and residents to find common ground and goals to work on together to identify solutions to meet the needs of the community. *In finding common ground, a commitment to the group process and the outcomes goal evolve into a solution.*

<u>Manage:</u> Solicit a cadre of individuals with expertise to enhance the assessment, planning, and implementation phases of the community health plan. *Advanced knowledge of the community health assessment and promotion process enables local leaders and residents to move steadily toward positive health outcomes.*

Engage local educators and community leaders to provide insight and recommendations into approaches for segments of the population. *Local experts can be translational leaders in bringing the right residents forward to benefit from the ideas and resources made available through the community health initiatives.*

SUGGESTED NIC INTERVENTIONS

Community Health Development; Program Development; Environmental Management: Community; Health Screening; Community Disease Management

REFERENCES

Chipp, C., & Roberts, L. W. (2010). Lessons learned from rural providers. *The Journal of Rural Health, 27*(2).

Kumaresan, J., Prasad, A., Alwan, A. & Ishikawa, N. (2010). Promoting health equity in cities through evidence based practice. *Journal of Urban Health: Bulletin of the New York Academy of Medicine, 87*(5), i16–i26.

DEFINITION

Impaired ability to modify lifestyle/behaviors in a manner consistent with a change in health status

DEFINING CHARACTERISTICS

- Demonstration of nonacceptance of health status to achieve optimal sense of control
- Failure to take action to prevent future health problems
- Failure to achieve optimal sense of control
- Denial of health status change

RELATED FACTORS

- Inadequate comprehension or social support
- Excess alcohol
- Low self-efficacy
- Multiple stressors
- Low socioeconomic status
- Negative attitude toward health care

ASSESSMENT FOCUS

(*Refer to comprehensive assessment parameters.*)

- Behavior
- Communication
- Coping
- Knowledge
- Self-perception

EXPECTED OUTCOMES

The patient will

- Identify inability to cope and will adjust adequately.
- Express understanding of the illness or disease.
- Participate in health care regimen including planning activities.
- Demonstrate ability to manage health problems.
- Help perform self-care activities.
- Show ability to accept and adapt to a new health status and integrate learning.
- Demonstrate new coping abilities.

SUGGESTED NOC OUTCOMES

Acceptance: Health Status; Adaptation to Physical Disability; Coping; Health Seeking Behavior; Participation in Healthcare Decisions; Psychosocial Adjustment: Life Change; Social Support; Treatment Behavior: Illness

INTERVENTIONS AND RATIONALES

Determine: Assess patient's present understanding of health status and treatment *to form the basis for any further planning.* Assess feelings about present health status. Do this in a safe, nonthreatening environment *to allow the patient to gain insight into and rationally define fears, goals, and potential problems.* Monitor patient involvement in care-related activities.

Perform: *Make changes in the environment that will encourage healthy behavior.*

Inform: Teach patient and caregiver the skills necessary to manage care adequately. *Teaching will encourage compliance and adjustment to optimum wellness.*

Teach patient how to find areas in which it is possible to maintain control *to avoid feelings of powerlessness and allow the patient to feel like a member of the team's effort to assist him or her.*

Teach caregivers to assist patient with self-care activities in a way that maximizes patient's potential. *This enables caregivers to participate in patient's care and encourages them to support patient's independence.*

Attend: Provide emotional support and encouragement by listening to the patient's feelings. *This will reassure the patient that you care.*

Allow patient to grieve. *Grieving is a normal and essential aspect of any kind of negative change in health status. After working through denial and isolation, anger, bargaining, and depression, the patient will progress toward acceptance.*

Provide reassurance that the patient's feelings, under the circumstances, are normal. *By realizing that it is acceptable to grieve, the patient will be willing to look for positive ways of coping.*

Involve patient in planning and decision making. *Having the ability to participate will encourage greater compliance with the plan for activity.*

Discuss health problems with family members *to encourage participation in the patient's care.*

Manage: Refer to a mental health specialist if patient develops severe depression or other psychiatric problem. *Although trauma or illness commonly causes some depression or other psychiatric disorders, consultation with a mental health professional may help minimize it.*

Arrange for an individual who has the same problem to meet with the patient. This exposes the patient to suitable role models and may encourage a supportive relationship to evolve.

SUGGESTED NIC INTERVENTIONS

Anxiety Reduction; Behavior Modification; Coping; Enhancement; Counseling; Decision-Making Support; Mutual Goal-Setting; Role Enhancement; Support System Enhancement

REFERENCE

Kravitz, M. (2010, May/June). Indoor tanning, skin cancer, and tanorexia: Development of U.S. indoor tanning policy. *Journal of the Dermatology Nurses' Association, 2*(3), 110–115.

DEFINITION
Inability to identify, manage, and/or seek out help to maintain health

DEFINING CHARACTERISTICS
- Demonstrated lack of adaptive behaviors (internal or external environmental changes)
- Demonstrated lack of knowledge regarding basic health practices
- History of lack of health-seeking behaviors
- Reported or observed impairment of personal support systems
- Reported or observed inability to take responsibility for meeting basic health practices in any or all functional pattern areas
- Reported or observed lack of equipment or financial and other resources

RELATED FACTORS
- Cognitive or perceptual impairment
- Complicated grieving
- Deficient communication skills
- Diminished fine or gross motor skills
- Insufficient resources
- Inability to make appropriate judgments
- Ineffective individual or family coping
- Spiritual distress
- Unachieved developmental tasks

ASSESSMENT FOCUS
(*Refer to comprehensive assessment parameters.*)
- Communication
- Coping
- Health care system
- Knowledge
- Risk management
- Values and beliefs

EXPECTED OUTCOMES
The patient will
- Maintain current health status.
- Sustain no harm or injury.
- Verbalize feelings and concerns.
- Explain health maintenance program.
- Identify available health resources.

SUGGESTED NOC OUTCOMES
Coping; Decision Making; Health Beliefs: Perceived Resources; Health-Promoting Behavior; Social Support; Spiritual Health; Knowledge: Treatment Regimen

INTERVENTIONS AND RATIONALES

Determine: Assess current health status; personal habits such as use of tobacco, drugs, and alcohol; level of knowledge about disease process; level of family and community assistance; coping mechanisms and communication skills (verbal and written); and degree of motivation to maintain health. *Assessment factors will assist the nurse in establishing interventions for this diagnosis.*

Perform: Provide assistance with self-care, as needed. Encourage increasing levels of independence. *The patient should be as independent in activities of living as possible.*

Administer medications as prescribed *to ensure continuation of therapy.*

Adapt environment to that which is best suited to the particular patient. Reorient the patient as needed. In the disoriented patient, *reorientation should take place frequently to keep the person as close to knowing person, place, and time as possible.*

Provide a consistent caretaker whenever possible *to promote stability for the patient.*

Plan a health maintenance program for patient and family members addressing current disabilities. Provide patient and family with a written copy. *Giving instructions in writing will reinforce the various aspects of the program and increase the possibility of compliance.*

Inform: Fully describe all aspects of the patient's care to the family *to elicit cooperation from them in continuing a plan.*

Instruct family members how to carry out health maintenance practices. Demonstrate skills such as bathing, feeding, and reality orientation; then, have family members return demonstration under supervision. *Involving family members allows them the opportunity to perform skills and solve problems with support and supervision.*

Provide specific instructions on how to maintain a safe environment for the patient *to avoid falls and other types of accidental injuries.*

Teach relaxation techniques (e.g., guided imagery, progressive muscle relaxation, and meditation) that can be done by the patient and the family *to enhance coping ability and restore psychological and physical equilibrium by decreasing autonomic response to anxiety.*

Attend: Encourage patient and family to verbalize feelings and concerns related to health maintenance. *This promotes better understanding and greater ease in managing challenging situations.*

Demonstrate willingness to repeat instruction and demonstrate skills needed *to care for the patients until they feel comfortable.*

<u>Manage:</u> Refer to social and community resources, such as stroke support group, and Alzheimer's family support group. *This helps the family gain support and receive factual information. It provides opportunity to express feeling in a group where others are experiencing similar issues.*

Making referrals is appropriate to mental health professional *to assist with prevention of burnout for the family.*

SUGGESTED NIC INTERVENTIONS

Anticipatory Guidance; Coping Enhancement; Counseling; Discharge Planning; Health Education; Health System Guidance; Physician Support; Referral; Support System Enhancement

REFERENCE

Bukhari, A., et al. (2011, September/October). Strategies to promote high school students' healthful food choices. *Journal of Nutrition Education Behavior,* *43*(5), 414–418.

DEFINITION
Inability to independently maintain a safe growth-promoting immediate environment

DEFINING CHARACTERISTICS
- Difficulty in maintaining home in a comfortable environment
- Outstanding debts or financial crises
- Request for assistance with home maintenance
- Disorderly surroundings
- Unwashed or unavailable cooking equipment, clothes, or linens
- Accumulation of dirt, food wastes, or hygienic wastes
- Offensive odors
- Inappropriate household temperatures
- Lack of necessary equipment or aids
- Presence of vermin
- Repeated hygienic disorders or infections

RELATED FACTORS
- Deficient knowledge
- Disease, illness, or injury
- Inadequate support systems
- Impaired functioning; lack of role model
- Insufficient finances, family organization, or family planning

ASSESSMENT FOCUS
(Refer to comprehensive assessment parameters.)
- Communication
- Coping
- Knowledge
- Roles/relationships
- Self-perception

EXPECTED OUTCOMES
The patient and family members will
- Express concern about poor home maintenance.
- Verbalize plans to correct health and safety hazards in home.
- Identify community resources available to help maintain home.

SUGGESTED NOC OUTCOMES
Family Functioning: Role Performance; Self-Care: IADLs; Comfort Status: Environment

INTERVENTIONS AND RATIONALES
<u>Determine:</u> Assess home environment, financial resources, patient's knowledge about self-care; and communication patterns in the family. *Assessment information will assist in identifying appropriate interventions.*

<u>Perform:</u> List obstacles to effective home maintenance management with patient and family *to develop understanding of potential and actual health and safety hazards.* Begin discussions at patient's level of comfort. *Adult learners learn best where they have specific needs to fulfill.*

Assist family members to assign daily and weekly responsibility for home maintenance activities. *Having a schedule will promote consistency in following the plan of care.*

<u>Inform:</u> Teach patient and family the importance of home maintenance *to ensure safety.* Provide written materials on environmental aspects of home maintenance.

Teach skills such as setting down and choosing from a list of options, and assertiveness skills *to enhance coping strategies.* Help patient and family develop a program by using relaxation strategies (i.e., meditation, guided imagery, yoga, exercise) *to reduce anxiety.*

<u>Attend:</u> Encourage weekly discussions about progress in maintaining home maintenance *schedule to develop family unity and allow members to address problems before they become overwhelming.*

<u>Manage:</u> Assist family members to contact community agencies *that can assist them in their efforts to improve home maintenance management, such as self-help groups, cleaning services, and exterminators. Community resources can lessen family's burden while members learn to function independently.*

SUGGESTED NIC INTERVENTIONS

Active Listening; Coping Enhancement; Counseling; Emotional Support; Family Integrity Promotion; Family Support; Home Maintenance Assistance; Environmental Management: Home Preparation & Safety; Referral

REFERENCE

Brady, T. (2012, March). Strategies to support self-management in osteoarthritis. *American Journal of Nursing, 112*(3, Suppl. 1), S54–S60.

DEFINITION

A pattern of expectations and desires that is sufficient for mobilizing energy on one's own behalf and can be strengthened

DEFINING CHARACTERISTICS

Expresses desire to enhance

- Ability to set personal goals
- Belief in possibilities
- Congruency of expectations with desires
- Hope
- Interconnectedness with others
- Problem solving to meet goals
- Sense of meaning to life
- Spirituality

ASSESSMENT FOCUS

(*Refer to comprehensive assessment parameters.*)

- Behavior
- Coping
- Emotional status
- Roles/responsibilities
- Self-perception

EXPECTED OUTCOMES

The patient will

- Express desire for positive health outcomes.
- Share personal goals to increase autonomy and personal satisfaction.
- Increase quality of life.
- Plan to promote maximal physical, mental, social, and psychological abilities.
- Share strategies to live a meaningful life.
- Express awareness of the need for developing and maintaining a positive attitude of hope.
- Seek spiritual support as needed.

SUGGESTED NOC OUTCOMES

Hope; Personal Well-Being; Quality of Life; Will to Live; Role Performance

INTERVENTIONS AND RATIONALES

Determine: Assess patient's perception of ability to set personal goals.

Assess expression of desire to build on possibilities for the future, and ability to align desires and expectations. Assess ability of patient to maintain and enhance relationships with others. Assess patient's and family's spiritual needs, including religious beliefs and affiliation. *Information from assessment will assist in determining appropriate interventions.*

<u>Perform:</u> Schedule time to meet with family and patient *to listen to ways in which they plan to enhance their coping skills in the present situation.*

Facilitate opportunities for spiritual nourishment and growth *to address patient's holistic needs for maximal therapeutic environment.*

<u>Inform:</u> Teach self-healing techniques to both the patient and family, such as meditation, guided imagery, yoga, and prayer, *to promote relaxation.*

Teach patient how to incorporate the use of self-healing techniques in carrying out usual daily activities. *Practicing will increase the chance that the patient will himself use these techniques.*

Teach caregivers to assist patient with self-care activities in a way that maximizes patient's comfort. *Comfort will reduce anxiety and help patient cooperate with his or her treatment.*

Demonstrate procedures and encourage participation in patient's care.

Provide patient with concise information about patient's condition. Be aware of what the family members have already been told.

<u>Attend:</u> Reinforce family's efforts to care for the patient. Let them know they are doing well *to ease adaptation to new caregiver roles.* Encourage family to support patient's independence.

Encourage patient's cooperation as you continue with healing techniques, such as therapeutic touch. *Cooperation will enhance the effect of the therapy.*

Provide emotional support to family and be available to answer questions. *Being available to answer questions and listen builds trust of the family.*

<u>Manage:</u> Refer family to community resources and support groups *to assist in managing patient's illness and providing emotional and financial assistance to caregivers.*

Refer to a member of the clergy or a spiritual counselor, according to the patient's preference, *to show respect for the patient's beliefs and provide spiritual care.*

SUGGESTED NIC INTERVENTIONS

Hope Facilitation; Self-Esteem Enhancement; Spiritual Growth Facilitation; Guided Imagery; Meditation Facilitation; Relaxation Therapy; Therapeutic Touch

REFERENCE

Digins, K. (2012, January–March). Hope yields health: Offering whole person care. *Journal of Christian Nursing, 29*(1), 11.

DEFINITION

Subjective state in which an individual sees few or no available alternatives or personal choices available and is unable to mobilize energy on own behalf

DEFINING CHARACTERISTICS

- Decreased appetite, affect, response to stimuli, verbalization
- Increased or decreased sleep
- Lack of involvement in self-care
- Nonverbal cues, such as closing eyes, shrugging in response to question, and turning away from speaker
- Passivity and lack of initiative

RELATED FACTORS

- Abandonment
- Deteriorating physical condition or long-term stress
- Lost belief in spiritual power
- Lost belief in transcendent power
- Social Isolation

ASSESSMENT FOCUS

(*Refer to comprehensive assessment parameters.*)

- Behavior
- Coping
- Roles/responsibilities
- Values/beliefs

EXPECTED OUTCOMES

The patient will

- Identify feelings of hopelessness regarding present situation.
- Demonstrate more effective communication skills.
- Resume appropriate rest and activity pattern.
- Participate in self-care activities and decisions regarding care planning.
- Begin to develop feelings of hope.

SUGGESTED NOC OUTCOMES

Acceptance: Health Status; Adaptation to Physical Disability; Depression Control; Hope; Quality of Life; Spiritual Health

INTERVENTIONS AND RATIONALES

Determine: Assess the following: nature of current medical diagnosis; patient's knowledge about medical diagnosis; actual or perceived self-care deficits; mental status; communication patterns and support systems; nutritional status and appetite; and sleep patterns. Also monitor heart rate and blood pressure; respiratory rate, quality and depth of respirations, and breath sounds. *Assessment factors will help identify appropriate interventions.*

<u>Perform:</u> Follow medical regimen *to manage the patient's physiologic condition.* Build non-care-related time into the daily schedule *to allow time to develop a trusting relationship with the patient.*

Provide comfort measures: adjust lighting and sound *to minimize irritating stimuli*; offer back rubs and space procedures *to promote relaxation.*

<u>Inform:</u> Keep patient informed about what to expect and when to expect it. *Accurate information reduces anxiety.*

Teach self-healing techniques to both the patient and the family, such as meditation, guided imagery, yoga, and prayer, *to enhance coping strategies.* Teach patient how to incorporate the use of self-healing techniques in carrying out usual daily activities.

<u>Attend:</u> Encourage patient to talk about personal assets and accomplishments and about improvements in his or her condition, no matter how small they may seem. Give positive feedback. *Conversation assists evaluation of patient's self-concept and adaptive abilities.*

Direct the patient's focus beyond the present state. For example, "Your nasogastric tube will come out tomorrow and you will feel more comfortable." *This helps instill hope.*

Encourage patient to talk about appropriate diversions and to participate in them. *Pleasurable activity decreases potential hazard of crisis.*

<u>Manage:</u> Refer patient and family to other professional caregivers, for example, dietitian, social worker, clergy, mental health professional, and support groups such as Ostomy Club, I Can Cope, and Reach for Recovery. Assist patient to utilize appropriate resources by contacting family and scheduling follow-up appointments. *These measures help give the patient a sense of direction and control over his or her future care.*

SUGGESTED NIC INTERVENTIONS

Coping Enhancement; Decision-Making Support; Energy Management; Mutual Goal Setting; Sleep Enhancement; Spiritual Growth Facilitation; Support Group; Relaxation Therapy

REFERENCE

Talseth, A. G., & Gilje, F. L. (2011, June). Nurses' responses to suicide and suicidal patients: A critical interpretive synthesis. *Journal of Clinical Nursing,* 20(11–12), 1651–1667.

DEFINITION
At risk for perceived loss of respect and honor

RISK FACTORS
- Cultural incongruity
- Disclosure of confidential information
- Exposure of the body
- Inadequate participation in decision making
- Loss of control of bodily functions
- Perceived dehumanizing treatment, humiliation, intrusion by clinicians, or invasion of privacy
- Stigmatizing label
- Use of undefined medical terms

ASSESSMENT FOCUS
(*Refer to comprehensive assessment parameters.*)
- Communication
- Behavior
- Values and beliefs
- Coping

EXPECTED OUTCOMES
The patient will
- Express satisfaction with level of respect
- Identify those things that will reduce feelings of powerlessness and vulnerability and increase perception of autonomy.

The patient and family will
- Agree on a plan to protect patient's privacy and respect patient's confidentiality; family members will evaluate the progress they are making in protecting the patient's right to confidentiality.
- Express satisfaction with the level of respect shown to patient's human dignity.

SUGGESTED NOC OUTCOMES
Client Satisfaction; Protection of Rights; Coping; Personal Autonomy; Self-Esteem

INTERVENTIONS AND RATIONALES
<u>Determine:</u> Assess patient's perception of the current health problem and problem-solving techniques he or she uses to cope. Determine level of family involvement and support. Ask about support systems, including family, friends, and clergy. Determine patient's legal status, including the authority to give consent for treatments or procedures. *Assessment of these factors will assist in identifying appropriate interventions.*

<u>Perform:</u> Schedule time to spend with the patient *to listen to concerns and feelings about current situation.*

Develop a plan visiting with patient *to ensure that the desirable level of privacy is being maintained.*

Incorporate questions into discussions with the patient that are open-ended, and start with such words as "what," "how," and "could," rather than "why." *Open-minded, nonthreatening questioning encourages the patient to discuss issues of concern and improve ability to articulate what he or she desires.*

Schedule team meetings with staff *to ensure that communication with the patient is consistent and truthful.*

<u>Inform:</u> Provide education on legal and ethical rights of the patient to have his human dignity respected, as well as the hospital's or agency's policies on respecting the rights of patients. Include family in this process. *Every patient is entitled to have a copy of the hospital's Bill of Patient's Rights.*

Arrange a team conference with the staff *to review with patient and family information on bioethics and moral rights of patients.* Role model or provide case studies with situations *to allow staff to design strategies for handling difficult issues associated with patient's rights.*

<u>Attend:</u> Encourage discussion of thoughts and feelings about the overuse of negative expressions on the part of the patient by suggesting strategies such as a rubber band on the wrist to snap every time negative expressions begin. *Negative expressions can impair the patient's progress toward a healthy lifestyle.*

Encourage role-playing of verbal and nonverbal communication techniques in a safe environment *to enhance communication skills.*

Provide support through active listening, appropriate periods of silence, reflection on feelings, and paraphrasing and summarizing comments. *Active listening techniques encourage patient participation in communication.*

Make sure that patient has clear explanations for everything that will happen to him. Ask for feedback to ensure that patient understands. *Anxiety may impair patient's cognitive abilities.*

<u>Manage:</u> Refer patient and/or family to a support network that will relate to them in regards to caregiving, the pressures of illness, and other issues related to respecting human dignity. *A support network will provide an outlet for the family members as they work through the various issues.*

SUGGESTED NIC INTERVENTIONS

Body Image Enhancement; Self-Awareness Enhancement; Self-Esteem Enhancement; Referral

REFERENCE

Condon, B. B., & Hegge, M. (2011, July). Human dignity: A cornerstone of doctoral education in nursing. *Nursing Science Quarterly, 24*(3), 209–214.

DEFINITION
Body temperature elevated above normal range

DEFINING CHARACTERISTICS
- Fever
- Flushed, warm skin
- Increased heart and respiratory rate
- Seizures

RELATED FACTORS
- Anesthesia
- Decreased perspiration
- Dehydration
- Exposure to hot environment
- Inappropriate clothing
- Increased metabolic rate
- Illness
- Medications
- Trauma
- Vigorous activity

ASSESSMENT FOCUS
(Refer to comprehensive assessment parameters.)
- Fluid and electrolytes
- Pharmacological function
- Physical regulation
- Neurocognition
- Respiratory function
- Tissue integrity

EXPECTED OUTCOMES
The patient will
- Remain afebrile.
- Maintain balance of intake and output within normal limits.
- Maintain urine specific gravity between 1.005 and 1.015
- Exhibit moist mucous membranes.
- Exhibit good skin turgor.
- Remain alert and responsive.

SUGGESTED NOC OUTCOMES
Hydration; Infection Severity; Thermoregulation; Vital Signs; Risk Control: Hyperthermia

INTERVENTIONS AND RATIONALES

<u>Determine:</u> Monitor heart rate and rhythm, blood pressure, respiratory rate, level of consciousness and level of responsiveness, and capillary refill time every 1 to 4 hours *to evaluate effectiveness of interventions and monitor for complications.*

Determine patient's preferences for oral fluids, and encourage patient to drink as much as possible, unless contraindicated. Monitor and record intake and output, and administer intravenous fluids, if indicated. *Because insensible fluid loss increases by 10% for every 1.8° F (1° C) increase in temperature, patient must increase fluid intake to prevent dehydration.*

<u>Perform:</u> Take temperature every 1 to 4 hours *to obtain an accurate core temperature.* Identify route and record measurements.

Administer antipyretics as prescribed and record effectiveness. *Antipyretics act on hypothalamus to regulate temperature.*

Use nonpharmacologic measures *to reduce excessive fever,* such as removing sheets, blankets, and most clothing; placing ice bags on axillae and groin; and sponging with tepid water. Explain these measures to patient. *Nonpharmacologic measures lower body temperature and promote comfort. Sponging reduces body temperature by increasing evaporation from skin. Tepid water is used because cold water increases shivering, thereby increasing metabolic rate and causing temperature to rise.*

Use a hypothermia blanket if patient's temperature rises above 103° F (39.4° C), if ordered. Monitor vital signs every 15 minutes for 1 hours and then as indicated. *Prolonged hyperthermia may lead to complications such as seizures.* Turn off blanket if shivering occurs. *Shivering increases metabolic rate, increasing temperature.*

<u>Manage:</u> Report lack of responses to interventions to physician *to prevent complications.*

SUGGESTED NIC INTERVENTIONS

Environmental Management; Fever Treatment; Fluid Management; Temperature Regulation

REFERENCE

Dai, Y. T., & Lu, S. H. (2012, May). What's missing for evidence-based fever management? Is fever beneficial or harmful to humans? *International Journal of Nursing Studies, 249*(5), 505–507.

DEFINITION
Body temperature below normal range

DEFINING CHARACTERISTICS
- Body temperature below normal range
- Cool, pale skin
- Cyanotic nail beds
- Increased blood pressure, heart rate, and capillary refill time
- Piloerection
- Shivering

RELATED FACTORS
- Aging
- Consumption of alcohol
- Damage to hypothalamus
- Decreased ability to shiver
- Decreased metabolic rate
- Evaporation from skin in cool environment
- Exposure to cool environment
- Illness
- Inactivity
- Inadequate clothing
- Malnutrition
- Medications
- Trauma

ASSESSMENT FOCUS
(*Refer to comprehensive assessment parameters.*)
- Fluid and electrolytes
- Pharmacological function
- Physical regulation
- Neurocognition
- Respiratory function
- Tissue integrity

EXPECTED OUTCOMES
The patient will
- Maintain body temperature within normal range.
- Have warm and dry skin.
- Maintain heart rate and blood pressure within normal range.
- Not shiver.
- Express feelings of comfort.
- Show no complications associated with hypothermia, such as soft-tissue injury, fracture, dehydration, and hypovolemic shock, if warmed too quickly.

- State an understanding of how to prevent further episodes of hypothermia.

SUGGESTED NOC OUTCOMES

Neurological Status: Autonomic; Thermoregulation; Vital Signs; Risk Control: Hypothermia

INTERVENTIONS AND RATIONALES

<u>Determine:</u> Monitor body temperature at least every 4 hours or more frequently, if indicated, *to evaluate effectiveness of interventions.*

Record temperature and route *to allow accurate data comparison.* Baseline temperatures vary, depending on route used. If temperature drops below 95° F (35° C), use a low-reading thermometer *to obtain accurate reading.*

Monitor and record neurologic status at least every 4 hours. *Falling body temperature and metabolic rate reduce pulse rate and blood pressure, which reduces blood perfusion to brain, resulting in disorientation, confusion, and unconsciousness.*

Monitor and record heart rate and rhythm, blood pressure, and respiratory rate at least every 4 hours. *Blood pressure and pulse decrease in hypothermia. During rewarming, patient may develop hypovolemic shock. During warming, ventricular fibrillation and cardiac arrest may occur, possibly signaled by irregular pulse.*

<u>Perform:</u> Provide supportive measures, such as placing patient in warm bed and covering with warm blankets, removing wet or constrictive clothing, and covering metal or plastic surfaces that contact patient's body. *These measures protect patient from heat loss.*

Follow prescribed treatment regimen for hypothermia: As ordered, administer medications *to prevent shivering to avoid overheating.* Monitor and record effectiveness. As ordered, administer analgesic *to relieve pain associated with warming.* Monitor and record effectiveness.

Use hyperthermia blanket, as ordered, *to warm patient* if temperature drops below 95° F (35° C). Warm patient to 97° F (36.1° C).

As appropriate, administer fluids during rewarming *to prevent hypovolemic shock.* If administering large volumes of intravenous fluids, consider using a fluid warmer to avoid heat loss.

<u>Inform:</u> Discuss precipitating factors with patient, if indicated. *Patient may require community outreach assistance with certain precipitating factors, including inadequate living conditions, insufficient finances, and abuse of medications (such as sedatives and alcohol).*

Instruct patient in precautionary measures to avoid hypothermia, such as dressing warmly even when indoors, eating proper diet, and remaining as active as possible. *Precautions help to prevent accidental hypothermia.*

<u>Manage:</u> Report lack of responses to interventions to physician *to prevent complications.*

SUGGESTED NIC INTERVENTIONS

Comfort Level; Fluid Management; Hypothermia Treatment; Temperature Regulation; Vital Signs Monitoring

REFERENCE

Davis, R. A. (2012, January). The big chill: Accidental hypothermia. *American Journal of Nursing, 112*(1), 38–46.

DEFINITION

A pattern of conforming to local, national, and/or international standards of immunization to prevent infectious disease(s) that is sufficient to protect a person, family, or community and can be strengthened

DEFINING CHARACTERISTICS

Expresses desire to enhance
- Behavior to prevent infectious disease
- Identification of possible problems associated with immunizations
- Identification of providers of immunizations
- Immunization status
- Knowledge of immunization standards
- Record keeping of immunizations

ASSESSMENT FOCUS

(*Refer to comprehensive assessment parameters.*)
- Health care system
- Self-perception

EXPECTED OUTCOMES

The patient will
- Express knowledge of health-seeking behaviors necessary to participate in immunization.
- Demonstrate adherence behavior to standard recommended immunization protocols.
- Develop an ongoing plan for maintaining records of immunizations.

SUGGESTED NOC OUTCOMES

Community Health Status: Immunity; Community Risk Control: Communicable Disease; Immunization Behavior; Knowledge: Infection

INTERVENTIONS AND RATIONALES

<u>Determine:</u> Assess patient's prior participation in immunization program. Determine patient's perception of the need for the prevention of infectious diseases and responsibility for controlling the spread of communicable disease. Assess patient's attitude toward health-seeking behavior that leads to immunization and knowledge of infection control through immunization for communicable disease. *Assessment factors help in determining appropriate interventions.*

<u>Perform:</u> Administer vaccines, as ordered, to ensure expected result will occur. Implement a mechanism or device for record keeping of immunizations *to prevent gaps and overlaps in patient immunizations.*

<u>Inform:</u> Help patient understand possible risks associated with immunizations *to assist patients identify reportable risks and complications resulting from immunizations.*

Attend: Encourage patients to have immunizations as close to due dates as possible *to ensure that protection from disease will be consistent* and continuous.

Listen attentively to what patient has to say about fear of vaccines. *Fear is often the factor that keeps people from being vaccinated.*

Manage: Request for a case manager to make a home visit *to help prepare the family for the patient's return to a safe environment.*

Refer patient to community resources *that may offer assistance to the patient when needed.*

Offer written information *that can be referred to when needed.*

Refer to home health nurse *for a follow-up visit in the home.*

SUGGESTED NIC INTERVENTIONS

Communicable Disease Management; Immunization/Vaccination Management; Infection Control

REFERENCE

Koch, J. A. (2012, February). Strategies to overcome barriers to pneumococcal vaccination in older adults: An integrative review. *Journal of Gerontology Nursing, 38*(2), 31–39.

DEFINITION

A pattern of performing rapid, unplanned reactions to internal or external stimuli without regard for the negative consequences of these reactions to the impulsive individual or to others

DEFINING CHARACTERISTICS

- Asking inappropriate questions of others despite their discomfort
- Disclosing inappropriate personal details with familiar persons and strangers
- Impulsive actions (e.g., gambling, setting fires, self-mutilation, sexual promiscuity, stealing, temper outbursts)
- Inability to manage finances
- Irritability
- Regret after impulsive actions
- Sensation seeking
- Violence

RELATED FACTORS

- Chronic low self-esteem
- Co-dependency
- Denial of responsibility regarding impulsive actions
- Disorder of development
- Economically disadvantaged
- Environment that might cause frustration or irritation
- Feelings of anger, fatigue, and hopelessness
- Insomnia
- Ineffective coping
- Organic brain disorders that affect cognition
- Psychiatric disorders (e.g., body image, depression, delusional, mood, personality, substance dependence)
- Social isolation
- Stress vulnerability
- Unpleasant physical symptoms

ASSESSMENT FOCUS

(*Refer to comprehensive assessment parameters.*)

- Behavior
- Communication
- Coping
- Emotional
- Pharmacological function
- Risk management

EXPECTED OUTCOMES

The patient will

- Identify triggers that lead to self-destructive actions.
- Identify appropriate coping mechanisms to prevent self-harm and minimize engaging in impulsive behaviors.

- Identify strategies that will aid in maintaining positive relationships.
- Report any thoughts of harming self or others to staff.
- Work with staff in planning ongoing treatment.

SUGGESTED NOC OUTCOMES

Aggression Control; Anxiety Control; Coping; Impulse Control; Self-Esteem; Self-Mutilation Restraint; Social Interaction Skills

INTERVENTIONS AND RATIONALES

Determine: Assess patient for thoughts of suicide, homicide, or self-mutilation. *Findings may require immediate safety precautions and psychological support.*

Assess for history of previous or current medical conditions and any pharmacological side effects that may be contributing to current symptoms *as brain trauma, organic brain disorders, or medications can present with impulse control symptoms.*

Perform: Decrease environmental stimuli if patient is feeling unsafe. *A quiet and nonstimulating environment will assist in decreasing level of anxiety.*

Assist the patient in identifying stressors that lead to inappropriate or harmful impulsive behaviors *as the patient is usually unaware of impulsive behaviors and will require assistance in identifying them.*

Inform: Educate the patient regarding cognitive therapies that can be used *to reinforce appropriate coping and social skills.*

Attend: Dedicate quality time to patient in a therapeutic and consistent manner *in order to help patient feel safe and allow an open and trusting relationship to develop.*

Encourage patient to attend milieu therapies. *Milieu therapies will offer the patient an opportunity to share feelings and learn/practice new coping and social skills with peers.*

Manage: Refer patient for treatment, which may include but is not limited to medication management, individual therapy sessions, peer support groups, and crisis center contacts *to ensure continuation of treatment.*

SUGGESTED NIC INTERVENTIONS

Anger Control Assistance; Anxiety Reduction; Cognitive Restructuring; Coping Enhancement; Impulse Control Training; Support Group

REFERENCE

Balarajah, S., & Cavanna, A. E. (2012, May 24). The pathophysiology of impulse control disorders in Parkinson disease. *Behavioral Neurology.*

DEFINITION
Change in normal bowel habits characterized by involuntary passage of stool

DEFINING CHARACTERISTICS
- Constant dribbling of soft stool
- Fecal odor
- Fecal staining of clothing or bedding
- Inability to delay defecation
- Inability to recognize urge to defecate
- Recognizes rectal fullness but reports inability to expel formed stool
- Inattention to urge to defecate
- Self-report of inability to recognize rectal fullness
- Red perianal skin
- Urgency

RELATED FACTORS
- Abnormally high abdominal pressure
- Abnormally high intestinal pressure
- Chronic diarrhea
- Colorectal lesions
- Dietary habits
- Environmental factors (e.g., inaccessible bathroom)
- General decline in muscle tone
- Immobility
- Impaired cognition
- Impaired reservoir capacity
- Incomplete emptying of bowel
- Laxative abuse
- Loss of rectal sphincter control
- Lower motor nerve damage
- Medications
- Rectal sphincter abnormality
- Impaction
- Stress
- Toileting self-care deficit
- Upper motor nerve damage

ASESSMENT FOCUS
(*Refer to comprehensive assessment parameters.*)
- Fluid and electrolytes
- Elimination
- Neurocognition

EXPECTED OUTCOMES
The patient will
- Experience a bowel movement every ___ day(s) when placed on commode or toilet at ___ a.m/p.m.
- Maintain clean and intact skin.
- Have improved control of incontinent episodes.
- State understanding of bowel routine.
- Demonstrate skill in using commode.
- Demonstrate skill in the use of suppository if indicated.

- Express an understanding of the relationship between food and fluid regulation and the promotion of continence.
- Maintain self-respect and dignity through participation and acceptance within group.

SUGGESTED NOC OUTCOMES

Bowel Continence; Bowel Elimination; Self-Care: Toileting

INTERVENTIONS AND RATIONALES

Determine: Establish a regular pattern for bowel care; for example, after breakfast every other day, place patient on the commode chair 1 hour, allow patient to remain upright for 30 minutes for maximum response, and then clean the anal area. *Procedure encourages adaptation and routine physiologic function.*

Monitor and record incontinent episodes; keep baseline record for 3 to 7 days *to track effectiveness of toileting routine.*

Perform: Clean and dry perianal area after each incontinent episode *to prevent infection and promote comfort.*

Inform: Demonstrate bowel care routine to family or caregiver *to reduce anxiety from lack of knowledge or involvement in care.*

Arrange for return demonstration of bowel care routine *to help establish therapeutic relationship with patient and family or caregiver.*

Establish a date when family or caregiver will carry out bowel care routine with supportive assistance; *this will ensure that patient receives dependable care.*

Discuss bowel care routine with family or caregiver *to foster compliance.*

Instruct family or caregiver on need to regulate foods and fluids that cause diarrhea or constipation *to encourage helpful nutritional habits.*

Attend: Maintain patient's dignity by using protective padding under clothing, by removing patient from group activity after incontinent episode, and by cleaning and returning patient to the group without undue attention. *These measures prevent odor, skin breakdown, and embarrassment and promote patient's positive self-image.*

Manage: Maintain diet log *to identify irritating foods,* and then eliminate them from patient's diet.

SUGGESTED NIC INTERVENTIONS

Bowel Incontinence Care; Bowel Management; Perineal Care; Skin Surveillance

REFERENCE

Landers, M., et al. (2011, December). Self-care strategies for the management of bowel symptoms following sphincter-saving surgery for rectal cancer. *Clinical Journal of Oncology Nursing, 15*(6), E105–113.

DEFINITION

Inability of usually continent person to reach toilet in time to avoid unintentional loss of urine

DEFINING CHARACTERISTICS

- Amount of time needed to reach toilet exceeding length of time between sensing urge to void and uncontrolled voiding
- Loss of urine before reaching toilet
- May be incontinent only in the morning
- Able to empty bladder completely
- Senses need to void

RELATED FACTORS

- Altered environmental factors
- Impaired cognition
- Impaired vision
- Neuromuscular limitations
- Psychological factors
- Weakened supporting pelvic structures

ASSESSMENT FOCUS

(*Refer to comprehensive assessment parameters.*)

- Activity/exercise
- Behavior
- Elimination
- Fluid and electrolytes
- Physical regulation
- Self-care

EXPECTED OUTCOMES

The patient will

- Void at appropriate intervals.
- Have minimal, if any, complications.
- Demonstrate skill in managing incontinence.
- Discuss impact of incontinence on him and family members.
- Identify resources to assist with care following discharge.

SUGGESTED NOC OUTCOMES

Coordinated Movement; Self-Care: Toileting; Symptom Control; Urinary Continence; Urinary Elimination

INTERVENTIONS AND RATIONALES

Determine: Monitor and record patient's voiding patterns *to ensure correct fluid replacement therapy.*

Perform: Stimulate patient's voiding reflexes (give patient drink of water while on toilet, stroke area over bladder, or pour water over perineum) to *trigger bladder's spastic reflex.* Provide hyperactive patient with distraction, such as a magazine, *to occupy attention while on toilet, reduce anxiety, and ease voiding.*

Maintain adequate hydration up to 3,000 mL daily, unless contraindicated. *Scheduling fluid intake promotes regular bladder distention and optimal time intervals between voidings.* Limit fluid intake to 150 mL after dinner *to reduce need to void at night.*

Assist with specific bladder elimination procedures, such as the following: **bladder training**—this involves muscle-strengthening exercises, adequate fluid intake, and carefully scheduled voiding times (encourage voiding every 2 hours while awake and once during night); **rigid toilet regimen**—place patient on toilet at specific intervals (every 2 hours or after meals) and note whether voiding occurred at each interval (*this helps patient adapt to routine physiologic function*); **behavior modification**—refrain from punishing unwanted behavior (e.g., voiding in wrong place), and reinforce positive behavior using social or material rewards (*this helps patient learn alternatives to maladaptive behaviors*); **use of external catheter**—apply according to established procedure and maintain patency, observe condition of perineal skin and clean with soap and water at least twice daily (*this ensures effective therapy and prevents infection and skin breakdown*); **application of protective pads and garments**—use only when interventions have failed to prevent infection and skin breakdown and allow at least 4 to 6 weeks for trial period (*establishing continence requires prolonged effort*).

Maintain continence based on patient's voiding patterns and limitations. Respond to call light promptly *to avoid delays in voiding routine.*

Orient patient to toileting environment: time, place, and activity *to offer security.* Provide privacy and adequate time to void *to allow patient to void easily without anxiety.*

Replace wet clothes immediately. Select clothing that promotes easy dressing and undressing (e.g., Velcro fasteners and gowns) *to reduce patient's frustration with voiding routine.*

Inform: Teach family members and support personnel *to reduce anxiety that results from noninvolvement.* Instruct patient and family members on continence techniques to use at home *to increase chances of successful bladder retraining.*

Attend: Encourage patient and family members to share feelings related to incontinence. This allows specific problems to be identified and resolved. *Attentive listening conveys recognition and respect.*

Manage: Refer patient/family to home health care agency, or support group *to provide access to additional community resources.*

SUGGESTED NIC INTERVENTIONS

Pelvic Muscle Exercise; Prompted Voiding; Self-Care Assistance; Urinary Elimination Management; Urinary Habit Training; Urinary Incontinence Care

REFERENCE

Cotterill, N. (2011, October). Quality of life issues in continence care. *Nursing Standard, 26*(8), 51.

DEFINITION
Involuntary loss of urine associated with overdistention of the bladder

DEFINING CHARACTERISTICS
- Bladder distention
- High postvoid residual volume
- Nocturia
- Reported and/or observed involuntary leakage of small volumes of urine

RELATED FACTORS
- Bladder outlet obstruction
- Detrusor external sphincter dyssynergia
- Detrusor hypocontractility
- Fecal impaction
- Severe pelvic prolapse
- Side effects of anticholinergic, calcium-channel blocker, or decongestant medications
- Urethral obstruction

ASSESSMENT FOCUS
(Refer to comprehensive assessment parameters.)
- Activity/exercise
- Behavior
- Elimination
- Fluid and electrolytes
- Physical regulation
- Self-care

EXPECTED OUTCOMES
The patient will
- Void 200 to 300 mL of clear, yellow urine every 3 to 4 hours while awake.
- Have postvoid residual of less than 50 mL.
- Have reduction in urinary incontinence episodes or complete absence of urinary incontinence.
- Experience relief of most bothersome aspect of urinary incontinence.
- Remain clean and dry without urine odor.
- Express understanding of condition and activities to prevent/reduce overflow incontinence.
- Express improvement in quality of life.

SUGGESTED NOC OUTCOMES
Knowledge: Treatment Regimen; Urinary Continence; Urinary Elimination

INTERVENTIONS AND RATIONALES

Determine: Monitor and record patient's voiding patterns *to determine existence and extent of overflow incontinence.*

Monitor and record patient's intake and output *to determine fluid balance.*

Perform: Ask patient to keep a bladder diary of continent and incontinent voids *to promote understanding of the extent of the problem of overflow incontinence.* Discuss voiding and fluid intake patterns. *Accurate understanding of patient's pattern provides a baseline for introducing new activities.*

Provide privacy and adequate time to void *to decrease anxiety and promote relaxation of sphincter.*

Assist patient to assume usual position for voiding. *Some patients are unable to void while lying in bed and may develop urinary retention and overflow incontinence.*

Massage (credé) the bladder area during urination *to increase pressure in the pelvic area to encourage drainage of urine from the bladder.*

Institute indwelling or intermittent catheterization, as ordered. Catheterization is used as a last resort *to empty the bladder preventing overflow incontinence.*

Assist with application of pads and protective garments (used only as a last resort) *to prevent skin breakdown and odor and to promote social acceptance*

Inform: Teach patient and/or family to catheterize patient with chronic overflow incontinence related to urinary retention using clean technique *to manage long-term overflow incontinence.*

Teach stress management and relaxation techniques. *Stress and anxiety interfere with sphincter relaxation, causing urinary retention and overflow incontinence.*

Attend: Encourage patient to share feelings related to incontinence *to reduce anxiety.*

Encourage patient to drink six to eight glasses of noncaffeinated, nonalcoholic, and noncarbonated liquid, preferably water, per day (unless contraindicated). *An intake of 1,500 to 2,000 mL/day promotes optimal renal function and flushes bacteria and solutes from the urinary tract. Caffeine and alcohol promote diuresis and may contribute to excess fluid loss and irritation of the bladder wall.*

Encourage patient to respond to the urge to void in a timely manner. *Ignoring the urge to urinate may cause incontinence.*

Encourage patient to participate in regular exercise, including walking and modified sit-ups (unless contraindicated). *Weak abdominal and perineal muscles weaken bladder and sphincter control.*

Encourage patient to avoid anticholinergics, opioids, psychotropics, α-adrenergic agonists, β-adrenergic agonists, and calcium-channel blockers (unless contraindicated), *which inhibit relaxation of the urinary sphincter and cause urinary retention.*

Manage: Provide referrals for physical therapy or psychological counseling as necessary *to enhance success.*

SUGGESTED NIC INTERVENTIONS

Urinary Incontinence Care; Urinary Retention Care; Urinary Elimination Management; Tube Care: Urinary; Teaching: Prescribed Activity/Exercise

REFERENCE

Chang, S. R., Chen, K. H., Chang, T. C., & Lin H. H. (2011). A Taiwanese version of the International Consultation on Incontinence Questionnaire—Urinary Incontinence Short Form for pregnant women: Instrument validation. *Journal of Clinical Nursing, 20*(5–6), 714–722.

DEFINITION

Involuntary loss of urine at somewhat predictable intervals when a specific bladder volume is reached

DEFINING CHARACTERISTICS

- Incomplete emptying (with lesion above sacral micturition center) of bladder
- Either inability to sense full bladder, urge to void, or voiding, or ability to sense urge to void without ability to voluntarily inhibit bladder contraction
- Inability to voluntarily inhibit or initiate voiding
- Predictable pattern of voiding
- Sensations associated with full bladder (sweating, restlessness, and abdominal discomfort)
- No sensation of bladder fullness

RELATED FACTORS

- Tissue damage (e.g., radiation therapy)
- Neurological impairment above level of pontine or sacral micturition center

ASSESSMENT FOCUS

(Refer to comprehensive assessment parameters.)

- Activity/exercise
- Behavior
- Elimination
- Fluid and electrolytes
- Physical regulation
- Self-care

EXPECTED OUTCOMES

The patient will

- Maintain fluid balance, with intake approximately equaling output.
- Have minimal, if any, complications.
- Achieve urinary continence.
- Demonstrate skill in managing urinary incontinence.
- Discuss impact of incontinence on himself and family.
- Identify resources to assist with care following discharge.

SUGGESTED NOC OUTCOMES

Knowledge: Treatment Regimen; Nutritional Status: Food & Fluid Intake; Tissue Integrity: Skin & Mucous Membranes; Urinary Continence; Urinary Elimination

INTERVENTIONS AND RATIONALES

<u>Determine:</u> Monitor intake and output *to ensure correct fluid replacement therapy.* Report output greater than intake.

<u>Perform:</u> Implement and monitor effectiveness of specific bladder elimination procedure, such as the following:

- Stimulate reflex arc. *Patient who voids at somewhat predictable intervals may be able to regulate voiding by reflex arc stimulation.* Trigger voiding at regular intervals (e.g., every 2 hours) by stimulating skin of abdomen, thighs, or genitals *to initiate bladder contractions.* Avoid stimulation at nonvoiding times. Stimulate primitive voiding reflexes by giving patient water to drink while he sits on toilet or pouring water over perineum. *External stimulation triggers bladder's spastic reflex.*
- Apply external catheter according to established procedure and maintaining patency. Observe condition of perineal skin and clean with soap and water at least twice daily. *Cleanliness prevents skin breakdown and infection.* External catheter protects surrounding skin, promotes accurate output measurement, and keeps patient dry. *Applying foam strip in spiral fashion increases adhesive surface and cuts risk of impaired circulation.*
- Insert indwelling catheter. Monitor patency and keep tubing free from kinks *to avoid drainage pooling and ensure accurate therapy.* Keep drainage bag below level of bladder *to avoid urine reflux into bladder.* Perform catheter care according to established procedure. Maintain closed drainage system *to prevent bacteriuria.* Secure catheter to leg (female) or abdomen (male) *to avoid tension on bladder and sphincter.*
- Apply suprapubic catheter. Change dressing according to established procedure *to avoid skin breakdown.* Monitor patency and keep tubing free from kinks *to avoid drainage pooling in loops of catheter.* Keep drainage bag below bladder level *to avoid urine reflux into bladder.* Maintain closed drainage system *to prevent bacteriuria.*
- Change wet clothes *to prevent patient from becoming accustomed to wet clothes.*

Inform: Instruct patient and family members on continence techniques to use at home. Have patient and family members return demonstrations until they can perform procedure well. *Patient education begins with assessment and depends on nurse's therapeutic relationship with patient and family.*

Attend: Encourage high fluid intake (3,000 mL daily, unless contraindicated) *to stimulate micturition reflex.* Limit fluid intake after 7 p.m. *to prevent nocturia.*

Encourage patient and family members to share feelings and concerns regarding incontinence. *A trusting environment allows nurse to make specific recommendations to resolve patient's problems.*

<u>Manage:</u> Refer patient and family members to psychiatric liaison nurse, home health care agency, support group, or other resources, as appropriate. *Community resources typically provide health care not available from other health care agencies.*

SUGGESTED NIC INTERVENTIONS

Pelvic Muscle Exercise; Urinary Bladder Training; Urinary Elimination Management; Urinary Incontinence Care; Urinary Catheterization; Urinary Catheterization: Intermittent

REFERENCE

Muller, N. (2011, September). Are you a bladder retraining coach? *Ostomy Wound Management, 57*(12), 18.

DEFINITION
Sudden leakage of urine with activities that increase intra-abdominal pressure

DEFINING CHARACTERISTICS
- Observed involuntary leakage of small amounts of urine without detrusor contraction, overdistended bladder, on exertion, with coughing or laughing, or with sneezing
- Reports involuntary leakage of small amounts of urine without detrusor contraction, overdistended bladder, on exertion, with coughing or laughing, or with sneezing

RELATED FACTORS
- Degenerative changes in pelvic muscles
- High intra-abdominal pressure
- Intrinsic urethral sphincter deficiency
- Weak pelvic muscles

ASSESSMENT FOCUS
(Refer to comprehensive assessment parameters.)
- Activity/exercise
- Behavior
- Elimination
- Fluid and electrolytes
- Physical regulation
- Self-care

EXPECTED OUTCOMES
The patient will
- Maintain continence.
- State increased comfort.
- State understanding of treatment.
- State understanding of surgical procedure.
- Demonstrate skill in managing urinary elimination problems.
- Identify resources to assist with care following discharge.

SUGGESTED NOC OUTCOMES
Tissue Integrity: Skin & Mucous Membranes; Urinary Continence; Urinary Elimination

INTERVENTIONS AND RATIONALES
<u>Determine:</u> Observe patient's voiding patterns, time of voiding, amount voided, and whether voiding is provoked by stimuli. *Accurate, thorough assessment forms basis of an effective treatment plan.*

<u>Perform:</u> Provide appropriate care for patient's urologic condition, monitor progress, and report patient's responses to treatment. Patient expects to receive adequate care and *to participate in decisions regarding care.*

Help patient to strengthen pelvic floor muscles by Kegel exercises for sphincter control. *Exercises increase muscle tone and restore cortical control.*

Promote patient's awareness of condition through education *to help patient understand illness as well as treatment.*

Help patient reduce intra-abdominal pressure by losing weight, avoiding heavy lifting, and avoiding chairs or beds that are too high or too low. *These measures reduce intra-abdominal pressure and bladder pressure.*

Provide supportive measures:

- Respond to call bell quickly, assign patient to bed next to bathroom, put night-light in bathroom, and have patient wear easily removable clothing (gown rather than pajamas and Velcro fasteners rather than buttons or zippers). *Early recognition of problems promotes continence; easily removed clothing reduces patient frustration and helps achieve continence.*
- Provide privacy during toileting *to reduce anxiety and promote elimination.*
- Have patient empty bladder before meals, at bedtime, and before leaving accessible bathroom area *to promote elimination, avoid accidents, and help relieve intra-abdominal pressure.*
- Limit fluids to 150 mL after dinner *to reduce need to void at night.*
- Encourage high fluid intake, unless contraindicated, *to moisten mucous membranes and maintain hydration.*
- Suggest patient eat increased amount of salty food before going on a long trip (unless contraindicated). *Increased sodium decreases urine production.*
- Make protective pads available for patient's undergarments, if needed, *to absorb urine, protect skin, and control odors.*

If surgery is scheduled, give attentive, appropriate preoperative and postoperative instructions and care *to reduce patient's anxiety and build trust in caregivers.*

Inform: Alert patient and family members about need for toilet schedule. Prepare for discharge according to individual needs *to ensure that patient will receive proper care.*

Attend: Encourage patient to express feelings and concerns related to urologic problems. *This helps patient focus on specific problem.*

Manage: Refer patient and family members to psychiatric liaison nurse, support group, or other resources, as appropriate. *Community resources typically provide health care not available from other health care agencies.*

SUGGESTED NIC INTERVENTIONS

Pelvic Muscle Exercise; Teaching: Individual; Urinary Elimination Management; Urinary Habit Training; Urinary Incontinence Care

REFERENCE

Keyok, K. L., & Newman, D. K. (2011, October). Understanding stress urinary incontinence. *Nurse Practitioner, 36*(10), 24–36.

DEFINITION
Involuntary passage of urine occurring shortly after a strong sense of urgency to void

DEFINING CHARACTERISTICS
- Involuntary loss of urine with bladder contraction or spasm
- Inability to reach toilet in time to avoid urine loss
- Urinary urgency

RELATED FACTORS
- Alcohol intake
- Atrophic urethritis
- Atrophic vaginitis
- Bladder infection
- Caffeine intake
- Decreased bladder capacity
- Detrusor hyperactivity with impaired bladder contractility
- Fecal impaction
- Use of diuretics

ASSESSMENT FOCUS
(Refer to comprehensive assessment parameters.)
- Activity/exercise
- Behavior
- Elimination
- Fluid and electrolytes
- Physical regulation
- Self-care

EXPECTED OUTCOMES
The patient will
- Have fewer episodes of incontinence.
- State increased comfort.
- State understanding of treatment.
- Have minimal, if any, complications.
- Discuss impact of disorder on himself and family members.
- Demonstrate skill in managing incontinence.

SUGGESTED NOC OUTCOMES
Tissue Integrity: Skin & Mucous Membranes; Urinary Continence; Urinary Elimination

INTERVENTIONS AND RATIONALES
Determine: Observe voiding pattern; document intake and output. *This ensures correct fluid replacement therapy and provides information about patient's ability to void adequately.*

Perform: Provide appropriate care for patient's urologic condition, monitor progress, and report patient's responses to treatment. *Patient should receive adequate care and take part in decisions about care as much as possible.*

Assist with specific bladder elimination procedures, such as the following:

bladder training—place patient on commode every 2 hours while awake and once during night, provide privacy, and gradually increase intervals between toileting (*these measures aim to restore a regular voiding pattern*). As well as **rigid toilet regimen**—place patient on toilet at specific times (*to aid adaptation to routine physiologic function*), and keep baseline micturition record for 3 to 7 days (*to monitor toileting effectiveness*).

Administer pain medication; discuss effectiveness with patient *to reinforce that pain can be alleviated, which reduces tension and anxiety.*

Place commode next to bed, or assign patient bed next to bathroom. *A bedside commode or convenient bathroom requires less energy expenditure than bedpan.* If using commode, keep bed and commode at same level *to facilitate patient's movements.* If using bathroom, provide good lighting from bed to bathroom *to reduce sensory misinterpretation*; remove all obstacles between bed and bathroom *to reduce chance of falling.* Prepare pleasant toilet environment that is warm, clean, and free from odors *to promote continence.*

Provide a clock *to help patient maintain voiding schedule through self-monitoring.*

Unless contraindicated, maintain fluids to 3,000 mL daily *to moisten mucous membranes and ensure hydration*; limit patient to 150 mL after dinner to reduce need to void at night.

Have patient wear easily removable clothes (gown instead of pajamas and Velcro fasteners instead of buttons or zippers) *to reduce frustration and delay in voiding routine.*

If patient loses control on way to bathroom, instruct patient to stop and take a deep breath. *Anxiety and rushing may strengthen bladder contractions.*

Inform: Explain urologic condition to patient and family members; include instructions on preventive measures and established bladder schedule. *Patient education begins with educational assessment and depends on establishing a therapeutic relationship with patient and family.* Prepare patient for discharge according to individual needs *to allow patient to practice under supervision.*

Instruct patient and family members on continence techniques for home use. *This reduces fear and anxiety resulting from lack of knowledge of patient's condition and reassures patient of continuing care.*

Attend: Encourage patient to express feelings and concerns related to his or her urologic problem *to identify patient's fears.*

Manage: Refer patient and family members to psychiatric liaison nurse, support group, or other resources, as appropriate. *Community resources typically provide health care not available from other health care agencies.*

SUGGESTED NIC INTERVENTIONS

Fluid Monitoring; Perineal Care; Self-Care Assistance: Toileting; Urinary Elimination Management; Urinary Habit Training; Urinary Incontinence Care; Referral

REFERENCE

Mangnall, J. (2012, February). Promoting patient safety in continence care. *Nursing Standard, 26*(23), 49–56.

DEFINITION

At risk for involuntary loss of urine associated occurring soon after a strong sensation of urgency to void

RISK FACTORS

- Effects of medication, caffeine, or alcohol
- Detrusor hyperactivity with impaired bladder contractility
- Impaired bladder contractility
- Fecal impaction
- Atrophic urethritis or vaginitis
- Ineffective toileting habits
- Involuntary sphincter relaxation
- Small bladder capacity

ASSESSMENT FOCUS

(Refer to comprehensive assessment parameters.)

- Activity/exercise
- Behavior
- Elimination
- Fluid and electrolytes
- Physical regulation
- Self-care

EXPECTED OUTCOMES

The patient will

- State ability to anticipate if incontinence is likely to occur.
- State understanding of potential causes of urge incontinence and its treatment.
- Avoid or minimize complications of urge incontinence.
- Discuss potential effects of urologic dysfunction on self and family members.
- Demonstrate skill in managing incontinence.
- Identify community resources to cope with alterations in urinary status.

SUGGESTED NOC OUTCOMES

Knowledge: Treatment Regimen; Urinary Continence; Urinary Elimination

INTERVENTIONS AND RATIONALES

<u>Determine:</u> Observe patient's voiding pattern and document intake and output *to ensure correct fluid replacement therapy and provide information about the patient's ability to void adequately.*

Determine patient's premorbid elimination status *to ensure that interventions are realistic and based on the patient's health status and goals.*

Assess patient's ability to sense and communicate elimination needs *to maximize self-care.*

<u>Perform:</u> Unless contraindicated, provide 2.5 to 3 L of fluid daily *to moisten mucous membranes and ensure adequate hydration.* Space out fluid intake through the day and limit it to 150 mL after supper *to reduce the need to void at night.*

Place commode next to bed, or assign patient bed next to bathroom. *A bedside commode or convenient bathroom requires less energy expenditure than bedpan.* If using commode, keep bed and commode at same level *to facilitate patient's movements.* If using bathroom, provide good lighting from bed to bathroom *to reduce sensory misinterpretation;* remove all obstacles between bed and bathroom *to reduce chance of falling.* Prepare pleasant toilet environment that is warm, clean, and free from odors *to promote continence.*

Have patient wear easily removed articles of clothing (a gown instead of pajamas, Velcro fasteners instead of buttons or zippers) *to facilitate the removal of clothing and foster independence.*

Have patient keep a diary recording episodes of incontinence to *use as a basis for planning bladder training interventions;* interventions may include voiding every 2 hours, avoiding high fluid intake, maintaining proper hygiene, or notifying a health care professional if urge incontinence occurs frequently. *Individualized interventions help promote self-care, foster motivation, and avoid incontinence.*

Incorporate patient's suggestions for managing incontinent episodes into a care plan *to foster motivation.*

Inform: Explain urge incontinence to patient and family members, especially preventive measures and potential underlying causes, *to foster compliance.*

Instruct patient to stop and take a deep breath if he or she experiences an intense urge to urinate before he can reach a bathroom. *Anxiety and rushing may increase bladder contraction.*

Attend: Encourage patient to express feelings about incontinence *to provide emotional support and identify needed areas for further patient teaching.*

Manage: Use an interdisciplinary approach to caring for incontinence. Incorporate recommendations from a urologist, urology nurse specialist, other health care providers, and the patient. Monitor progress and report the patient's response to interventions. *An interdisciplinary approach helps ensure that the patient receives adequate care. Encouraging patient participation on the team will help foster motivation.*

Note if patient expresses concern about the effect of incontinence on sexuality. If appropriate, refer him to a sex therapist *to promote sexual health.*

Refer patient and family members to community resources such as support groups, as appropriate, *to help ensure continuity of care.*

SUGGESTED NIC INTERVENTIONS
Fluid Monitoring; Urinary Elimination Management; Urinary Habit Training; Urinary Incontinence Care; Journaling; Urinary Bladder Training

REFERENCE
Basak, T., Uzun, S., & Arslan, F. (2012, January–February). Incontinence features, risk factors, and quality of life in Turkish women presenting at the hospital for urinary incontinence. *Journal of Wound, Ostomy, and Continence Nursing, 39*(1), 84–89.

DEFINITION

At risk for being invaded by pathogenic organisms

RISK FACTORS

- Chronic disease (e.g., diabetes mellitus, obesity)
- Environmental exposure to pathogens
- Invasive procedures
- Lack of knowledge about causes of infection
- Inadequate vaccination
- Inadequate primary (such as broken skin, prolonged rupture of amniotic membranes, smoking, traumatized tissue) or secondary (such as suppressed inflammatory response, immunosuppression, leukopenia) defenses
- Malnutrition

ASSESSMENT FOCUS

(Refer to comprehensive assessment parameters.)

- Fluid/electrolytes
- Neurocognition
- Risk management
- Sensation/perception

EXPECTED OUTCOMES

The patient will

- Have normal temperature, WBC count, and differential.
- Maintain good personal and oral hygiene.
- Have clear and odorless respiratory secretions.
- Have normal urine and be free from evidence of diarrhea.
- Exhibit wounds and incisions that show no signs of infection; and intravenous sites with no signs of inflammation.
- Take ___ mL of fluid and ___ g of protein daily.
- Identify infection risk factors, and signs and symptoms of infection.

SUGGESTED NOC OUTCOMES

Immune Status; Infection Severity; Knowledge: Treatment Procedure(s) and Infection Management; Nutritional Status; Risk Control: Infectious Process; Risk Detection; Wound Healing: Primary and Secondary Intention

INTERVENTIONS AND RATIONALES

Determine: Monitor and record temperature after surgery at least every 4 hours; report elevations immediately *as this may signal onset of pulmonary complications, wound infection or dehiscence, urinary tract infection, or thrombophlebitis.*

Monitor WBC count, as ordered. Report elevations or depressions. *Elevated total WBC count indicates infection. Markedly decreased WBC count may indicate decreased production resulting from extreme debilitation or severe lack of vitamins and amino acids. Any damage to bone marrow may suppress WBC formation.*

Monitor culture results of urine, respiratory secretions, wound drainage, or blood according to facility policy and physician's order. *This identifies pathogens and guides antibiotic therapy.*

<u>Perform:</u> Perform hand hygiene before and after providing care, and direct patient to do this before and after meals and after using bathroom, bedpan, or urinal *to avoid spread of pathogens;* also, use strict sterile technique when handling dressings *to maintain asepsis.*

Offer frequent oral hygiene *to prevent colonization of bacteria and reduce risk of descending infection. Disease and malnutrition may reduce moisture in mucous membranes of mouth and lips.*

Change intravenous tubing and give site care every 24 to 48 hours or as facility policy dictates *to help keep pathogens from entering body.* Rotate intravenous sites every 48 to 72 hours or as facility policy dictates *to reduce chances of infection at individual sites.*

Have patient cough and deep-breathe every 4 hours after surgery *to help remove secretions and prevent pulmonary complications.* Provide tissues to *encourage expectoration* and convenient disposal bags for expectorated sputum *to reduce spread of infection.*

Help patient turn every 2 hours. Provide skin care, particularly over bony prominences to *help prevent venous stasis and skin breakdown.*

Assist patient when necessary to ensure that perianal area is clean after elimination. *Cleaning perineal area by wiping from the area of least contamination (urinary meatus) to the area of most contamination (anus) helps prevent genitourinary infections.*

Use sterile water for humidification or nebulization of oxygen. *This prevents drying and irritation of respiratory mucosa, impaired ciliary action, and thickening of secretions within respiratory tract.*

<u>Inform:</u> Instruct patient to immediately report loose stools or diarrhea *which may indicate need to discontinue or change antibiotic therapy; or to test for Clostridium difficile.*

Instruct patient about good hand hygiene, factors that increase infection risk, and signs and symptoms of infection *to encourage patient to participate in care and modify lifestyle to maintain optimum health.*

<u>Attend:</u> Unless contraindicated, encourage fluid intake of 3,000 to 4,000 mL daily *to help thin mucus secretions;* and offer high-protein supplements *to help stabilize weight, improve muscle tone and mass, and aid wound healing.*

<u>Manage:</u> Arrange for protective isolation if patient has compromised immune system. Monitor flow and number of visitors. *These measures protect patient from pathogens in environment.*

SUGGESTED NIC INTERVENTIONS

Incision Site Care; Infection Protection; Teaching: Procedure/Treatment; Wound Care; Surveillance

REFERENCE

Eseonu, K. C., et al. (2011, May). A retrospective study of risk factors for poor outcomes in methicillin-resistant Staphylococcus aureus (MRSA) infection in surgical patients. *Journal of Orthopedic Surgery and Research, 6*, 25.

DEFINITION

At risk for injury as a result of environmental conditions interacting with the individual's adaptive and defensive resources

RISK FACTORS

External
- Biological: Community immunization level; microorganisms
- Chemical: Cosmetics; drugs, pharmaceutical agents; dyes; alcohol, nicotine, preservatives; poisons
- Human: Nosocomial agents; staffing patterns; cognitive, affective, psychomotor factors
- Nutritional: Food types, vitamins
- Physical: Design, structure, and arrangement of community, building, and/or equipment
- Mode of transport

Internal
- Abnormal blood profile: Altered clotting factors; decreased hemoglobin; leukocytosis/leucopenia; sickle cell; thalassemia; thrombocytopenia
- Biochemical dysfunction
- Immune or autoimmune disorder
- Developmental age: physiological and/or psychosocial
- Tissue hypoxia

ASSESSMENT FOCUS

(Refer to comprehensive assessment parameters.)
- Behavior
- Emotional
- Knowledge
- Risk management

EXPECTED OUTCOMES

The patient will
- Acknowledge presence of environmental hazards in their everyday surroundings.
- Take safety precautions in and out of home.
- Instruct children in safety habits.
- Childproof house to ensure safety of young children and cognitively impaired adults.

SUGGESTED NOC OUTCOMES

Immune Status; Risk Control; Safety Home Environment; Personal Safety Behavior; Falls Occurrence; Falls Prevention Behavior; Physical Injury Severity; Risk Detection

INTERVENTIONS AND RATIONALES

Determine: Help patient identify situations and hazards that can cause accidents *to increase patient's awareness of potential dangers.*

Perform: Arrange environment of patient with dementia *to minimize risk of injury:*

- Place furniture against walls.
- Avoid use of throw rugs.

Maintain lighting so that patient can find her way around room and to bathroom. *Poor lighting is a major cause of falls.*

Prevent iatrogenic harm to hospitalized patient by following the 2007 National Patient Safety goals. *This resource provides comprehensive measures designed to prevent harm.*

Follow agency policy regarding the use of restraints—they are generally used as a last resort after other measures have failed. *Agency policies will provide clear direction to use restraints safely.*

Inform: Encourage adult patient to discuss safety rules with children *to foster household safety.* For example:

- Don't play with matches.
- Use electrical equipment carefully.
- Know location of the fire escape route.
- Don't speak to strangers.
- Dial 911 in an emergency.

Attend: Encourage patient to make repairs and remove potential safety hazards from environment *to decrease possibility of injury.*

Manage: Refer patient to appropriate community resources for more information about identifying and removing safety hazards. *This enables patient and family to alter environment to achieve optimal safety level.*

SUGGESTED NIC INTERVENTIONS

Environmental Management; Fall Prevention; Health Education; Parent Education: Adolescent; Parent Education: Childrearing Family; Risk Identification; Surveillance: Safety; Environmental Management: Home Preparation and Safety; Fire-Setting Precautions

REFERENCE

Forest, G., et al. (2012, March). Falls on an inpatient rehabilitation unit: Risk assessment and prevention. *Rehabilitation Nursing, 37*(2), 56–61.

DEFINITION
A disruption in the amount and quality of sleep that impairs functioning

DEFINING CHARACTERISTICS
- Observed changes in affect
- Observed lack of energy, difficulty concentrating
- Increased work or school absenteeism
- Reports changes in mood
- Reports decreased health status, quality of life
- Reports difficulty falling asleep and staying asleep
- Reports dissatisfaction with sleep
- Reports early morning awakening
- Reports nonrestorative sleep

RELATED FACTORS
- Activity pattern
- Anxiety
- Depression
- Environmental factors
- Fear
- Gender-related hormonal shifts
- Grief
- Inadequate sleep hygiene
- Intake of stimulants
- Intake of alcohol
- Medication
- Physical discomfort

ASSESSMENT FOCUS
(Refer to comprehensive assessment parameters.)
- Coping
- Emotional
- Sleep/rest
- Values/beliefs

EXPECTED OUTCOMES
The patient will
- Identify factors that prevent or promote sleep.
- Achieve sleep for ___ hours without interruption.
- Report feeling well-rested.
- Be free from signs of sleep deprivation.
- Alter diet and habits to promote sleep, such as reducing caffeine and alcohol intake before bedtime.

- Not exhibit sleep-related behavioral symptoms, such as restlessness, irritability, lethargy, and disorientation.
- Perform relaxation exercises at bedtime.

SUGGESTED NOC OUTCOMES

Anxiety Level; Anxiety Self Control; Fear Level; Mood Equilibrium; Personal Well-Being; Rest; Sleep

INTERVENTIONS AND RATIONALES

<u>Determine:</u> Assess patient's daytime activity and work patterns; travel history; normal bedtime; problems associated with sleep; quality of sleep; sleeping environment; personal beliefs about sleep; use of alcohol, caffeine, hypnotics, and nicotine. *Assessment information will assist in selecting appropriate interventions.*

<u>Perform:</u> Ask patient to help make changes in the environment that would promote sleep. *This allows patient to have an active role in treatment.*

Administer medications on a schedule that will allow for maximum rest. *Disturbing for medication administration during rest periods will disrupt sleep patterns.* If the patient requires diuretics in the evening, give far enough in advance *to allow peak effect before bedtime.* Other medications that may interfere with sleep are β-blockers, MAO inhibitors, and phenytoin.

Provide patient with sleep aids, such as pillows, bath before sleep, food or drink, and reading *materials to promote ease in falling asleep.* Milk and some high-protein snacks, such as cheese and nuts, contain L-tryptophan, a sleep promoter. Personal hygiene and prebedtime rituals promote sleep in some patients.

Develop a sleep log with the patient describing sleep disturbances and the effect on daytime functioning. *The log will help both patient and nurse to evaluate progress in evaluating sleep patterns.*

<u>Inform:</u> Teach patient relaxation techniques such as guided imagery, deep breathing, meditation, aromatherapy, and progressive muscle relaxation. Practice with the patient at bedtime. *Purposeful relaxation efforts usually help promote sleep.*

Instruct patient to eliminate or reduce caffeine and alcohol intake and avoid foods that interfere with sleep (e.g., spicy foods). *Foods and beverages containing caffeine consumed fewer than 4 hours before bedtime may interfere with sleep. Alcohol disrupts normal sleep, especially when ingested immediately before retiring.*

When anxiety is a factor in sleep deprivation, teach coping techniques *to reduce the frustration of being unable to sleep.*

Attend: Listen to the patient's description of insomnia. Allow time for the patient to talk about his frustration. *Being able to have a sensitive listener may help reduce some of the frustration and may lead to new ideas about how to help the patient resolve his sleep* issues.

Ask the patient each day to describe the quality of his sleep. *Patients are sometimes unaware of the periods in which they do sleep.*

Manage: Refer to case manager/social worker *to ensure that follow-up is provided.*

SUGGESTED NIC INTERVENTIONS

Biofeedback; Calming Techniques; Coping Enhancement; Energy Management; Security Enhancement; Relaxation Therapy; Sleep Enhancement; Journaling; Aromatherapy

REFERENCE

Hedges, C., & Ruggiero, J. S. (2012, January). Treatment options for insomnia. *Nurse Practitioner, 37*(1), 14–19.

DEFINITION

Intracranial fluid dynamic mechanisms that normally compensate for increases in intracranial volumes are compromised, resulting in repeated disproportionate increases in intracranial pressure (ICP) in response to a variety of noxious and non-noxious stimuli

DEFINING CHARACTERISTICS

- Baseline ICP $\geq$ 10 mm Hg
- Disproportionate increase in ICP following stimulus
- Elevated P_2 ICP wave form
- Repeated increase of >10 mm Hg for more than 5 minutes following external stimuli
- Volume pressure response test variation (volume–pressure ratio >2, pressure–volume index <10)
- Wide amplitude ICP waveform

RELATED FACTORS

- Brain injuries
- Decreased cerebral perfusion $\leq$50 to 60 mm Hg
- Sustained increased ICP of 10 to 15 mm Hg
- Sustained hypotension with intracranial hypertension

ASSESSMENT FOCUS

(Refer to comprehensive assessment parameters.)

- Cardiac functioning
- Comfort
- Elimination
- Fluid and electrolytes
- Neurocognition
- Pharmacologic function
- Respiratory functioning
- Values/beliefs

EXPECTED OUTCOMES

The patient will

- Maintain patent airway, effective breathing pattern and normal arterial blood gas (ABG) levels.
- Show no evidence of fever.
- Modify environment to eliminate noxious stimuli.
- Maintain regular bowel function.
- Maintain skin integrity.
- Remain free of signs and symptoms of infection.
- Not show evidence of neurological compromise.

SUGGESTED NOC OUTCOMES

Electrolyte & Acid/Base Balance; Fluid Balance; Neurological Status: Central Motor Control, Consciousness, Cranial Sensory/Motor Function, Peripheral, and Spinal Sensory/Motor Function; Wound Healing: Primary Intention; Bowel Elimination; Infection Severity; Tissue Perfusion: Cerebral

INTERVENTIONS AND RATIONALES

Determine: Assess vital signs, temperature, pulses, heart sounds, jugular vein distension; electrocardiogram, history of hypertension; mental status, reflexes, response to pain, papillary size and response to light; respiratory rate, depth, and pattern of respiration, ABG, pulse oximetry; monitor ICP wave forms for trends over time. Monitor for damped waves. Assess cerebral perfusion pressure. *Assessment information will assist in identifying appropriate interventions.*

Perform: Maintain ICP monitoring systems if used. *Careful attention must be paid to ensure that the system is functioning to provide accurate information.* Use sterile technique for dressing changes *to prevent contamination of equipment and infection.*

Maintain a patent airway and suction only if needed. *Suctioning stimulates coughing and Valsalva maneuver; Valsalva increases intrathoracic pressure, decreases cerebral venous drainage, and increases cerebral blood volume, resulting in increased ICP.* Elevate head of the bed 15° to 30° or as ordered, and use sandbags, rolled towels, or small pillows *to keep head in a neutral position. Reposition patient by using a draw sheet to prevent friction.* Use minimal amount of stimuli when caring for the patient. Turn and reposition patient every 2 hours *to prevent atelectasis.*

Perform range of motion exercises *to maintain muscle tone.*

Provide uninterrupted rest periods as much as possible. Avoid awakening patient during rapid eye movement (REM) sleep. *Cerebral blood flow increases during REM sleep.*

Inform: Teach patient and family those aspects of care in which they can participate without feeling anxious. Instruct family members in gentle stroking of patient's face, arms, or hand. *Touch by family members may lower the ICP in some cases.*

Attend: Provide nursing care in a calm, reassuring manner. Avoid discussion of upsetting topics near the bedside. *This helps prevent emotional upset that can increase ICP.* Encourage patient and family to express feelings associated with diagnosis, treatment, and recovery. *Expression of feelings helps patient and family cope with treatment.*

Manage: Arrange for frequent multidisciplinary/family care conference *in order to keep care goal-oriented.* Refer patient and family to support group *to help deal with the injury, diagnosis, or recovery.* Refer to social worker/case manager *for follow-up care, home assessment, home visits, and referral to community agencies.*

SUGGESTED NIC INTERVENTIONS

Acid–Base Management; Bedside Laboratory Testing; Cerebral Edema Management; Fluid/Electrolyte Management; Intracranial (ICP) Monitoring; Cerebral Perfusion Monitoring; Consultation; Referral; Presence; Surveillance; Technology Management

REFERENCE

Brosche, T. M. (2011, August). Intracranial pressure and cerebral perfusion pressure ranges. *Critical Care Nurse, 31*(4), 18–19.

DEFINITION

The yellow-orange tint of the neonate's skin and mucous membranes that occurs after 24 hours of life as a result of unconjugated bilirubin in the circulation

DEFINING CHARACTERISTICS

- Abnormal skin bruising
- Yellow-orange skin
- Yellow sclera
- Yellow mucous membranes
- Abnormal blood profile (e.g., hemolysis; total serum bilirubin >2 mg/dL; total serum bilirubin in high-risk range on age in hour-specific nomogram)

RELATED FACTORS

- Abnormal weight loss (>7% to 8% in breastfeeding newborn, 15% in term infant)
- Feeding pattern not well established
- Infant experiences difficulty making transition to extrauterine life
- Stool (meconium) passage delayed
- Neonate age 1 to 7 days

ASSESSMENT FOCUS

(Refer to comprehensive assessment parameters.)
- Elimination
- Fluid and electrolytes
- Growth and development
- Nutrition

EXPECTED OUTCOMES

The neonate will
- Establish effective feeding pattern (breast or bottle) that enhances stooling.
- Not experience injury as a result of increasing bilirubin levels.
- Receive bilirubin assessment and screening within the first week of life to detect increasing levels of serum bilirubin.
- Receive appropriate therapy to enhance bilirubin excretion.
- Receive nursing assessments to determine the risk for severity of jaundice.

SUGGESTED NOC OUTCOMES

Bowel Elimination; Breast-Feeding Establishment: Infant; Nutritional Status; Risk Control; Risk Detection

INTERVENTIONS AND RATIONALES

Determine: Evaluate maternal and delivery history for risk factors for neonatal jaundice (Rh, ABO, G6PD deficiency, direct Coombs, prolonged labor, maternal viral illness, medications) *to anticipate which neonates are at higher risk for jaundice.*

Perform: Collect and evaluate laboratory blood specimens as ordered or per unit protocol *to permit accurate and timely diagnosis and treatment of neonatal jaundice.*

Inform: Educate parents regarding newborn care at home in relation to appearance of jaundice in association with any of the following: no stool in 48 hours, lethargy with refusal to nurse or bottle feed, less than one wet diaper in 12 hours, abnormal infant behavior. *Parent education is crucial for the time after the neonate is discharged. Parents are the major decision makers concerning whether and when to bring the neonate back for medical and nursing assessments after being discharged from the hospital.*

Attend: Provide caring support to the family if a breastfed neonate must receive supplementation. *It can be upsetting and result in feelings of inadequacy to a breastfeeding mother for her neonate to require supplementation.*

Manage: Coordinate care and facilitate communication between family, nursing staff, pediatrician, and lactation specialist. *A multidisciplinary approach that includes the family enhances communication and improves outcomes.*

SUGGESTED NIC INTERVENTIONS

Attachment Promotion; Bottle Feeding; Bowel Management; Breast-Feeding Assistance; Capillary Blood Sample; Discharge Planning; Infant Care; Kangaroo Care; Newborn Monitoring; Nutritional Monitoring; Risk Identification: Childbearing Family; Surveillance; Teaching: Infant Nutrition; Vital Signs Monitoring; Lactation Counseling

REFERENCE

Brethauer, M , et al. (2010, January–February). Maternal experience with neonatal jaundice. MCN. *The American Journal of Maternal Child Nursing, 35*(1), 8–14.

DEFINITION

At risk for the yellow-orange tint of the newborn's skin and mucous membranes that occurs after 24 hours of life as a result of unconjugated bilirubin in the circulation

RISK FACTORS

- Abnormal weight loss (>7% to 8% in breastfeeding newborn, 15% in term infant)
- Feeding pattern not well established
- Infant experiences difficulty making transition to extrauterine life
- Neonate aged 1 to 7 days
- Stool (meconium) passage delayed
- Prematurity

ASSESSMENT FOCUS

(Refer to comprehensive assessment parameters.)
- Growth and development
- Nutrition
- Tissue Integrity
- Roles/relationships
- Risk Management

EXPECTED OUTCOMES

The parents will
- Identify factors that place infant at risk for neonatal jaundice.
- Will identify potential signs of neonatal jaundice in infant.

The neonate will
- Establish effective feeding pattern (breast or bottle) that enhances stooling.
- Not experience injury as a result of increasing bilirubin levels.
- Will receive bilirubin assessment and screening within first week of life to detect increasing levels of serum bilirubin.

SUGGESTED NOC OUTCOMES

Bowel Elimination; Breast-Feeding Establishment: Infant; Nutritional Status; Risk Control; Risk Detection; Newborn Adaptation; Knowledge: Infant Care

INTERVENTIONS AND RATIONALES

Determine: Review history of mother and prior obstetrical and medical histories in determining risk factors leading to neonatal jaundice. *Utilizing the knowledge about the maternal factors and blood type incompatibilities that can lead to neonatal jaundice aids the provider team preparations.*

At birth assess the neonate for gestational age. *Neonates less than 38 weeks are at higher risk for jaundice.*

At birth, assess the neonate for birthing trauma such as excessive bruising. *Bruising is indicative of increased bleeding which results in hemolysis and leading to increased bilirubin.*

At birth, place the neonate to the breast for initial feeding. *This stimulates the production of milk initiating the process to produce sufficient milk for the infant over the next days.*

Rely on laboratory analysis for total serum bilirubin (TSB) or calibrated trans-cutaneous bilirubin (TcB) graphed on the Bhutani nomogram. *Accurate clinical observations of the neonate's skin color for jaundice is difficult in varying lighting settings and varying skin tone pigmentation. Laboratory and calibrated cutaneous readings provide consistent accurate measures and interpreted using the nomogram.*

Adhere to nursery protocol on time intervals to obtain readings/ heel-stick blood. *Clinical protocols are critical for assessment and treatment of hyperbilirubinemia since there are specific time-rate increase factors. This differentiates "normal physiologic" hyperbilirubinemia from more serious hemolytic forms.*

Perform: Inject vitamin K (phylloquinone) into the vastus lateralus muscle of the newborn. *Newborns lack vitamin K and cannot produce sufficient amounts for several weeks; injecting vitamin K provides a primary chemical for the clotting factors.*

Examine the skin and head of the neonate carefully to determine bruising or the presence of cephalohematoma. *Presence of bruising/ hematoma indicates bleeding and increases the risk for jaundice as the RBCs are reabsorbed.*

If the neonate is less than 38 weeks, at 12 hours postpartum, obtain a heel-stick blood sample for TSB; graph results to the Bhutani nomogram; continue every 12 hours per protocol or provider orders. *At risk premature neonates have elevated TSB in comparison to 38 week neonates; the rate of TSB rise will determine the treatment plan and therapies I.*

Maintain the nursery protocol on assessing vital signs, bilirubin, weight, intake, diaper output, and other parameters. *Close vigilance by the caregivers will inform the providers of progress in the neonate's health status and hydration status.*

Institute the treatment plan—aggressive breastfeeding and/or phototherapy. *Sufficient breast milk intake by the neonate prevents dehydration and assists in the eliminate of bilirubin; exposure to therapeutic photo-light converts insoluble bilirubin to a water soluble form easily eliminated.*

Inform: Provide information to the mother/family unit of the identified factors that may lead to neonatal jaundice. *Understanding information and expectations reduces anxiety.*

Breastfeeding 8 to 12 times a day (every 2 to 3 hours), beginning immediately at birth, with adequate amounts of milk decreases the incidence of hyperbilirubinemia. *Understanding information and expectations allows the mother to participate in the care of her newborn.*

Provide detailed information to the family unit regarding the interventions to prevent bleeding and increased bilirubin, assessment findings, the lab values and treatments for the neonate. *Understanding expectations improves confidence and reduces anxiety.*

<u>Attend:</u> Support the family when they receive the knowledge that risk factors exist. *Understanding information and expectations reduces anxiety and allows the family to prepare for their participation in the treatment plan.*

Encourage the mother to breastfeed her newborn. *This allows the mother to be the active agent intervening for her newborn by breastfeeding.*

Support bonding of the neonate and mother/family unit if the neonate receives phototherapy. *Understanding information and expectations of how the neonate will appear during therapy reduces anxiety and reduces barriers to bonding.*

Support the bonding of the neonate and mother/family unit if the neonate receives aggressive therapies that include blood exchange transfusions. *Understanding information and expectations of the implications and how the neonate appears during therapy reduces anxiety and reduces barriers to bonding.*

<u>Manage:</u> Refer to lactation consultant to manage breastfeeding and methods to enhance milk production. *Expertise and support provide the confidence to achieve success in breastfeeding.*

Emphasize the importance of follow-up at discharge for any level of hyperbilirubinemia; adhere to the clinical protocols and clinical pathways. *Newborns are frequently discharged after 24 hours and need to have professional evaluation to assure the bilirubin levels follow a predicted decrease.*

SUGGESTED NIC INTERVENTIONS

Attachment Promotion; Kangaroo Care; Newborn Monitoring; Vital Signs Monitoring; Infant Care; Breast-feeding Assistance; Bottle-Feeding; Teaching: Infant Nutrition; Capillary Blood Sample; Surveillance; Risk Identification: Childbearing Family; Bowel Management; Discharge Planning

REFERENCE

Stokowski, L. (2011, October). Reviewing the needs of jaundice management. *Advances in Neonatal Care, 11*(5, Suppl.), S1–S2.

DEFINITION

Absence or deficiency of cognitive information related to a specific topic

DEFINING CHARACTERISTICS

- Inaccurate follow-through of instruction
- Inaccurate performance of test
- Inappropriate or exaggerated behaviors (hysteria, hostility, agitation, apathy)
- Verbalization of the problem

RELATED FACTORS

- Cognitive limitation
- Information misinterpretation
- Lack of exposure
- Lack of interest in learning
- Lack of recall
- Unfamiliarity with information resources

ASSESSMENT FOCUS

(Refer to comprehensive assessment parameters.)

- Activity
- Communication
- Coping
- Knowledge
- Nutrition
- Sleep
- Values/beliefs

EXPECTED OUTCOMES

The patient will

- Communicate desire to understand disease state and need for treatment.
- Demonstrate ability to perform new health-related procedures.
- Set realistic learning goals within target dates.
- State intention to make needed modifications in lifestyle.

SUGGESTED NOC OUTCOMES

Cognition; Communication; Concentration; Information Processing; Knowledge: Disease Process; Knowledge: Health Behaviors; Knowledge: Health Resources; Knowledge: Illness Care; Stress Level; Memory

INTERVENTIONS AND RATIONALES

<u>Determine:</u> Determine level of knowledge and skills patient already possesses about his or her health status; motivation to understand what is needed to improve health status; obstacles to learning; support systems; usual coping patterns; beliefs about health and treatment of disease;

ethnicity; financial resources. *Assessment information will assist in identifying appropriate interventions.*

<u>Perform:</u> Establish an environment of mutual trust and respect *to enhance learning. Consistency between action and words, combined with the patient's self-awareness ability to share this awareness with others, and receptiveness to new experiences form the basis of a trusting relationship.*

Develop with patient specific learning goals with target dates. *Involving patient in planning meaningful goals encourages compliance.*

Select teaching strategies *that will enhance teaching/learning effectiveness,* such as discussion, demonstration, role-playing, and visual materials. Provide all the equipment needed for the patient to learn. *This reduces frustration, aids learning, and minimizes dependence by promoting self-care.*

<u>Inform:</u> Teach those skills that the patient must incorporate into daily living. Have patient do return demonstration of each skill *to aid in gaining confidence.*

When teaching, go slowly and repeat frequently. Offer small amounts of information and present it in various ways. *By building cognition, patient will be better able to complete self-care measures.*

Demonstrate to family members how each self-care measure is broken down into simple tasks *to enhance patient's success and foster a sense of control.*

<u>Attend:</u> Encourage family members to participate in and have patience toward learning process (patient may need to repeat new skills multiple times) *to help create a therapeutic environment after discharge.*

<u>Manage:</u> Have patient incorporate learned skills into care while still in the hospital. *This allows practice and time for feedback.*

Provide patient and/or family with names and telephone numbers of resource people or community agencies *so that care is continuous and follow-up is possible after discharge.*

If financial hardship interferes with the ability of the family to provide equipment and supplies, offer a referral to a social worker *to improve the family's access to financial assistance.*

SUGGESTED NIC INTERVENTIONS

Behavior Management; Behavior Modification; Decision-Making Support; Energy Management; Family Support; Financial Resource Assistance; Health Education; Healthcare Information Exchange: Risk Identification; Learning Facilitation; Support System Enhancement; Teaching Procedure/Treatment

REFERENCE

Yetzer, E. A., Goetsch, N., St. Paul, M. (2011, November–December). Teaching adults SAFE medication management. *Rehabilitation Nursing, 36*(6), 255–260.

DEFINITION

The presence or acquisition of cognitive information related to a specific topic that is sufficient for meeting health-related goals and can be strengthened

DEFINING CHARACTERISTICS

- Expresses an interest in learning
- Explains knowledge of topic
- Behaviors congruent with expressed knowledge
- Describes previous experience related to topic

ASSESSMENT FOCUS

(Refer to comprehensive assessment parameters.)

- Communication
- Knowledge
- Risk management
- Values and beliefs

EXPECTED OUTCOMES

The patient will

- Identify new sources for enhancing knowledge in the topic of interest.
- Make use of all relevant resources to enhance knowledge.
- Ask questions where new information needs clarification.
- Begin practicing new behaviors gleaned from enhanced knowledge.

SUGGESTED NOC OUTCOMES

Knowledge: Health Promotion; Client Satisfaction: Teaching; Health Promoting Behavior; Health Seeking Behavior

INTERVENTIONS AND RATIONALES

Determine: Assess current health status; problems, restrictions, limitations; personal habits, such as the use of tobacco, drugs, alcohol consumption, level of knowledge about disease process; communication skills (verbal and written), degree of motivation to maintain health; familiarity with technology as a source of learning. *Assessment information will help identify appropriate interventions.*

Perform: Plan a health maintenance program for the patient and family members addressing current problems. *Developing a plan with the family will increase the probability of compliance by giving them information to review each day.* Provide the family and patient with a written copy. *A written copy can be posted in the patient's home where it is always available for review.*

Inform: Provide books and videos that will help the patient's quest for enhanced knowledge. *Supplying some materials directly may be a motivation for the patient to search further.*

Direct patient and family to use other sources such as libraries, the Internet, or professional organizations. *An independent search results in the patient developing confidence in his or her ability to go much deeper into the area of interest.*

Attend: Encourage patient and family to verbalize feelings and concerns related to the knowledge and skills that patient needs. *This promotes greater ease in managing challenging situations.*

Demonstrate willingness to repeat instruction and demonstrations of skills needed by the patient. *Repetition will reinforce learning and give the patient added confidence in his or her ability to comply.*

Be available to answer questions and correct misconceptions for the patient/family *to enhance the effectiveness of learning.*

Introduce the patient and/or family to individuals who may have had experience with the health problems in question if that is advisable. *In many cases, having the opportunity to talk to another person that has coped well with the same problem will provide support and encouragement to the patient.*

Manage: Refer to social worker/case manager early in the patient's hospitalization. *This person will begin identifying the types of support and resources the family and patient will need to prepare for follow on care.*

Refer to social and community resources, such as stroke support group, and Alzheimer's family support group, American Cancer Society. *The patient can contact these sources for additional information as needed.*

SUGGESTED NIC INTERVENTIONS

Discharge Planning; Teaching: Individual; Learning Readiness Enhancement; Learning Facilitation; Referral; Teaching

REFERENCE

Coulter, A. (2012, June). Patient engagement—What works? *Journal of Ambulatory Care Management, 35*(2), 80–89.

DEFINITION
A hypersensitive reaction to natural latex rubber products

DEFINING CHARACTERISTICS
Immediate reactions (<1 hours of exposure) can be life-threatening
- Contact urticaria progressing to generalized symptoms: Edema of the lips, eyelids, sclera, tongue, uvula, and/or throat
- Shortness of breath or tightness in the chest, wheezing or broncho-spasm leading to respiratory arrest
- Hypotension, syncope, and cardiac arrest
- Gastrointestinal characteristics (e.g., abdominal pain or nausea)
- Generalized characteristics (e.g., increasing body warmth flushing, discomfort, edema, and/or restlessness)
- Orofacial characteristics (e.g., erythema, edema, itching, and/or tearing of the eyes and/or face, nasal congestion, itching, or erythema)
- Nasal congestion, erythema, itching, and/or rhinorrhea

type IV reactions (>1 hours after exposure)
- Generalized discomfort
- Eczema, irritation, and/or redness

RELATED FACTORS
- Hypersensitivity to natural latex rubber

ASSESSMENT FOCUS
(Refer to comprehensive assessment parameters.)
- Cardiac function
- Respiratory function
- Tissue integrity

EXPECTED OUTCOMES
The patient will
- Maintain normal vital signs, respiratory status, and laboratory values.
- Exhibit skin that is moist, clear, and free of erythema, edema, itching, urticaria, and breakdown.
- Express awareness of allergic response to latex-containing products.
- State intention to avoid contact with products containing latex.

SUGGESTED NOC OUTCOMES
Comfort Level; Immune Hypersensitivity Response; Knowledge: Infection Control; Tissue Integrity: Skin and Mucous Membrane

INTERVENTIONS AND RATIONALES
<u>Determine:</u> Determine whether patient has had past episodes of latex allergy; food, pollen, or drug allergy. Report contacts with latex products including when, where, and what. *History will lead to more precise assessment.*

Monitor respiratory status; include rate, rhythm, skin color, and breath sounds. Be particularly alert for signs of bronchospasms and complaints of dyspnea. Assess heart rate, rhythm, and blood pressure. Check skin carefully for urticaria. Document findings. *These measures detect changes in status to more accurately determine interventions.*

Remove all latex products from immediate proximity of patient and staff treating the patient *to prevent inadvertent use of products by staff or patient, increasing the risk for contact and allergic reaction.*

<u>Perform:</u> Administer prescribed drugs and treatments as ordered. *Wheezing and shortness of breath can quickly deteriorate to respiratory distress and failure. Skin with urticaria and itching is uncomfortable and unsightly so patients appreciate timely administration of treatment.*

<u>Inform:</u> Teach patient and his or her family to avoid latex products *to prevent future contact and allergic reactions.* Provide instruction about household items that contain latex (provide a written list) and tell them about nonlatex substitutes. *Prevention is the foundation of treatment of latex allergies.*

Instruct patient and his or her family about importance of seeking immediate medical treatment of allergic reactions *to foster timely intervention.*

<u>Attend:</u> Provide emotional support and encouragement *to help* improve patient's self-concept.

Involve patient in planning and decision making, and have him or her perform self-care activities. *Having the ability to participate will encourage greater compliance with the plan for activity.*

<u>Manage:</u> When latex allergy is confirmed, document and label record clearly *to prevent future contact with the allergen.*

Emphasize need to inform all health care providers about patient's sensitivity to latex. Stress the importance of wearing a medical identification bracelet that specifies latex allergy *to prevent future contact and allergic reactions.*

Provide documentation of latex allergy for the patient to take to employer; with the patient's permission, communicate with employee health department and discuss patient's need to avoid contact with latex products *to prevent further contamination.*

SUGGESTED NIC INTERVENTIONS

Allergy Management; Anaphylaxis Management; Environmental Risk Protection; Latex Precautions; Risk Identification; Teaching: Individual

REFERENCE

Ismail, N. A., Hoosen, A. A., & Mehtar, S. (2010, January). Latex allergies in health care workers: Prevalence and knowledge at a tertiary teaching hospital in a developing country. *International Journal of Infection Control, 6*(1), 1–4.

DEFINITION

Risk of hypersensitivity to natural latex rubber products that may compromise health

RISK FACTORS

History of food allergies, such as allergy to bananas, kiwi, avocados, chestnuts, or pineapples

- Professions with daily exposure to latex
- Multiple surgical procedures, especially beginning in infancy
- History of reaction to latex
- Allergy to poinsettia plants or tropical fruits
- History of allergies and asthma

ASSESSMENT FOCUS

(Refer to comprehensive assessment parameters.)

- Activity/exercise
- Nutrition
- Tissue integrity

EXPECTED OUTCOMES

The patient will

- Regain normal vital signs, respiratory status, and laboratory values.
- Exhibit moist, clear skin that is free of erythema, edema, itching, urticaria, and breakdown.
- Express awareness of allergic response to latex-containing products.

SUGGESTED NOC OUTCOMES

Allergy Response: Localized; Immune Hypersensitivity Response; Risk Control

INTERVENTIONS AND RATIONALES

Determine: Determine whether patient has had past episodes of latex allergy; food, pollen, or drug allergy. Report contacts with latex products including when, where, and what. *History will lead to more precise assessment.*

Monitor respiratory status; include rate, rhythm, skin color, and breath sounds. Be particularly alert for signs of bronchospasms and complaints of dyspnea. Assess heart rate, rhythm, and blood pressure. Check skin carefully for urticaria. Document findings. *These measures detect changes in patient's response to latex or other substances that cause allergic reactions status.*

Remove all latex products from the immediate proximity of the patient and staff treating the patient *to prevent inadvertent use of latex products by the staff or patient, increasing the risk for contact and allergic reaction.*

Perform: Administer prescribed drugs and treatments as ordered. *Wheezing and shortness of breath can quickly deteriorate to respiratory distress and failure. Skin with urticaria and itching is uncomfortable and unsightly so patients appreciate timely administration of treatment.*

Inform: Educate patient and family about allergic reaction *to latex products to prevent future contact and allergic reactions.* Provide a list of household items containing latex, emphasize importance of avoiding these, and tell them about nonlatex substitutes. *Prevention is the foundation of treatment of latex allergies.*

Educate patient and his or her family about importance of seeking immediate medical treatment of allergic reactions *to foster timely intervention.*

Attend: Involve patient in planning and decision making, and have the patient perform self-care activities. *Having the ability to participate will encourage greater compliance with the plan for activity.*

Manage: Emphasize need to inform all health care providers about sensitivity to latex. Stress importance of wearing a medical identification bracelet that specifies possible latex allergy *to prevent contact and allergic reactions.*

Provide documentation of the risk of latex allergy for the patient to take to employer. With patient's permission, communicate with employee health department and discuss patient's need *to avoid contact with latex products to prevent further contamination.*

SUGGESTED NIC INTERVENTIONS

Allergy Management; Anaphylaxis Management; Environmental Risk Protection; Latex Precautions; Risk Identification; Teaching: Individual

REFERENCE

Galindo, M. J., Quirce, S., & Garcia, O. L. (2011, June). Latex allergies in primary care providers. *Journal of Clinical Immunology, 21*(6), 459–465.

DEFINITION
Reports a habit of life that is characterized by a low physical activity level

DEFINING CHARACTERISTICS
- Chooses a daily routine lacking physical exercise
- Demonstrates physical deconditioning
- Verbalizes preference for activities low in physical activity

RELATED FACTORS
- Deficient knowledge of health benefits of physical exercise
- Lack of interest, motivation, resources, and/or training

ASSESSMENT FOCUS
(Refer to comprehensive assessment parameters.)
- Activity/exercise
- Growth and development
- Knowledge
- Nutrition
- Risk management

EXPECTED OUTCOMES
The patient will
- Maintain independent living status with reduced risk for falling.
- Identify barriers to increasing physical activity level.
- Identify health benefits to increasing physical activity level.
- Increase physical activity and limit inactive forms of diversion, such as television and computer games.
- Seek professional consultation to develop an appropriate plan to increase physical activity.
- Identify factors that enhance readiness for sleep.
- Demonstrate readiness for enhanced sleep through the use of appropriate sleep hygiene measures.
- Have amount of sleep congruent with developmental needs and experience rapid-eye-movement sleep.
- Express a feeling of being rested after sleep.
- Increase lean muscle and bone strength and decrease body fat.
- Demonstrate weight control and, if appropriate, weight loss.
- Exhibit enhanced psychological well-being and reduced risk of depression.
- Have reduced depression and anxiety and an improved mood.
- Demonstrate increased ability to perform activities of daily living within limits of chronic, disabling conditions.

SUGGESTED NOC OUTCOMES
Activity Tolerance; Endurance; Energy Conservation; Health Promoting Behavior; Immobility Consequences: Physiologic; Adherence Behavior Immobility Consequences: Physiologic and Psycho-Cognitive; Compliance Behavior; Endurance; Health Seeking Behavior

INTERVENTIONS AND RATIONALES

<u>Determine:</u> Identify barriers and enhancers to increasing physical activity, including time management, diet, lifestyle, access to facilities, and safe environments in which to be active. *Breaking down barriers and building opportunities for activity increase the probability of consistent physical activity.*

<u>Perform:</u> Develop a behavior modification plan based on patient's condition, history, and precipitating factors *to maximize physical activity and compliance.*

<u>Inform:</u> Instruct patient to keep a daily activity and dietary log to help him or her achieve a more objective view of his or her behavior.

Educate patient about how sedentary lifestyle affects cardiovascular risk factors (such as hypertension, dyslipidemia, hyperinsulinemia, insulin resistance) *to motivate patient to be more active.*

Teach exercises for increasing strength and endurance to maintain mobility and prevent musculoskeletal degeneration.

Educate patient about using the bedroom only for sleep or sexual activity and avoiding other activities such as watching television, reading, and eating *to increase sleep efficiency.*

<u>Attend:</u> Provide counseling tailored to patient's risk factors, needs, preferences, and abilities *to enhance emotional well-being and motivation for physical activity.*

Discuss the need for activity that will improve psychosocial well-being *to encourage compliance with activities.*

Discuss behavioral risk factors in lack of motivation such as ingestion of carbohydrates, caffeine, nicotine, alcohol, sedatives, hypnotics, and fluid intake, *to focus behavior on positive outcomes of increased physical activity.*

<u>Manage:</u> Provide education about community resources available *to increase physical activity to decrease barriers to activity.*

SUGGESTED NIC INTERVENTIONS

Activity Therapy; Energy Management; Teaching: Prescribed Activity/ Exercise; Body Mechanics Promotion; Exercise Promotion

REFERENCE

Matthews, C. E., George S. M., et al. (2012, February). Amount of time spent in sedentary behaviors and cause-specific mortality in US adults. *American Journal of Clinical Nutrition, 95*(2), 437–445.

DEFINITION
At risk for a decrease in liver function that may compromise health

RISK FACTORS
- Hepatotoxic medications (e.g., acetaminophen, statins)
- HIV coinfection
- Substance abuse (e.g., alcohol, cocaine)
- Viral infection (e.g., hepatitis A, B, or C, Epstein-Barr)

ASSESSMENT FOCUS
(Refer to comprehensive assessment parameters.)
- Risk management
- Pharmacological function
- Fluids/electrolytes

EXPECTED OUTCOMES
The patient will
- State effects of environmental and ingested chemicals and substances on health and liver function.
- Work with industry managers and with public health officials to lower or eliminate the presence of environmental chemicals and substances in their work or living environment.
- Have liver function indicators within normal limits.
- Modify lifestyle and risk behaviors to avoid behaviors leading to hepatic dysfunction and inflammation.
- Maintain long-term follow-up for chronic illness with health care provider.
- Manage concurrent disease processes that impact hepatic function.
- Optimize nutritional intake for needs.
- Acknowledge the impact of medications on hepatic function.
- Observe measures to avoid the spread of infection to self and to others.

SUGGESTED NOC OUTCOMES
Health Promoting Behavior; Risk Control; Risk Control: Alcohol Use; Risk Control: Drug Use; Safe Home Environment; Substance Addiction Consequences; Nutritional Status

INTERVENTIONS AND RATIONALES
<u>Determine:</u> Assist patient and family to assess workplace and home environments for potential substances *to increase patient's awareness of hazards in the environment and to lower potential for hepatic injury.*

Monitor for clinical manifestations of hepatic inflammation and dysfunction *to notify physician in order to initiate treatment if liver function is compromised.* Clinical manifestations may include fatigue, depression or mood changes, anorexia, Right-upper-quadrant tenderness, pruritus, jaundice, bruising, or nontraumatic bleeding.

Monitor customary clinical laboratory tests *to alert the health care provider of the status of the immune/inflammatory response, the degree of hepatic metabolic dysfunction, and the impact of concurrent disorders on liver function.* Clinical laboratory tests include complete blood cell (CBC) count: lower red blood cell count, elevated WBC (increased immunocyte and inflammatory responses); basic metabolic panel—altered electrolyte balance, elevated glucose, elevated blood urea nitrogen and creatinine level, elevated HbA_{1c}; hepatic plasma markers: elevated liver enzymes (alanine aminotransferase, aspartate aminotransferase, and γ-glutamyltranspeptidase); positive immunoassays *for pathogen and viral antigens*; elevated ammonia; elevated bilirubin; low coagulation factors; low total protein/albumin; elevated lipid panel.

Perform: Carry out postprocedure measures, as ordered, *to identify and/or minimize complications.*

Inform: Teach patient about the following: perform hand hygiene before and after personal hygiene and care; cover draining and nonhealing wounds; report to care provider; inform others of infectious condition *so that each observes barrier precautions*; adhere to prescribed plan of care and treatment with immune system modifiers (antibiotics, antivirals, interferon, others); maintain a balanced nutritional diet intake. *These measures minimize patient's risk for self-infection and spread of infection and allow the patient to help modify lifestyle to maintain optimum health level for self and for others.*

Along with health care team, prepare the patient for and later evaluate the results of liver biopsy and provide explanation to patient and family.

The patient and family need understanding of purpose for and implications of results obtained from a liver biopsy. This support and education helps the patient understand rationale for plan of treatment and genetic counseling for genetically linked hepatic disorders.

Attend: Provide a nonjudgmental attitude toward patient's lifestyle choices *to promote feelings of self-worth.*

Manage: Refer patient to counseling and therapy to address lifestyle choices and risk behaviors. *Modification of behaviors will provide risk avoidance for drug and alcohol abuse and exposure to body-substance pathogen infection.*

SUGGESTED NIC INTERVENTIONS

Behavior Modification; Environmental Risk Protection; Infection Protection; Risk Identification; Risk Identification: Genetic; Self-Modification Assistance; Surveillance; Referral

REFERENCE

Wu, L. J., Wu, M. S., Lien, G. S., Chen, F. C., & Tsai, J. C. (2012, January). Fatigue and physical activity levels in patients with liver cirrhosis. *Journal of Clinical Nursing, 21*(1–2), 129–138.

DEFINITION

At risk for experiencing discomfort associated with a desire or need for more contact with others

RISK FACTORS

- Affectional deprivation
- Cathectic deprivation
- Physical isolation
- Social isolation

ASSESSMENT FOCUS

(Refer to comprehensive assessment parameters.)

- Coping
- Emotional
- Roles/relationships
- Values/beliefs

EXPECTED OUTCOMES

The patient will

- Identify feelings of loneliness and express desire to socialize more.
- Identify behaviors that lead to loneliness.
- Identify people who will likely support and accept him.
- Spend time with others.
- Be comfortable in social settings, interact with peers, and receive support from others.
- Make specific plans to continue involvement with others, such as through recreational activities or social interaction groups.

SUGGESTED NOC OUTCOMES

Decision-Making; Loneliness Severity; Risk Control; Social Involvement; Social Support; Social Interaction Skills

INTERVENTIONS AND RATIONALES

Determine: Work with patient to identify factors and behaviors that have contributed to loneliness *to begin changing behaviors that may have alienated others.*

Help patient identify feelings associated with loneliness. *This lessens the impact of feelings and mobilizes energy to counteract them.*

Perform: Spend sufficient time with patient to allow him to express his feelings of loneliness *to establish trusting relationship.*

Work with patient to establish goals for reducing feelings of loneliness after he leaves health care setting *to focus energy on specific objectives.*

Inform: Inform patient that assistance is available to help him express feelings of loneliness and identify ways to increase social activity *to bring issue into open and help patient understand that you want to help him.*

Help patient curb feelings of loneliness by encouraging one-on-one interaction with others who are likely to accept him (e.g., church members or patients with similar health problems) *to promote feelings of acceptance and support.*

Help patient identify social activities he can initiate, such as becoming active in a support group or volunteer organization. *This fosters feelings of control and increase social contacts.*

Help patient accept that other people may view him differently because of his illness, and explore ways of coping with their reactions *to help patient learn to cope with stigma associated with illness.*

Attend: Encourage patient to address his needs assertively. *By being assertive, patient assumes responsibility for meeting his needs without anger or guilt.*

As patient's comfort level improves, encourage him to attend group activities and social functions *to promote the use of social skills.*

Manage: Refer patient and family to social service agencies, mental health center, and appropriate support groups *to ensure continued care and maintain social involvement.*

SUGGESTED NIC INTERVENTIONS

Activity Therapy, Anxiety Reduction, Emotional Support; Socialization Enhancement; Spiritual Support; Visitation Facilitation; Family Integrity Promotion; Behavior Management

REFERENCE

Playfair, C. (2011, February). Human relationships: And exploration of loneliness and touch. *British Journal of Nursing, 19*(2), 122–124.

DEFINITION

At risk for disruption of the symbiotic maternal–fetal dyad as a result of comorbid or pregnancy-related conditions

RISK FACTORS

- Complications of pregnancy (e.g., premature rupture of membranes, placenta previa or abruption, late prenatal care, multiple gestation)
- Compromised O_2 transport (e.g., anemia, cardiac disease, asthma, hypertension, seizures, premature labor, hemorrhage)
- Impaired glucose metabolism (e.g., diabetes, steroid use)
- Physical abuse
- Substance abuse (e.g., tobacco, alcohol, drugs)
- Treatment-related side effects (e.g., medications, surgery, chemotherapy)

ASSESSMENT FOCUS

(Refer to comprehensive assessment parameters.)

- Behavior
- Emotional
- Roles/relationships

EXPECTED OUTCOMES

The patient will

- Be compliant with recommendations for self care activities to minimize prenatal complications and optimize maternal–fetal health.
- Verbalize fears and uncertainty related to prenatal condition.
- Actively involve significant other/support systems with pregnancy expectations and plan of care.
- Demonstrate the "maternal tasks of pregnancy" culminating in an unconditional acceptance of the fetus before delivery.

SUGGESTED NOC OUTCOMES

Prenatal Health Behavior; Knowledge: Pregnancy; Role Performance; Family Integrity

INTERVENTIONS AND RATIONALES

<u>Determine:</u> At each prenatal visit, assess physical condition, psychosocial well-being, and cultural beliefs *to be able to counsel and/or refer as needed.*

<u>Perform:</u> Encourage support/involvement of significant other(s) during course of pregnancy *to enhance maternal role adaptation.*

Incorporate the cultural beliefs, rites, and rituals of the childbearing family into the plan of care *to foster feelings of normalcy with pregnancy.*

<u>Inform:</u> Educate patient/significant other on role transition and maternal tasks of pregnancy *to provide anticipatory guidance on expected psychosocial changes.*

Teach trimester-specific risks/danger signs and emphasize importance of self-monitoring *to empower the patient and reduce potential for adverse fetal effects.*

Attend: Encourage patient to express disappointment/concerns related to relationships, physical condition, and fetal well-being *to promote therapeutic communication.*

Manage: Refer to community resources as needed (e.g., prenatal classes, psychological counseling, pastoral care, social services) *to facilitate appropriate role adaptation.*

SUGGESTED NIC INTERVENTIONS

Anticipatory Guidance; Childbirth Preparation; Coping Enhancement; Role Enhancement; Cultural Brokerage

REFERENCE

Watson, G. (2011, May). Parental liminality: A way of understanding the early experiences of parents who have a very preterm infant. *Journal of Clinical Nursing, 20*(9–10), 1462–1471.

DEFINITION
Inability to remember or recall bits of information or behavioral skills

DEFINING CHARACTERISTICS
- Inability to determine whether a behavior was performed
- Inability to learn new skills or information or to perform previously learned skills
- Inability to recall factual information and recent or past events
- Incidences of forgetting, including forgetting to perform a behavior at a scheduled time

RELATED FACTORS
- Anemia
- Decreased cardiac output
- Excessive environmental disturbances
- Fluid and electrolyte imbalance
- Hypoxia
- Neurological disturbances

ASSESSMENT FOCUS
(Refer to comprehensive assessment parameters.)
- Cardiac function
- Emotional
- Fluids and electrolytes
- Neurocognition
- Self-care

EXPECTED OUTCOMES
The patient/family will
- Express feelings about memory impairment.
- Acknowledge need to take measures to cope with memory impairment.
- Identify coping skills to deal with memory impairment.
- State specific plans to modify lifestyle.
- Establish realistic goals to deal with further memory loss.

SUGGESTED NOC OUTCOMES
Cognition; Cognitive Orientation; Concentration; Coping; Memory; Neurological Status: Consciousness

INTERVENTIONS AND RATIONALES
<u>Determine:</u> Observe patient's thought processes during every shift. Document and report any changes. *Changes may indicate progressive improvement or a decline in patient's underlying condition.*

<u>Perform:</u> Implement appropriate safety measures *to protect patient from injury. He or she may be unable to provide for his or her own safety needs.*

Call patient by name and tell him or her your name. Provide background information (place, time, and date) frequently throughout the day *to provide reality orientation*. Use a reality orientation board *to visually reinforce reality orientation*.

Spend sufficient time with patient *to allow her to become comfortable discussing memory loss and establish a trusting relationship.*

Be clear, concise, and direct in establishing goals *to promote maximal use of patient's remaining cognitive skills.* Offer short, simple explanations to patient each time you carry out any medical or nursing procedure *to avoid confusion.*

Label patient's personal possessions and photos, keeping them in the same place as much as possible, *to reduce confusion and create a secure environment.*

<u>Inform:</u> Inform patient that you are aware of his or her memory loss and that you will help him or her cope with his or her condition *to bring the issue into the open and help patient understand that your goal is to help him or her.*

Teach patient ways to cope with memory loss (e.g., using a beeper to remind her when to eat or take medications; using a pillbox organized by days of the week; keeping lists in notebooks or a pocket calendar; having family members or friends remind her of important tasks). *Reminders help limit the amount of information patient must maintain in her memory.*

Help patient and family members establish goals for coping with memory loss. Discuss with family members the need to maintain the least restrictive environment possible. Instruct them on how to maintain a safe home environment for patient. *This helps ensure that patient's needs are met and promotes his or her independence.*

Demonstrate reorientation techniques to family members and provide time for supervised return demonstrations *to prepare them to cope with patient with memory impairment.*

<u>Attend:</u> Encourage patient to develop a consistent routine for performing activities of daily living *to enhance his self-esteem and increase his self-awareness and awareness of his environment.*

Encourage patient to interact with others *to increase social involvement, which may decline with memory loss.*

Encourage patient to express the feelings associated with impaired memory *to reduce the impact of memory impairment on patient's self-image and lessen anxiety.*

<u>Manage:</u> Help family members identify appropriate community support groups, mental health services, and social service agencies *to assist in coping with the effects of patient's illness or injury.*

SUGGESTED NIC INTERVENTIONS

Anxiety Reduction; Calming Technique; Cerebral Perfusion Promotion; Dementia Management; Memory Training; Neurologic Monitoring; Reality Orientation; Home Maintenance Assistance; Referral

REFERENCE

Marchant, J. A., & Williams, K. N. (2011, March–April). Memory matters in assisted living. *Rehabilitation Nursing, 36*(2), 83–88.

DEFINITION

Limitation of independent movement from one bed position to another

DEFINING CHARACTERISTICS

Impaired ability to perform the following actions while in bed

- Move from supine to long sitting or long sitting to supine
- Move from supine to prone or prone to supine
- Move from supine to sitting or sitting to supine
- "Scoot" or reposition body
- Turn from side to side

RELATED FACTORS

- Cognitive impairment
- Deconditioning
- Deficient knowledge
- Environmental constraints
- Insufficient muscle strength
- Musculoskeletal and/or neuromuscular impairment
- Obesity
- Pain
- Sedating medications

ASSESSMENT FOCUS

(Refer to comprehensive assessment parameters.)

- Activity/exercise
- Pharmacological function
- Physical regulation

EXPECTED OUTCOMES

The patient will

- Have no complications associated with impaired bed mobility, such as altered skin integrity, contractures, venous stasis, thrombus formation, depression, altered health maintenance, and falls.
- Maintain or improve muscle strength and joint range of motion (ROM).
- Achieve the highest level of bed mobility possible (independence, independence with device, verbalization of needs for assistance with bed mobility, requires assistance of one person or two people).
- Demonstrate ability to use equipment or devices to assist with moving about in bed safely.
- Adapt to alteration in ability to move about in bed.
- Participate in social, physical, and occupational activities to the extent possible.

SUGGESTED NOC OUTCOMES

Body Positioning: Self-Initiated; Immobility Consequences: Physiological; Immobility Consequences: Psycho-Cognitive; Joint Movement; Mobility; Neurological Status: Consciousness

INTERVENTIONS AND RATIONALES

Determine: Identify patient's level of independence using functional mobility scale and document findings *to provide continuity of care.*

Monitor and record daily evidence of complications related to impaired bed mobility (contractures, venous stasis, skin breakdown, thrombus formation, depression, altered health maintenance or self-care skills, falls). Assess patient's skin every 2 hours *to maintain skin integrity.*

<u>Perform:</u> Perform ROM exercises to affected joints, unless contraindicated, at least once per shift. Progress from passive to active ROM, as tolerated, *to prevent joint contractures and muscle atrophy.*

Assist patient in maintaining anatomically correct and functional body positioning *to relieve pressure, thereby preventing skin breakdown and fluid accumulation in dependent extremities.* Encourage repositioning every 2 hours while in bed.

Establish a turning schedule for immobile patient. Encourage progressive mobility within patient's limits *to maintain muscle tone, prevent complications, and promote self-care.*

If you are uncertain about your ability to move the patient, request help from colleagues *to maintain safety.*

<u>Inform:</u> Instruct patient and family members in techniques to improve bed mobility and ways to prevent complications *to help prepare the patient and family members for discharge.*

Demonstrate patient's bed mobility regimen and note the date. Have patient and family members perform a return demonstration *to ensure continuity of care and use of proper technique.*

<u>Attend:</u> Encourage patient to participate in physical and occupational therapy sessions. Incorporate equipment, devices, and techniques used by therapists into your care. Request written instructions from the patient's therapists to use as a reference *to help ensure continuity of care and reinforce learned skills.*

<u>Manage:</u> Refer patient to a physical therapist *to continue improvement in bed mobility and rehabilitate musculoskeletal deficits;* and an occupational therapist *to continue to maximize self-care skills.*

Assist patient in identifying and contacting resources for social and spiritual support *to promote the patient's reintegration into the community and help him maintain psychosocial health.*

SUGGESTED NIC INTERVENTIONS

Bed Rest Care; Body Mechanics Promotion; Exercise Promotion: Strength Training; Exercise Therapy: Joint Mobility; Exercise Therapy: Muscle Control; Positioning; Referral

REFERENCE

Lindemann, U., Reicherz, A., Nicolai, S., & Becker, C. (2010, August). Evaluation of an ergonomically modified bed to enhance mobilization in geriatric rehabilitation: A pilot study. *Zeitschrift für gerontologie und geriatrie, 43*(4), 235–238.

DEFINITION

Limitation in independent, purposeful physical movement of the body or of one or more extremities

DEFINING CHARACTERISTICS

- Gait changes, postural instability; difficulty turning
- Limited range of motion (ROM); ability to perform fine and gross motor skills
- Movement-induced tremor, uncoordinated or jerky movements
- Slowed and/or uncoordinated movements; reaction time
- Substitution of other behaviors for impaired mobility (for instance, increased attention to other's activity and controlling behavior)

RELATED FACTORS

- Activity intolerance
- Altered cellular metabolism
- Body mass index above 75th percentile
- Cognitive impairment
- Contractures
- Cultural beliefs regarding age-appropriate activity
- Deconditioning
- Decreased endurance; muscle control, mass or strength
- Depressive mood state
- Deficient knowledge about value of exercise
- Developmental delay
- Discomfort
- Disuse
- Joint stiffness

ASSESSMENT FOCUS

(Refer to comprehensive assessment parameters.)
- Activity/exercise
- Neurocognition

EXPECTED OUTCOMES

The patient will
- Maintain muscle strength and joint ROM.
- Be free from complications (e.g., contractures, venous stasis, thrombus formation, skin breakdown, and hypostatic pneumonia).
- Achieve the highest level of mobility (will transfer independently, will be wheelchair-independent, or will ambulate with assistive devices such as walker, cane, and braces).
- Carry out mobility regimen.
- Use resources to help maintain level of functioning.

SUGGESTED NOC OUTCOMES

Ambulation; Ambulation: Wheelchair; Joint Movement: Hip; Joint Movement: Passive; Mobility; Transfer Performance; Discharge Readiness: Independent Living; Discharge Readiness: Supported Living

INTERVENTIONS AND RATIONALES

<u>Determine:</u> Identify level of functioning using a functional mobility scale. Communicate patient's skill level to all staff members *to provide continuity and preserve identified level of independence.*

Monitor and record daily any evidence of immobility complications as they *may be more prone to develop complications.*

<u>Perform:</u> Perform ROM exercises to joints, unless contraindicated, at least once every shift *to prevent joint contractures and muscular atrophy.* Turn and reposition patient every 2 hours. Establish a turning schedule and post at bedside. Monitor frequency of turning *to prevent skin breakdown by relieving pressure. Place joints in functional position.* Use trochanter roll along the thigh, abduct thighs, use high-top sneakers, and pull a small pillow under patient's head *to maintain joints in a functional position and prevent musculoskeletal deformities.*

Place items within reach of the unaffected arm if patient has one-sided weakness or paralysis *to promote patient's independence.*

Carry out medical regimen to manage or prevent complications (e.g., administer prophylactic heparin for venous thrombosis). *This promotes patient's health and well-being.*

Provide progressive mobilization to the limits of patient's condition (bed mobility to chair mobility to ambulation) *to maintain muscle tone and prevent complications of immobility.*

<u>Inform:</u> Instruct patient and family members in ROM exercises, transfers, skin inspection, and mobility regimen *to help prepare for discharge and promote continuity of care.* Request return demonstration *to ensure use of proper technique.*

<u>Attend:</u> Help patient use a trapeze and side rails to *encourage independence in mobility.* Instruct him to perform self-care activities *to increase muscle tone.*

Encourage physical therapy sessions and support activities on the unit by using the same equipment and technique. Request written mobility plans for reference. Ensure all members of the health care team are reinforcing learned skills in the same manner.

<u>Manage:</u> Refer patient to a physical therapist for development of mobility regimen *to help rehabilitate musculoskeletal deficits.*

Assist patient in identifying resources such as American Heart Association to provide *a comprehensive approach to rehabilitation.*

SUGGESTED NIC INTERVENTIONS

Activity Therapy; Exercise Promotion: Strength Training; Exercise Therapy: Joint Mobility; Exercise Therapy: Muscle Control; Positioning: Wheelchair; Positioning; Energy Management

REFERENCE

Yor, S. C., Shumway-Cook, A., Silver, I. F., & Morrison, A. C. (2011). A translational research evaluation of the Stay Active and Independent for Life (SAIL) community-based fall prevention exercise and education program. *Health Promotion Practice,* 12(6), 832–839.

DEFINITION
Limitation of independent operation of wheelchair within environment

DEFINING CHARACTERISTICS
- Impaired ability to operate a manual or power wheelchair on curbs, even surfaces, uneven surfaces, and/or an incline or a decline

RELATED FACTORS
- Cognitive impairment
- Deconditioning
- Deficient knowledge
- Depressed mood
- Environmental constraints
- Impaired vision
- Limited endurance
- Musculoskeletal or neuromuscular impairment
- Obesity
- Pain

ASSESSMENT FOCUS
(Refer to comprehensive assessment parameters.)
- Activity/exercise
- Pharmacological function
- Physical regulation
- Neurocognition

EXPECTED OUTCOMES
The patient will
- Have no complications associated with impaired wheelchair mobility, such as skin breakdown, contractures, venous stasis, thrombus formation, depression, alteration in health maintenance, and falls.
- Maintain or improve muscle strength and joint range of motion (ROM).
- Achieve the highest level of independence and safety possible with regard to wheelchair use.
- Express feelings regarding alteration in ability to use wheelchair.
- Participate in social and occupational activities to the greatest extent possible.
- Demonstrate understanding of techniques to improve wheelchair mobility.

SUGGESTED NOC OUTCOMES
Ambulation: Wheelchair; Balance; Mobility Level; Muscle Function; Joint Movement Immobility Consequences: Physiological; Immobility Consequences: Psycho-Cognitive

INTERVENTIONS AND RATIONALES
Determine: Assess wheelchair status: Seat is wide and deep enough to support thighs, low enough for feet to touch the floor, yet high enough to allow easy transfer from bed to chair; the back is tall enough to support upper body; brakes on wheels lock; and seat belt is present (may attach at waist, hips, or chest). *Assessment ensures chair meets patient's physical needs (identifies need for modification), promotes comfort, and prevents injuries (e.g., falls).*

Assess patient's level of strength in arms, and if chair is easy for patient to operate when weak. *This determines the need for a motorized wheelchair to help maintain mobility and independence.*

Identify patient's level of independence using the functional mobility scale. Communicate findings to staff *to promote continuity of care and preserve the documented level of independence.*

Monitor and record daily evidence of complications related to impaired wheelchair mobility. *Patients with neuromuscular dysfunction are at risk for complications.*

Assess patient's skin on return to bed and request a wheelchair cushion, if necessary, *to maintain skin integrity.*

<u>Perform:</u> Perform ROM exercises for affected joints, unless contraindicated, at least once per shift. Progress from passive to active ROM as tolerated. *This prevents joint contractures and muscle atrophy.*

<u>Inform:</u> Explain to patient location of vulnerable pressure points and instruct to shift and reposition weight *to prevent skin breakdown.* Ensure patient maintains anatomically correct and functional body positioning *to promote comfort.*

Demonstrate techniques to promote wheelchair mobility to the patient and family members and note the date; have them perform a return demonstration *to ensure continuity of care and use of proper technique.*

<u>Attend:</u> Encourage patient to operate her wheelchair independently to the limits imposed by her condition *to maintain muscle tone, prevent complications of immobility, and promote independence in self-care and health maintenance skills.*

Encourage attendance at physical therapy sessions and reinforce prescribed activities on the unit by using equipment, devices, and techniques used in the therapy session. *To maintain continuity of care and promote patient safety.*

<u>Manage:</u> Refer patient to a physical therapist *to enhance wheelchair mobility and rehabilitation of musculoskeletal deficits.*

Help patient identify resources for maintaining highest level of mobility (e.g., community stroke program, sports associations for people with disabilities, and the National Multiple Sclerosis Society) *to promote reintegration into the community.*

SUGGESTED NIC INTERVENTIONS

Exercise Promotion: Strength Training; Exercise Therapy: Balance; Exercise Therapy: Muscle Control; Positioning: Wheelchair

REFERENCE

Mortenson, W. B., Miller, W. C., Backman, C. L., & Oliffe, J. L. (2011, October). Predictors of mobility among wheelchair using residents in long-term care. *Archives of Physical Medicine and Rehabilitation, 92*(10), 1587–1593.

DEFINITION
Response to the inability to carry out one's chosen moral/ethical decision/action

DEFINING CHARACTERISTICS
- Expresses anguish (e.g., powerlessness, guilt, frustration, anxiety, self-doubt, fear) over difficulty acting on moral choice

RELATED FACTORS
- Conflict among decision makers
- Conflicting information guiding ethical and/or moral decision making
- Cultural conflicts
- Decisions involving end-of-life matters
- Loss of autonomy
- Physical distance of decision maker
- Time constraints for decision making
- Treatment decisions

ASSESSMENT FOCUS
(Refer to comprehensive assessment parameters.)
- Roles/relationship
- Communication
- Coping
- Values/beliefs

EXPECTED OUTCOMES
The patient and family will
- Understand medical diagnosis, treatment regimen, and limitations related to extent of illness.
- Identify ethical/moral dilemma.
- Describe personal and family values and conflict with current situation.
- Identify health care ethics resources to assist in resolution of conflict.
- Verbalize relief from anguish, uneasiness, or distress.

SUGGESTED NOC OUTCOMES
Acceptance: Health Status; Client Satisfaction: Communication; Decision Making; Family Integrity; Family Functioning; Family Health Status; Family Integrity; Knowledge: Health Resources; Spiritual Health

INTERVENTIONS AND RATIONALES
<u>Determine:</u> Assess patient's and family's understanding of the diagnosis and prognosis, limitations, treatment options; description of their personal values; and their physical expressions of suffering. *Assessment factors assist in identifying appropriate interventions.*
<u>Perform:</u> Establish an environment in which family members can share comfortably and openly their issues and concerns.

Enlist assistance of health care ethics resources such as ethics committee or consultants. *Including experts in health care ethics will assist in identifying the patient/family values and reason for the dilemma. By identifying the source of the conflict, the process of resolution may begin, thus leading to better understanding by all parties and partial or full relief from moral suffering.*

Enlist assistance of chaplain or personal clergy *to assist in the process of resolution through clarification of values related to religious views. Chaplains and personal clergy may provide a more neutral "third party" that can help defuse the situation. Personal trusted clergy might recognize or facilitate patient/family verbal and physical expressions of suffering or relief.*

Inform: Educate patient and family about medical diagnosis, treatment regimen, and limitations involved in *to help both patient and family understand the limits of and read on for medical treatment related to medical diagnosis.*

Attend: Provide or set aside ample time for patient and family to express their feelings about the current situation. *Open, honest communication may clear misconceptions on both sides and facilitate relief from suffering in the mid of dilemma.*

Acknowledge ethical/moral position of the patient/family who may feel that their positions or views will go unrecognized in the mid of serious illness and high-tech treatments; they may not want to "bother" nurses and physicians with these concerns. *Acknowledging their concerns, values, and moral position allows for holistic care.*

Manage: Refer, where requested, for follow-up for a family member who needs exercise, weight management, diet assistance, health screenings, and so forth. *Assisting patient to make referrals will help ensure continued efforts on the part of the patient to live a healthier lifestyle.*

SUGGESTED NIC INTERVENTIONS

Active Listening; Anger Control Assistance; Anxiety Reduction; Conflict Mediation; Consultation; Counseling; Family Integrity Promotion; Multidisciplinary Care Conference; Spiritual Support; Family Support; Family Integrity Promotion; Family Maintenance; Truth Telling; Spiritual Growth Facilitation

REFERENCE

Wocial, L. D., & Weaver, M. T. (2012). Development and psychometric testing of a new tool for detecting moral distress: The Moral Distress Thermometer. *Journal of Advanced Nursing*, 69(1): 167–174.

DEFINITION
A subjective unpleasant, wavelike sensation in the back of the throat, epigastrium, or abdomen that may lead to the urge or need to vomit

DEFINING CHARACTERISTICS
- Gagging sensation
- Aversion toward food
- Increased salivation, swallowing
- Sour taste in the mouth
- Reports "nausea" or "sour taste in mouth"

RELATED FACTORS
Biophysical
- Biochemical disorders
- Esophageal disease
- Gastric distention, irritation
- Increased intracranial pressure
- Motion sickness
- Pain
- Pancreatic disease
- Tumors, intra-abdominal or localized tumors

Situational
- Anxiety
- Fear
- Noxious odors, taste, visual stimulation
- Pain
- Physiological factors

Treatment
- Gastric distention, irritation
- Pharmaceuticals

ASSESSMENT FOCUS
(Refer to comprehensive assessment parameters.)
- Nutrition
- Fluid and electrolytes
- Pharmacological function
- Knowledge
- Comfort

EXPECTED OUTCOMES
The patient will
- State reasons for nausea and vomiting.
- Take steps to manage episodes of nausea and vomiting.
- Ingest sufficient nutrients to maintain health.
- Take steps to ensure adequate nutrition when nausea abates.
- Maintain weight within specified limits.

SUGGESTED NOC OUTCOMES
Appetite; Comfort Status: Physical; Fluid Balance; Hydration; Nausea & Vomiting Control; Nutritional Status: Food & Fluid Intake; Suffering Severity; Symptom Control; Nausea & Vomiting Severity; Nausea & Vomiting: Disruptive Effects

INTERVENTIONS AND RATIONALES
<u>Determine:</u> Assess for illness, pregnancy, medication use (prescription and over-the-counter); exposure to tainted foods, chemicals, occupational

hazards; weight (fluctuation in last 6 months); food preferences and usual dietary patterns; history of gastric/esophageal problems. *Assessment information will help in identifying appropriate interventions.*

Monitor direct observation of food and fluid intake *to ensure whether or not the patient is receiving adequate nutritional intake.*

Perform: Provide comfort measures (e.g., back massage, warm bath) *to promote feelings of comfort for the patient.*

Reduce noise, control odors, and adjust light in the environment to help the patient relax and *to reduce environmental factors that produce nausea.*

Allow periods of uninterrupted sleep between procedures. *Procedures and medication administration sometimes trigger periods of nausea.*

Offer small amount of cool liquids or ice chips *to provide some fluid* to reduce the possibility of dehydration.

Suggest frequent mouth care *to reduce unpleasant taste in the mouth.*

Give dry, bland foods, such as dry toast or crackers, during periods of nausea *to make it possible to eat. These foods have been found to be effective.*

Administer antinausea medications, as prescribed.

Inform: Teach relaxation techniques and encourage patient to use these techniques during mealtime *to reduce stress and divert attention from the nausea.*

Teach patient how to use food and fluid during periods of nausea *to avoid dehydration and lack of nutrients. Food should be taken in small, frequent feedings. Avoid drinking with meals.*

Attend: When nausea abates, encourage patient to increase food intake *to assist with adequate intake of nutrients.*

Assist patient to make a list of best tolerated and poorly tolerated foods *so he or she can choose quickly and wisely when nausea abates.*

Manage: If nausea persists, refer patient to a nutritionist to assist after discharge *to ensure that adequate nutrients will be ingested.*

Stress the importance of follow-up appointments with the physician. *Nausea is a preventable problem and should respond to appropriate measures.*

SUGGESTED NIC INTERVENTIONS

Diet Staging; Fluid and Electrolyte Management; Fluid Monitoring; Medication Management; Nausea Management; Nutrition Management; Massage; Relaxation Therapy

REFERENCE

Buck, H. G. (2012, March). Real-world of symptom management: Nausea. *Nursing*, 42(3), 18–19.

DEFINITION

Behavior of person and/or caregiver that fails to coincide with a health-promoting or therapeutic plan agreed on by the person (and/or family and/or community) and health care professional. In the presence of an agreed upon, health-promoting or therapeutic plan, person's or caregiver's behavior is fully or partially nonadherent and may lead to clinically ineffective or partially ineffective outcomes

DEFINING CHARACTERISTICS

- Behavior indicative of failure to progress
- Complications or evidence of exacerbation of signs and symptoms
- Failure to keep appointments and adhere to treatment regimen
- Objective indications (e.g., laboratory tests, physiologic markers)

RELATED FACTORS

Health system
- Access to, convenience of care
- Client–provider relationships
- Individual health coverage
- Provider communication skills, credibility; continuity; teaching skills; reimbursement

Health care plan
- Complexity, intensity
- Cost, financial flexibility, and duration of plan

Individual
- Cultural/spiritual values
- Developmental and personal abilities
- Health beliefs
- Knowledge of regimen
- Motivational forces

Network
- Involvement of members in health plan
- Social value regarding plan

ASSESSMENT FOCUS

(Refer to comprehensive assessment parameters.)
- Behavior
- Beliefs/values
- Coping
- Emotional status
- Knowledge
- Roles/responsibilities
- Self-perception

EXPECTED OUTCOMES

The patient will
- Identify factors that influence noncompliance.
- Demonstrate level of compliance that maintains safety.
- Contract to perform specific behaviors.
- Use support systems to modify noncompliant behaviors.

SUGGESTED NOC OUTCOMES

Acceptance: Health Status; Adherence Behavior; Compliance Behavior; Symptom Control; Treatment Behavior: Illness or Injury

INTERVENTIONS AND RATIONALES

Determine: Assess patient's perception of health problem, treatment regimen and history of compliance, obstacles to compliance, financial resources, ethnicity, and religious influences. *Assessment information may help select appropriate interventions.*

Perform: Provide an environment that is nonjudgmental. *This demonstrates unconditional respect for the patient.*

Contract with the patient to practice only nonthreatening behaviors. *This involves the patient in a formal commitment and gives the patient a sense of personal control.*

Inform: Teach self-healing techniques to both the patient and family such as meditation, guided imagery, yoga, and prayer. *These techniques promote self-reliance.*

Teach principles of good nutrition for patient's specific condition. *Understanding importance of nutrition will encourage compliance.*

Inform patient about diagnosis. *Understanding essential information needed to perform skills or give self-care increases compliance.* Demonstrate skills needed by patient to comply with treatment regimen *to reinforce patient's confidence in ability to replicate.*

Attend: Provide opportunities for the patient to discuss reasons for noncompliance. *The willingness of the nurse to listen allows the patient the ability to listen to his or her own reasoning.*

Help patient clarify his or her values about the importance of following a treatment plan *to determine appropriate interventions.*

Acknowledge patient's right to choose not to comply with prescribed regimen *to respect autonomy. Control over patient's actions is legitimate only when dangerous to self or others.* Offer positive reinforcement.

Use support systems to reinforce negotiated behaviors. *Support from the family and friends help foster compliance.*

Manage: When medically appropriate, support patient's cultural beliefs towards medical practices to demonstrate respect; and refer to a member of the clergy or a spiritual counselor.

Refer family to community resources and support groups *to promote compliance with modification of behavior.* If patient's situation is complicated by lack of financial resources, contact agencies that may offer help with costs of medical treatment.

SUGGESTED NIC INTERVENTIONS

Coping Enhancement; Counseling; Decision-Making Support; Health Education; Patient Contracting; Self-Modification Assistance; Self-Responsibility Facilitation

REFERENCE

Townsend, M. S. (2011, September). Patient-driven education materials: Low-literate adults increase understanding of health messages and improve compliance. *Nursing Clinics of North America, 46*(3), 367–378.

DEFINITION

Intake of nutrients insufficient to meet metabolic needs

DEFINING CHARACTERISTICS

- Abdominal pain, cramping
- Altered taste sensation; aversion to or lack of interest in eating
- Body weight >20% under ideal weight
- Diarrhea or steatorrhea
- Excessive hair loss
- Fragile capillaries
- Hyperactive bowel sounds
- Lack of information, misconceptions, or misinformation
- Loss of body weight despite adequate food intake
- Pale conjunctiva and mucous
- Perceived inability to digest or ingest food
- Satiety immediately after ingesting food
- Weakness of muscle required for chewing or swallowing

RELATED FACTORS

- Biological factors
- Economic factors
- Inability to absorb nutrients
- Inability to digest/ingest food
- Psychological factors

ASSESSMENT FOCUS

(Refer to comprehensive assessment parameters.)

- Behavior
- Coping
- Nutrition
- Elimination
- Fluids and electrolytes
- Values/beliefs

EXPECTED OUTCOMES

The patient will

- Consume _____ calories daily.
- Gain __ lb/week and show no further evidence of weight loss.
- Communicate understanding of dietary needs.
- Demonstrate ability to plan meals that will help patient gain weight.

SUGGESTED NOC OUTCOMES

Nutritional Status; Nutritional Status: Food & Fluid Intake; Nutritional Status: Nutrient Intake; Weight Gain Behavior; Weight: Body Mass; Weight Maintenance Behavior; Knowledge: Diet

INTERVENTIONS AND RATIONALES

<u>Determine:</u> Assess height, weight, meal preparation, serum albumen, usual dietary pattern, weight fluctuation over the last 10 years, psychosocial status, and coping behavior. *Assessment of these factors will allow the nurse to choose appropriate interventions.*

<u>Perform:</u> Obtain and record patient's weight everyday at the same time *to ensure keeping an accurate record of weight.*

Monitor fluid intake and output every 8 hours *to provide adequate fluid replacement.*

Provide a diet prescribed for the patient's specific condition and preferences *to ensure that the patient's dietary restrictions are followed as much as possible.* Keep snacks at the bedside *to allow the patient to eat small amounts frequently.*

Approach patient in a nonjudgmental manner. *This demonstrates unconditional positive respect for the patient.* Facilitate opportunities for spiritual nourishment and growth *to address patient's holistic needs for maximal therapeutic environment.*

Inform: Teach self-healing techniques to both the patient and family such as meditation, guided imagery, yoga, and prayer. Teach patient how to incorporate the use of self-healing techniques in carrying out usual daily activities. *These techniques can be used to reduce anxiety and increase self-reliance.*

Provide patient with concise information about the diagnosis, and teach principles of good nutrition for specific condition. *Understanding encourages compliance with treatment and nutritional regimen.*

Attend: Provide opportunities for the patient to discuss reasons for not eating and to clarify values about the importance of food *in order to determine appropriate interventions.*

After obtaining patient's food preferences, attempt to obtain desired foods for the patient. Offer food that appeal to olfactory, visual, and tactile senses *to enhance patient's appetite.* Whenever possible, sit with patient for a predetermined time during each meal. *This inhibits patient from dawdling during the meal.*

Acknowledge patient's right to choose not to comply with prescribed regimen. *Patient's autonomy must be respected. Control over patient's actions is legitimate only when danger is posed to patient or others.*

Use support systems to reinforce negotiated behaviors. *Support from the family helps foster compliance.*

Manage: Refer patient to a dietitian or nutritional support team *for dietary management.* Refer family to community resources and support groups available *to assist patient in complying with modification of behavior.* If patient's situation is complicated by a lack of financial recourses, contact agencies *that may offer help with the cost of medical treatment.* Refer to a member of the clergy or a spiritual counselor, according to the patient's preference, *to show respect for the patient's beliefs and provide spiritual care.*

SUGGESTED NIC INTERVENTIONS

Eating Disorders Management; Fluid Monitoring; Mutual Goal-Setting; Weight Goal-Setting; Nutrition Management; Nutritional Monitoring

REFERENCE

Walz, D. A. (2010, June). Cancer-related anorexia-cachexia syndrome. *Clinical Journal of Oncology Nursing, 14*(3), 283–287.

DEFINITION

Intake of nutrients that exceed metabolic needs

DEFINING CHARACTERISTICS

- Body weight >20% above ideal body weight
- Dysfunctional eating patterns, such as concentrating food intake at the end of the day, eating in response to internal cues other than hunger, eating in response to external cues, and pairing food with other activities
- Sedentary lifestyle
- Triceps skin fold greater than 15 mm in men and 25 mm in women

RELATED FACTORS

- Excessive intake related to metabolic needs or physical activity

ASSESSMENT FOCUS

(Refer to comprehensive assessment parameters.)

- Behavior
- Communication
- Coping
- Emotional
- Knowledge
- Nutrition
- Values and beliefs

EXPECTED OUTCOMES

The patient will

- Voice feelings about present weight.
- Identify internal and external cues that increase food consumption.
- Verbalize need to lose weight.
- Set a goal of losing ____ lb a week.
- Adhere to prescribed diet, and plan menus appropriate to diet.
- Set target weight before discharge.
- State plan to monitor and maintain target weight.
- Participate in an exercise plan ___ times per week.

SUGGESTED NOC OUTCOME

Adherence Behavior; Knowledge: Diet; Motivation; Nutritional Status; Nutritional Status: Nutrient Intake; Risk Detection; Stress Level; Weight Control

INTERVENTIONS AND RATIONALES

Determine: Assess height, weight, usual dietary patterns, food preference, understanding of risk factors, heredity influences, activity level, usual coping patterns, and body image. *Information from assessment will help identify appropriate interventions.*

Perform: Weigh patient weekly, or as ordered to evaluate patient's progress toward reaching goal and provide feedback.

Help patient set realistic goal for weight loss. Goal should be in the ideal range considering the patient's height and age, but the patient needs to be reminded that slow weight loss will help him or her reach his or her goal more effectively.

Inform: Teach patient about low-calorie, nutritious foods. This encourages patient to eat foods that provide energy without causing weight gain.

Have patient keep a food diary in order to keep track of what is actually eaten. Without this, foods are sometimes eaten and not included in daily food consumption. This will act a self-monitoring tool.

Teach coping skills. Have patient role-play to provide practical experience. Provide instructional material on healthy eating habits, coping skills, self-esteem, and so forth.

Attend: Listen to patient's personal values and beliefs, but remain nonjudgmental, even if his or her values and beliefs differ from your own. Remaining nonjudgmental, but attentive, shows your support. Explore personal identity issues distressing to the patient to isolate issues into small, more solvable units.

Help patient identify his or her values, beliefs, hopes, dreams skills, and interest. The patient's deficits may lie in a lack of self-exploration or problem-solving methods used.

Promote choices with the most likeliness of success. Specific instructions can help the patient gain problem-solving ability and maturity.

Manage: Refer patient to a mental health professional for behavior modification to help change poor eating habits and ensure permanent weight loss.

Have a dietitian calculate the caloric intake the patient will require to reach a desirable weight to allow for planning.

Refer to peer support group, and promote outpatient counseling and family meetings to reinforce progress and reduce regression.

SUGGESTED NIC INTERVENTIONS

Behavior Management; Behavior Modification; Coping Enhancement; Eating Disorders Management; Exercise Promotion; Limit Setting; Nutrition Management; Weight Reduction Assistance; Journaling

REFERENCE

Mieres, J., & Christie, C. (2011, September). Contemporary approaches to adult treatment of obesity. Nurse Practitioner, 36(9), 37–46.

DEFINITION

A pattern of nutrient intake that is sufficient for meeting metabolic needs and can be strengthened

DEFINING CHARACTERISTICS

- Attitude toward drinking and eating is congruent with health goals
- Consumes adequate fluid and food on regular basis
- Expresses knowledge of healthy fluid and food choices
- Expresses willingness to enhance nutrition
- Follows an appropriate standard for intake
- Safely prepares fluids and foods
- Safely stores fluids and foods

ASSESSMENT FOCUS

(Refer to comprehensive assessment parameters.)
- Knowledge
- Nutrition
- Risk management
- Values/beliefs

EXPECTED OUTCOMES

The patient will
- Articulate present understanding of factors that enable and hinder enhanced nutritional status.
- Evaluate each of the barriers to enhancing nutritional status.
- Articulate the personal value of practicing positive behaviors.
- Plan modifications of environment to reinforce change in eating habits.
- Express positive feelings about himself.

SUGGESTED NOC OUTCOMES

Adherence Behavior: Healthy Diet; Knowledge: Diet; Knowledge: Weight Management; Nutritional Status: Fluid and Food Intake; Health Promoting Behavior

INTERVENTIONS AND RATIONALES

<u>Determine:</u> Assess height, weight, body mass index; self-esteem, attitude toward food and eating; moral or health concerns about eating; financial status; cultural background and influences of same on food; ability to read food labels, numbers of take-out meals per week; cost of food in particular geographic area. *Assessment information about these factors will help identify appropriate interventions.*

<u>Perform:</u> Help patient list the internal and external barriers to improving nutritional status. *Lack of understanding of the patient's individual barriers, such as unclear goals, lack of skill, or lack of motivation will prevent change from occurring.*

<u>Inform:</u> Provide materials that are intellectually and culturally appropriate for enhancing nutritional knowledge. *It is important to engage the patient in information gathering before beginning to develop a plan to change behavior.*

Teach patient to read food labels, to plan meals using a standard method such as the meals in the Food Guide (American Diabetic Association) and to stop and stock the refrigerator and pantry with smart food choices. *New behaviors require practice in a practical sense for the kind of reinforcement that will produce the desired change.*

Teach patient about the importance of exercise. Assist patient to outline a realistic program that provides adequate exercise on a weekly basis. *Having a schedule that is realistic for the individual will assist the patient with personal compliance.*

<u>Attend:</u> Encourage patient to list realistic goals with target dates for meeting. *Goal-directed behavior will increase the chance of positive outcomes.*

Have patient make a list of the positive outcomes of changing behaviors (e.g., wearing smaller size clothing, feeling better about being with others who are health conscious, enjoying feelings of physical and emotional well-being). *Positive reinforcers make changes more appealing.*

<u>Manage:</u> Refer patient to a nutrition group and an exercise group in the community, and community resources that may offer assistance to the patient when needed. *Patients often do better when they are participating with others who are working toward similar goals.*

Offer written information that can be referred to when needed. *Having written instructions reinforces learning.*

SUGGESTED NIC INTERVENTIONS

Nutrition Management; Nutritional Monitoring; Nutritional Counseling; Weight Management; Teaching: Prescribed Diet

REFERENCE

Dunstan, K. (2012, June). Maintaining nutritional intake in adults admitted to an acute medical ward in a tertiary hospital: A best practice implementation project. *PACEsetterS, 9*(2), 30–35.

DEFINITION
At risk for intake of nutrients that exceeds metabolic needs

RISK FACTORS
- Consumption of solid food as a major source before 5 months of age
- Dysfunctional eating patterns, such as concentrating food intake at the end of the day, using food as a reward, eating in response to external cues
- High baseline weight at the beginning of pregnancy
- Obesity of one or more parents
- Rapid movement across growth percentiles
- Sedentary lifestyle

ASSESSMENT FOCUS
(Refer to comprehensive assessment parameters.)
- Activity
- Knowledge
- Nutrition
- Risk management

EXPECTED OUTCOMES
The patient will
- Express need to stabilize weight within 5 to 10 lb of target weight.
- Plan to monitor weight and sustain target weight.
- Express feelings regarding dietary regimen and current weight.
- Identify internal and external cues that lead to increased food consumption.
- Plan menus that are appropriate for prescribed diet.
- Participate in selected exercise program every week.

SUGGESTED NOC OUTCOMES
Knowledge: Diet; Nutritional Status; Nutritional Status: Nutrient Intake; Risk Control; Stress Level; Weight Control

INTERVENTIONS AND RATIONALES
<u>Determine:</u> Assess nutritional history, usual dietary habits, frequency and size of meals, snacks, meal preparation; meals eaten out or take-out per week. Assess weight, weight fluctuation over past year; activity level, body image; motivation to modify lifestyle. *Information from the assessment will help identify appropriate interventions.*

<u>Perform:</u> Weigh patient weekly or as prescribed *to monitor the effectiveness of the diet and provide feedback to the patient.*

Establish, with the patient, a realistic target weight, and help patient take an active role in health care decisions. *The greater the role the patient takes, the more likely he will succeed in reaching the goal.*

Determine food preferences to evaluate eating habits and to include preferred food on the patient's list if they are nutritious. *This will help the patient make healthful choices.*

Inform: Teach the basics of meal planning using the Food Guide Pyramid found at www.MYPyramid.gov *to help patients find food types and calories needed to remain on target.*

Give written materials and use visuals, discussion, and role-playing to help the patient learn to make healthy food selection. *Use a variety of media to make important points.*

Teach the importance of incorporating exercise into lifestyle. Help patient select a program with various activities (such as swimming, walking, cycling, aerobics) appropriate for age and physical condition. *Exercise burns calories, offers an alternative to eating to alleviate stress, and fosters a sense of accomplishment.*

Attend: Give patient emotional support and positive feedback for adhering to the prescribed diet. *This will foster compliance and help ensure adherence to weight program.*

Manage: Refer patient to an appropriate resource for behavior modification and cognitive therapy *to prevent relapse into high-risk eating behaviors.*

If patient has new insights in his or her motivation to reduce his weight, encourage him or her to share this information with his primary health care practitioner *to foster a sense of responsibility for obtaining health care.*

Suggest that patient present practitioner with a summary of his or her goals and the strategies to meet them. *As patients move from one physician to another, information about the patients' problems and goal to resolve and progress in doing the same often get lost. In this way the patient takes responsibility for bringing his or her primary care practitioner up to date with his or her progress.*

Recommend that the patient explore group diet therapies, such as Weight Watchers and Overeaters Anonymous, *to provide additional sources of information and encouragement.*

SUGGESTED NIC INTERVENTIONS

Behavior Management; Exercise Promotion; Nutritional Counseling; Nutrition Management; Teaching; Prescribed Diet

REFERENCE

Burke, L. E., & Wong, J. (2011, December). Treatment strategies for overweight and obesity. *Journal of Nursing Scholarship, 43*(4), 368–375.

DEFINITION
Disruption of the lips and/or soft tissue of the oral cavity

DEFINING CHARACTERISTICS
- Bleeding
- Coated tongue
- Desquamation
- Difficulty eating, speaking, or swallowing
- Diminished, absent, or bad taste
- Dry mouth
- Edema
- Enlarged tonsils
- Fissures and cheilitis
- Gingival hyperplasia or recession (pockets deeper than 4 mm)
- Gingival or mucosal pallor
- Halitosis
- Mucosal denudation
- Oral lesions, ulcers, pain, or discomfort
- Purulent drainage or exudate; presence of pathogens
- Smooth, atrophic, sensitive tongue
- Spongy patches or white, curdlike exudate
- Stomatitis
- Vesicles, nodules, or papules
- White patches and plaque

RELATED FACTORS
- Barriers to oral self or professional care
- Chemical irritants (e.g., alcohol, drugs, regular use of inhalers)
- Chemotherapy
- Cleft lip and/or palate
- Mechanical factors (braces, dentures)
- Ineffective oral hygiene
- Malnutrition
- Dehydration
- Stress
- Trauma

ASSESSMENT FOCUS
(Refer to comprehensive assessment parameters.)
- Coping
- Fluid and electrolytes
- Nutrition
- Tissue integrity

EXPECTED OUTCOMES

The patient will
- Maintain fluid balance (intake equals output).
- State increased comfort.
- Have pink, moist oral mucous membranes.
- Have minimal, if any, complications of the oral mucosa.
- Correlate precipitating factors with appropriate oral care.
- Demonstrate oral hygiene practices.

SUGGESTED NOC OUTCOMES

Oral Hygiene; Tissue Integrity: Skin & Mucous Membranes

INTERVENTIONS AND RATIONALES

<u>Determine:</u> Inspect patient's oral cavity every shift. Describe and document condition; report any change in status. *Regular assessments can anticipate or alleviate problems.*

Monitor progress, reporting favorable and adverse responses to the treatment regimen *to evaluate effectiveness.*

<u>Perform:</u> Perform the prescribed treatment regimen, including administering intravenous or oral fluids, *to improve the condition of patient's mucous membranes.*

Provide supportive measures, as indicated:

- Assist with oral hygiene before and after meals *to promote a feeling of comfort and well-being.*
- Use a toothbrush with suction if patient can't spit out water *to minimize risk of aspiration.*
- Provide mouthwash or gargles, as ordered, *to increase patient comfort and maintain moisture in his or her mouth.*
- Lubricate patient's lips frequently with water-based lubricant *to prevent cracked, irritated skin. These measures improve oral health.*

<u>Inform:</u> Instruct patient in oral hygiene practices, if necessary. Have patient return a demonstration of the oral care routine.

- Use a soft-bristled toothbrush.
- Brush with a circular motion away from the gums.
- Include the tongue when brushing.
- Review the need for routine visits to a dentist (annually for adults).

These measures increase patient's awareness of oral hygiene practices and reduce discomfort, resulting in increased nutrition and hydration.

Tell patient to chew gum or suck on sugarless hard candy *to stimulate salivation.*

Discuss precipitating factors, if known, and work to prevent future episodes. For example, encourage patient to avoid exercising in heat and to report effects of medication. *Patient's increased awareness of causative factors will help prevent recurrence.*

Attend: Encourage adherence to other aspects of health care management (controlling diabetes, changing dietary habits, and avoiding alcoholic beverages) *to control or minimize effects on mucous membranes.*

Manage: Refer patient to a dentist, dental hygienist, or other appropriate resource to correct ill-fitting dentures, modify braces, and adjust jaw wires as needed. *Regularly scheduled dental follow-up reduces the risk of trauma to oral mucous membranes.*

SUGGESTED NIC INTERVENTIONS

Fluid and Electrolyte Management; Oral Health Maintenance; Oral Health Restoration; Oral Health Promotion

REFERENCES

Bisset, S., & Preshaw, P. (2011, December). Guide to providing mouth care for older people. *Nursing Older People, 23*(10), 14–21.

Prendergast, V., et al. (2012, June). Effects of a standard versus comprehensive oral care protocol among intubated neuroscience ICU patients: Results of a randomized controlled trial. *Journal of Neuroscience Nursing, 44*(3), 134–146.

DEFINITION

At risk for behaviors in which an individual demonstrates that he or she can be physically, emotionally, and/or sexually harmful to others

RISK FACTORS

- Availability of weapons
- Body language
- Cognitive impairment
- Cruelty to animals
- Fire setting
- History of childhood abuse
- History of substance abuse
- History of threats of violence against person or personal property
- History of violence, including hitting, kicking, scratching, throwing objects at someone, attempting rape, sexual molestation
- History of violence against others
- History of violent antisocial behavior
- Impulsivity
- Motor vehicle offenses
- Neurological impairment
- Suicidal behavior

ASSESSMENT FOCUS

(Refer to comprehensive assessment parameters.)

- Behavior
- Coping
- Emotional
- Knowledge
- Neurocognition
- Risk factor management
- Self-perception

EXPECTED OUTCOMES

The patient will

- Maintain control over anger.
- Successfully rechannel hostility into socially acceptable behaviors.
- Discuss angry feelings and verbalize appropriate ways to tolerate frustration.
- Express need for long-term treatment.

SUGGESTED NOC OUTCOMES

Abuse Cessation; Abusive Behavior Self-Restraint; Aggression Self-Control; Impulse Self-Control

INTERVENTIONS AND RATIONALES

<u>Determine:</u> Assess recent stressors; substance abuse history; previous episodes of violence; reaction of family members to episodes of violence;

neurological examination; toxicology examination and blood chemistry. *Assessment information will help identify appropriate intervention.*

Perform: Remove all objects from the environment that the patient could use to harm himself or herself *in order to provide safety and protect potential victims of violence.*

Administer prescribed medications *to help patient control aggressive behavior and remain calm.* Monitor for effectiveness. *When used appropriately, medications will remove the need for physical restraint.*

Inform: Explain medication program to patient *to promote compliance.* Make sure that medication is swallowed, as prescribed, *to ensure compliance and produce calmness.*

Teach coping strategies and self-healing techniques to patient and family members, including meditation, guided imagery, and prayer.

Teach patient how to incorporate the use of self-healing techniques in carrying out usual daily activities. *These techniques help calm the mind and promote ability to cooperate with the difficulties associated with violent behavior.*

Attend: Explain to patient in a firm, calm voice that you will help him or her maintain control. *Communicating a willingness to help encourages the patient to take control of his or her behavior.*

Encourage patient to begin discussing hostile feelings gradually *to help him or her develop more appropriate ways of dealing with hostility.*

Discuss situations that provoke feelings of anxiety, anger, and powerlessness *to identify areas of patient concern and to prevent anger from being inappropriately directed at self.*

Manage: Set limits on patient's behavior *to reinforce the expectation that the patient will act in a responsible controlled manner.*

Provide patient with telephone numbers and other information about crisis centers, hotlines, and counselors. *Alternatives may ease anxiety about the perceived threat of long-term psychotherapy.*

SUGGESTED NIC INTERVENTIONS

Anger Control Assistance; Behavior Management; Environmental Management: Violence Prevention; Impulse Control Training

REFERENCE

Bailey, L. D. (2012, April). Professional growth and development: Adolescent girls: A vulnerable population. *Advances in Neonatal Care, 12*(2), 102–106.

DEFINITION

Unpleasant sensory and emotional experience arising from actual or potential tissue damage or described in terms of such damage (International Association for the Study of Pain); sudden or slow onset of any intensity from mild to severe with an anticipated or predictable end and a duration of less than 6 months

DEFINING CHARACTERISTICS

- Alteration in muscle tone
- Autonomic responses
- Changes in appetite and eating
- Communication (verbal or coded) of pain
- Distracting behavior (such as pacing, seeking out other people, and performing repetitive activities)
- Expression of pain (such as moaning or crying)
- Facial mask of pain
- Guarding or protective behavior
- Narrowed focus
- Self-focusing
- Sleep disturbance

RELATED FACTORS

- Injury agents (biological, chemical, physical, psychological)

ASSESSMENT FOCUS

(Refer to comprehensive assessment parameters.)

- Communication
- Coping
- Emotional
- Sleep/rest
- Values/beliefs

EXPECTED OUTCOMES

The patient will

- Rate pain on a scale of 1 to 10.
- Articulate factors that intensify pain and will modify behaviors accordingly.
- State and carry out appropriate interventions for relief of pain.
- Decrease amount and frequency of pain medication needed.
- Express feeling of comfort and relief from pain.
- Perform relaxation exercises at bedtime.

SUGGESTED NOC OUTCOMES

Comfort Status; Pain Control; Pain: Disruptive Effects; Pain Level; Sleep; Client Satisfaction: Pain Management; Knowledge: Pain Management

INTERVENTIONS AND RATIONALES

Determine: Assess descriptive characteristics of pain, including location, quality and intensity on a scale of 1 to 10, temporal factors and sources of relief; pain tolerance; ethnicity; attitude and values. *Descriptions about the particulars of pain will help determine what goals are realistic for the patient.*

<u>Perform:</u> Make changes in the environment at the patient's suggestion that will promote sleep. *This allows patient to have an active role in treatment.*

Apply heat or cold as prescribed *to minimize or relieve pain.* Reposition patient and use pillows to splint or support painful areas, as appropriate *to reduce muscle spasm and to redistribute pressure on body parts.* Administer analgesic medications in a collaborative mode with the patient when alternative methods are not sufficient to make the pain tolerable. *Gaining the patient's trust and involvement helps ensure compliance and make reduce medication intake.*

Provide patient with sleep aids, such as pillows, bath before sleep, and reading materials. Milk and some high-protein snacks, such as cheese and nuts, contain L-tryptophan and are also sleep promoters. *Personal hygiene and prebedtime rituals promote sleep in some patients. Comfort measures act as distracters from pain, reduce muscle tension or spasm, and redistribute pressure on body parts.*

<u>Inform:</u> Teach patient relaxation techniques such as guided imagery, deep breathing, meditation, aromatherapy, and progressive muscle relaxation. Practice with the patient frequently and especially at bedtime. *Purposeful relaxation efforts usually help promote sleep.*

Instruct patient to eliminate or reduce caffeine and alcohol intake and avoid foods that interfere with sleep (e.g., spicy foods). *Foods and beverages containing caffeine consumed fewer than 4 hours before bedtime may interfere with sleep. Alcohol disrupts normal sleep, especially when ingested immediately before retiring.*

<u>Attend:</u> Listen to patient's description of pain. Allow time for the patient to talk about his or her frustration. *Listening attentively gives the patient a feeling that the nurse is interested. It also helps determine progress in alleviating the pain.*

Ask patient each day to describe the quality of his or her sleep. *Discomfort associated with pain may prevent the patient from sleeping well.*

Encourage activities that provide distraction, such as reading, crafts, television, and visits *to help patient focus on non-pain-related matters.*

<u>Manage:</u> When possible, allow patient to use alternative pain treatments common in his or her culture (such as acupuncture) as a substitute or a complement to Western treatments *to promote nonpharmacologic pain management.*

Refer to case manager/social worker *to ensure that follow-up is provided.*

SUGGESTED NIC INTERVENTIONS

Analgesic Administration; Coping Enhancement; Emotional Support; Medication Management; Pain Management; Positioning; Sleep Enhancement; Environmental Management; Guided Imagery, Aromatherapy; Massage; Relaxation Therapy; Biofeedback; Referral

REFERENCE

Marmo, L., & Fowler, S. (2010, September). Pain assessment tool in the critically ill post-open heart surgery patient population. *Pain Management Nurse, 11*(30), 134–140.

DEFINITION

Unpleasant sensory and emotional experience arising from actual or potential tissue damage or described in terms of such damage (International Association for the Study of Pain); sudden or slow onset of any intensity from mild to severe, constant or recurring without an anticipated or predictable end and a duration of more than 6 months

DEFINING CHARACTERISTICS

- Altered ability to continue usual activity
- Atrophy of involved muscle group
- Changes in sleep pattern
- Depression
- Facial mask (e.g., beaten look, grimace)
- Fatigue
- Fear of reinjury
- Irritability
- Protective or guarding behavior
- Reduced social action
- Restlessness
- Self-focusing
- Sympathetic-mediated responses (such as change in temperature and hypersensitivity)
- Verbal report of pain

RELATED FACTORS

- Chronic physical disability
- Chronic psychological disability

ASSESSMENT FOCUS

(Refer to comprehensive assessment parameters.)
- Cardiac functioning
- Comfort
- Coping
- Emotional
- Neurocognitive functioning
- Pharmacologic function
- Respiratory functioning
- Values/beliefs

EXPECTED OUTCOMES

The patient will
- Identify characteristics of pain and pain behaviors.
- Develop pain management program that includes activity and rest, exercise, and medication regimen that isn't pain contingent.
- Carry out resocialization behaviors and activities.

- State relationship of increasing pain to stress, activity, and fatigue.
- State importance of self-care behavior or activities.

SUGGESTED NOC OUTCOMES

Comfort Status; Depression Level; Depression Self-Control; Pain Control; Pain Level; Quality of Life; Sleep; Symptom Control; Knowledge: Pain Management; Pain: Adverse Psychological Response

INTERVENTIONS AND RATIONALES

<u>Determine:</u> Assess descriptive characteristics of pain, including location, quality, intensity on a scale of 1 to 10, temporal factors and sources of relief; pain tolerance; ethnicity; self-image, coping behaviors, sleep patterns, activity level, attitude, and values. *Assessment will provide information to help identify interventions for that specific patient.*

<u>Perform:</u> Set up a behavior-oriented plan; for instance, set up a plan to follow the activity schedule. *Behavioral–cognitive measures can help patient modify learned pain behaviors.*

Contract with patient to increase probability that he or she will follow the plan for pain management that has been developed with him. *A contract is an agreement that can always be referred to when the patient attempts to make decisions outside the provisions of the plan.*

Schedule self-care activities for the patient. *This reduces dependence on caregivers and others in the patient's environment.*

Administer analgesic pain medication as outlined in the plan. *When a patient requests more than the plan allows, reiterate the terms of the plan in order not to overmedicate.*

<u>Inform:</u> Teach patient relaxation techniques such as guided imagery, deep breathing, meditation, aromatherapy, and progressive muscle relaxation. Practice with the patient frequently and especially at bedtime. *Purposeful relaxation efforts may help promote sleep.*

Instruct patient to eliminate or reduce caffeine and alcohol intake and avoid foods that interfere with sleep (e.g., spicy foods). *Foods and beverages containing caffeine consumed fewer than 4 hours before bedtime may interfere with sleep. Alcohol disrupts normal sleep, especially when ingested immediately before retiring.*

<u>Attend:</u> Work closely with staff and family *to achieve pain management goals and maximize the patient's cooperation.*

Encourage patient and family to express feelings associated with diagnosis, treatment, and recovery *to help patient and family cope with treatment.* Schedule time to spend with the patient's family. *They need time with health care providers to ask questions.*

Encourage activities that provide distraction, such as reading, crafts, television, and visits *to help patient focus on non-pain-related matters.*

<u>Manage:</u> When possible, allow patient to use alternative pain treatments common in his or her culture (such as acupuncture) as a substitute or a

complement to Western treatments *to promote nonpharmacologic pain management.*

Arrange for frequent multidisciplinary/family care conference *to keep care goal-oriented.* Refer patient to support group *to help deal with pain, depression, and so forth.* Refer to social worker/case manager *for follow-up care.*

SUGGESTED NIC INTERVENTIONS

Analgesic Administration; Behavior Modification; Emotional Support; Mood Management; Pain Management; Patient Contracting; Massage; Biofeedback; Relaxation Therapy

REFERENCE

Cornally, N., & McCarthy, G. (2011, December). Chronic Pain: The health seeking behavior, attitudes, and beliefs of older adults living in the community. *Pain Management Nursing, 12*(4), 206–207.

DEFINITION

A pattern of providing an environment for children or other dependent person(s) that is sufficient to nurture growth and development and can be strengthened

DEFINING CHARACTERISTICS

- Willingness to enhance parenting
- Satisfaction with home environment (children or other dependent persons)
- Emotional and tacit support of children or other dependent persons; bonding or attachment
- Fulfillment of physical and emotional needs (children or other dependent persons)
- Realistic expectations of children or other dependent persons

ASSESSMENT FOCUS

(Refer to comprehensive assessment parameters.)
- Communication
- Coping
- Knowledge
- Roles/responsibilities
- Values/beliefs

EXPECTED OUTCOMES

The parents will
- Express satisfaction with and confidence in parental role.
- Discuss signs of safe and functional environment in the home setting and state or demonstrate an understanding of teaching.
- Demonstrate consistency and effectiveness related to discipline.

The family will
- Appear to be physically and emotionally healthy.
- Express belief in a higher spiritual power.
- Express enjoyment of spending time together.
- Express confidence in social and community resources available related to family needs.

SUGGESTED NOC OUTCOMES

Parent–Infant Attachment; Parenting: Psychosocial Safety; Family Health Status; Family Social Climate; Knowledge: Parenting; Parenting Performance

INTERVENTIONS AND RATIONALES

Determine: Assess age and maturity of the parents; parental role-models during childhood; role satisfaction; social support; educational needs of parents, present parenting skills, coping mechanism utilized, knowledge of child growth and development, disciplinary methods used by parents. Family status, including relationship between parents and parents to children, sibling relationships, and spirituality. Psychological status, including financial, educational level, and consistency and reliability of parenting techniques. *A thorough assessment will help identify appropriate interventions for this diagnosis.*

<u>Perform:</u> Explore family's value systems as well as their spiritual beliefs and practices. *Spirituality and values provide a basis for ethical and moral reasoning and an enhanced meaning to life.*

Explore parents' idea of social support and community resources available to the family *to prepare for later referrals.*

Establish an environment of mutual trust and respect *to enhance learning. Consistency between action and words combined with the parents' self-awareness forms the basis of a trusting relationship.*

<u>Inform:</u> Select teaching strategies that will enhance teaching/learning effectiveness, such as discussion, demonstration, role-playing, and visual materials. Teach those skills that the patient must incorporate into daily living. Have patient do return demonstration of each skill *to aid in gaining confidence.*

When teaching, go slowly and repeat frequently. Offer small amounts of information and present it in various ways. *By building cognition, parents will be better prepared to cope.* Include family members in teaching. Demonstrate to family members how each coping strategies can be used *to deal with challenging incidents.*

<u>Attend:</u> Engage parents in a discussion of discipline practices and offer suggestions *to enhance their present skills.* Discipline needs to be consistent and loving and have reasonable guidelines. *Children want and need to have limits in order to feel safe.*

Encourage family to "play" together. *Laughter and joy increase enjoyment and bonding as well as growth as a family unit.*

Praise family for activities and traditions they honor together. *Sharing meaningful activities increases loyalty, security, and a sense of belonging for family members.* Encourage family members to participate in patient's learning process *to help create a therapeutic environment after discharge.*

Demonstrate patience in helping the patient repeat new skills multiple times. Offer parents opportunities to express their doubts or convictions about the adequacy of their parenting skills. *An open and receptive attitude provides an atmosphere for increased trust and enhanced learning.*

<u>Manage:</u> Have patient incorporate learned skills into care while still in the hospital *to allow practice and time for feedback.*

Provide patient and/or family with names and telephone numbers of resource people or community agencies *so that care is continuous and follow-up is possible after discharge.*

If financial hardship interferes with the family's ability to provide equipment and supplies, offer a referral to a social worker *to improve the family's access to financial assistance.*

SUGGESTED NIC INTERVENTIONS

Attachment Promotion; Developmental Enhancement: Child and Adolescent; Family Integrity Promotion: Childbearing Family; Environmental Management: Attachment Process; Family Integrity Promotion; Role Enhancement

REFERENCE

McGrath, J., et al. (2011, April–June) Family-centered developmental care practices and research: What will the next century bring? *Journal of Perinatal and Neonatal Nursing, 25*(2), 165–179.

DEFINITION

Inability of the primary caretaker to create, maintain, or regain an environment that promotes the optimum growth and development of the child

DEFINING CHARACTERISTICS

Infant or child

- Behavioral disorders, failure to thrive, frequent accidents and illness
- History of trauma or abuse
- Lack of attachment, no separation anxiety, poor social competence

Parental

- Parents' inflexibility in meeting child's needs
- Evidence of negligent behavior toward or abandonment of child
- Expressed frustration over inability to control child
- Expressed inability to meet child's needs
- Poor or inappropriate caregiving skills
- Poor parent–child interaction
- Rejection or hostility toward child

RELATED FACTORS

- Altered perceptual abilities
- Attention-deficit/hyperactivity disorder
- Deficient knowledge about parenting skills
- Developmental delay
- Lack of education
- Maladaptive coping strategies
- Multiple births
- Premature birth
- Separation from parent
- Sleep disruption

ASSESSMENT FOCUS

(Refer to comprehensive assessment parameters.)

- Communication
- Coping
- Knowledge
- Risk management
- Roles/responsibilities
- Self-perception
- Values and beliefs

EXPECTED OUTCOMES

The parents will

- Make appropriate physical, verbal, and eye contact when interacting with infant or a child.
- Make statements indicating satisfaction with infant or child.
- Demonstrate correct feeding, bathing, and dressing techniques.
- Express willingness to maintain their relationship with each other.
- Bring infant for routine well-child care.

SUGGESTED NOC OUTCOMES

Coping Enhancement; Family Process Maintenance; Family Coping; Family Health Status; Family Functioning; Knowledge: Infant Care and Parenting; Parent–Infant Attachment; Parenting: Adolescent

INTERVENTIONS AND RATIONALES

<u>Determine:</u> Assess developmental state; interaction between parent and child; financial status; work demands; support systems, parents' knowledge of child. *Assessment of these factors will help identify appropriate interventions for this diagnosis.*

<u>Perform:</u> Act as a role model for parenting when caring for the child in the presence of the parents. *Lack of knowledge of routine child care practices, as well as growth and developmental norms, significantly contributes to child abuse.*

Involve parents in the care of the child immediately *to promote attachment to the child.*

<u>Inform:</u> Provide books and videos that will help the patient's quest for enhanced knowledge. *Supplying some materials directly may be a motivation for the parents to search further.*

Direct patient to use other sources such as libraries, Internet, or professional organizations. *An independent search results in the parents' developing confidence.* Select teaching strategies *that will enhance teaching/learning effectiveness,* such as discussion, demonstration, role-playing, and visual materials.

Teach those skills that the patient must incorporate into ability *to go much deeper into the area of interest.*

<u>Attend:</u> Encourage patient and family to verbalize feelings and concerns related to the knowledge and skills that parents need. *This promotes greater ease in managing challenging situations.*

Demonstrate willingness to repeat instruction and demonstrations of skills needed by parents. Be available to answer questions and correct misconceptions for parents *to enhance the effectiveness of learning.*

<u>Manage:</u> Refer to social and community resources *for ongoing assistance with parenting. The parents can contact these sources for additional information as needed.*

SUGGESTED NIC INTERVENTIONS

Attachment Promotion; Coping Enhancement; Family Process Maintenance; Family Support; Mutual Goal-Setting; Infant Care; Learning Enhancement; Role Enhancement; Family Integrity Promotion: Childbearing Family; Environmental Management: Attachment Process; Parent Education: Infant

REFERENCE

Darvill, R., et al. (2010, June). Psychological factors that impact on women's experiences of first-time motherhood: A qualitative study of the transition. *Midwifery, 26*(3), 357–366.

DEFINITION

Risk for inability of the primary caretaker to create, maintain, or regain an environment that promotes the optimum growth and development of the child

RISK FACTORS

- Social (e.g., change in family unit, low self-esteem, father of child not involved, financial difficulties, history of being abused, lack of poor parental role model or social support network)
- Infant (e.g., developmental delay, illness, multiple births, not gender desired, prolonged separation from parent, attention deficit hyperactivity disorder
- Knowledge (e.g., low educational level, poor communication skills, preference for physical punishment, unrealistic expectations of child)
- Physiological (e.g., physical illness)
- Psychological (e.g., closely spaced pregnancies, depression, difficult birthing process, history of mental illness, sleep disruption, young parental age

ASSESSMENT FOCUS

(Refer to comprehensive assessment parameters.)
- Coping
- Communication
- Roles/responsibility
- Behavioral
- Emotional
- Knowledge

EXPECTED OUTCOMES

The parent or caregiver will
- Establish eye, physical, and verbal contact with infant or child.
- Demonstrate correct feeding, bathing, and dressing techniques.
- State plans to bring the infant or child to clinic for routine physical and psychological examinations.
- Express understanding of developmental norms.
- Provide age-related play activities.

SUGGESTED NOC OUTCOMES

Caregiver Emotional Health; Caregiver Physical Health; Knowledge: Health Resources; Knowledge: Parenting; Parenting Performance; Role Performance; Social Support; Caregiver Performance: Direct and Indirect Care; Family Coping; Family Functioning

INTERVENTIONS AND RATIONALES

<u>Determine:</u> Assess caregiver's psychosocial status, including developmental state, educational level, presence or absence of spouse or significant other,

financial stressors, previous parenting. *Information of assessment factors helps identify appropriate interventions.*

Perform: Act as a role model for parenting when caring for the child in the presence of the parents. *Lack of knowledge of routine childcare practices, as well as growth and developmental norms, significantly contributes to child abuse.*

Involve parents in the care of the child immediately *to promote attachment to the child.*

Inform: Teach caregiver in the basics of infant and childcare. *Research shows that the primary source of information about care giving is the caregiver's own family. If a caregiver lacks an effective role model, you may need to supply basic information.*

Provide written materials on environmental aspects of home maintenance. *Written materials provide a resource for parents to refer to when problems arise.*

Teach additional skills that enhance coping strategies. Help caregiver and other family members develop a program using relaxation strategies such as meditation, guided imagery, yoga, exercise, and so forth. *These strategies reduce stresses associated with parenting.*

Teach problem-solving skills.

Attend: Encourage weekly discussions about progress in parenting *to develop family unity and allow members to address problems before they become overwhelming.*

Manage: Assist family members to contact community agencies to assist in efforts to improve parenting skills, such as self-help groups. *Community resources can lessen family's burden while parents learn to function independently.*

SUGGESTED NIC INTERVENTIONS

Counseling; Family Integrity Promotion; Family Support; Childbearing Family; Parenting Promotion; Active Listening; Coping Enhancement

REFERENCE

Appelbaum, M. G., & Smolowicz, J. L. (2012). Appreciating life: Being the father of a child with severe cerebral palsy. *Journal of Neuroscience Nursing, 44*(1), 36–44.

DEFINITION

At risk for inadvertent anatomical and physical changes as a result of posture on equipment used during an invasive/surgical procedure

RISK FACTORS

- Disorientation
- Edema
- Emaciation
- Immobilization
- Muscle weakness
- Obesity
- Sensory–perceptual disturbances from anesthesia

ASSESSMENT FOCUS

(Refer to comprehensive assessment parameters.)

- Activity/exercise
- Fluid/electrolytes
- Pharmacological function
- Physical regulation
- Risk management

EXPECTED OUTCOMES

The patient will

- Maintain effective breathing patterns.
- Maintain adequate cardiac output.
- Have surgical positioning that facilitates gas exchange.
- Not show evidence of neurologic, musculoskeletal, or vascular compromise.
- Maintain tissue integrity.

SUGGESTED NOC OUTCOMES

Blood Coagulation; Circulation Status; Neurological Status; Respiratory Status: Ventilation; Thermoregulation; Tissue Integrity: Skin & Mucous Membranes; Tissue Perfusion: Peripheral

INTERVENTIONS AND RATIONALES

<u>Determine:</u> Document and report the results of the preoperative nursing assessment. Identify factors predisposing patient to tissue injury. *This information guides interventions.*

<u>Perform:</u> Use the appropriate mode of patient transportation (stretcher, patient bed, wheelchair, or crib) *to ensure patient safety.*

Make sure an adequate number of staff members assist with transferring patient—obtain at least two for moving patient onto an operating room bed and at least four for moving anesthetized patient off operating room bed. *Adequate staffing enhances safety.*

Check the operating room bed before surgery for proper functioning. *Intraoperative bed malfunction can result in increased anesthesia time and a more difficult surgical approach.*

Ensure proper positioning (follow institutional policies):

- Check patient's neck and spine for proper alignment *to avoid trauma.*
- Check that patient's legs are straight and ankles uncrossed. *Crossed ankles cause pressure on tissue, vessels, and nerves.*
- Place a safety strap 29 (5 cm) above patient's knees, tight enough to restrain without compromising superficial venous return. *Applied too tightly, the safety strap may cause venous thrombosis or compression of tibial, peroneal, or sciatic nerves.*
- Secure patient's arms at his sides with a draw sheet, with palms down, making sure that no part of the arm or hand extends over the mattress. *Hyperextension can cause injury to the brachial plexus. Supination of palms minimizes pressure.*

Apply eye pads if patient's eyelids don't remain closed or if surgery is being performed on his head, neck, or chest. *If allowed to remain open, the eyes may dry out and become infected. Corneal abrasions may result from drapes and other foreign material rubbing against the eyes.*

If surgery is expected to last more than 2 hours or if patient is predisposed to a pressure injury, place padding under his occiput, scapulae, olecranon, sacrum, coccyx, and calcaneus *to protect potential pressure points.* Apply a padded footboard *to support patient's feet.* Avoid plantar flexion, and prevent stretching of the tibial nerve and subsequent foot drop.

Assess patient position following each positional change *to ensure proper body alignment and adequate padding and support.*

Inform: Tell patient about positioning measures planned *to reduce preoperative anxiety.*

Attend: Assure patient that careful positioning of the body will be carried *to reduce worry about possible injury.*

Manage: Consult with a physical or occupational therapist if special protective equipment is needed *to ensure safety for the patient.*

SUGGESTED NIC INTERVENTIONS

Circulatory Care: Mechanical Assist Device, Circulatory Care: Arterial Insufficiency; Circulatory Care: Venous Insufficiency; Circulatory Precautions; Infection Control: Intraoperative; Positioning: Intraoperative; Skin Surveillance; Surgical Precautions; Temperature Regulation: Intraoperative; Surgical Precautions

REFERENCE

Waters, T., et al. (2011, April). AORN ergonomic tool 2: Positioning and repositioning the supine patient on the OR bed. *AORN Journal, 93*(4), 445–449.

DEFINITION
At risk for disruption in circulation, sensation, or motion of an extremity

RISK FACTORS
- Burns
- Fractures
- Mechanical compression (such as tourniquet, cast, brace, dressing, and restraint)
- Immobilization
- Orthopedic surgery
- Trauma
- Vascular obstruction

ASSESSMENT FOCUS
(Refer to comprehensive assessment parameters.)
- Physical regulation
- Sensation/perception
- Cardiac function
- Comfort

EXPECTED OUTCOMES
The patient/family will
- Have no evidence of disability related to peripheral neurovascular dysfunction after injury or treatment.
- Maintain circulation in extremities.
- Feel and move each toe or finger after application of cast, brace, or splint.
- Demonstrate correct body positioning techniques.
- Express understanding of risk of altered neurovascular status and need to report symptoms of impaired circulation.
- Enroll in smoking-cessation program, as appropriate.
- Exhibit no symptoms of neurovascular compromise.

SUGGESTED NOC OUTCOMES
Circulation Status; Neurological Status: Peripheral; Risk Control: Tobacco Use; Risk Detection; Tissue Perfusion: Peripheral; Knowledge: Substance Abuse Control

INTERVENTIONS AND RATIONALES
<u>Determine:</u> Note if patient will undergo surgery or a procedure that increases his or her risk of peripheral neurovascular dysfunction *to anticipate complications.*

As appropriate, assess circulation before and after application of the cast, brace, or splint *to detect signs of impaired circulation.*

<u>Perform:</u> Immobilize the joints directly above and below the suspected fracture site, leaving room for pulse assessment *to facilitate monitoring of circulatory status.*

Remove the clothing around the suspected fracture site, clean the site, apply sterile dressings to open wounds, and carefully apply a cast, brace, or splint *to avoid further infection and trauma.*

Follow facility guidelines for the application of such devices as tourniquets, restraints, and tape *to ensure adequate circulation in affected extremity.*

If you suspect nerve compression, assess the position of the extremity that has a cast, brace, or splint. *Positioning of the extremity may affect circulation.*

Elevate the limb above heart level after surgery or trauma *to reduce the risk of edema.* If increased intracompartmental pressure is evident, maintain the affected limb at heart level *to reduce pressure.*

If edema appears in the affected extremity, split, bivalve, slit, or cut a window in the cast and padding according to facility protocol *to avoid neurovascular impairment.*

Inject prescribed neurotoxic agents (such as penicillin G, hydrocortisone, tetanus toxoid, and diazepam) away from the affected extremity and major nerves *to avoid injury.*

Avoid flexing the affected extremity. *Flexion may reduce venous circulation, increasing the risk of neurovascular complications.*

Administer and monitor the effectiveness of vasodilators, as ordered, *to control vasospasm.*

Inform: If patient requires a fasciotomy to restore circulation, provide educational material that explains this emergency procedure *to reduce patient anxiety.*

Instruct patient and family members in proper positioning when lying in bed and when sitting and in methods of obtaining pressure relief *to avoid pooling of blood and pressure ulcers.*

If appropriate, discuss the cause of the injury and safety precautions *to avoid further injury.*

Instruct patient and family members in recognizing and reporting symptoms of peripheral neurovascular dysfunction, including numbness, pain, and tingling *to prevent onset of neurovascular damage after discharge.*

Attend: If patient smokes, encourage him or her to enroll in a smoking-cessation program. *Quitting smoking may enhance oxygenation, decreasing the risk of peripheral neurovascular dysfunction.*

Take measures to ease anxiety *which could lead to vasoconstriction.*

Manage: Refer patient to appropriate community resources related to safety precautions *to achieve optimal safety level.*

SUGGESTED NIC INTERVENTIONS

Circulatory Precautions; Exercise Promotion: Strength Training; Exercise Therapy: Joint Mobility; Peripheral Sensation Management; Positioning: Neurologic; Pressure Ulcer Prevention; Skin Surveillance; Splinting; Smoking Cessation Assistance

REFERENCE

Johnston-Walker, E., & Hardcastle, J. (2011, July–August). Neurovascular assessment in the critically ill patient. *Nursing in Critical Care, 16*(4), 170–177.

DEFINITION

Inability to maintain an integrated and complete perception of self

DEFINING CHARACTERISTICS

- Disturbed body image
- Fluctuating feelings about self
- Gender confusion
- Unable to distinguish between inner and outer stimuli
- Delusional description of self
- Feelings of emptiness
- Feelings of strangeness
- Contradictory personal traits
- Ineffective role performance
- Ineffective coping
- Uncertainty about ideological and cultural values
- Uncertainty about goals
- Disturbed relationships

RELATED FACTORS

- Organic brain syndrome
- Dissociative identity disorder
- Psychiatric disorders
- Low self-esteem
- Manic states
- Social role change
- Stage of growth
- States of development
- Situational crisis
- Dysfunctional family processes
- Cultural discontinuity
- Cult indoctrination
- Discrimination or prejudice
- Use of psychoactive drugs
- Ingestion of toxic chemicals
- Inhalation of toxic chemicals

ASSESSMENT FOCUS

(Refer to comprehensive assessment parameters.)

- Safety
- Mental status
- Self-care
- Sexual practices
- Cultural beliefs
- Relationships

EXPECTED OUTCOMES

The patient will

- Contract for safety.
- Identify internal versus external stimuli.
- Maintain adequate nutritional intake.
- Identify personal goals and realistic steps toward those goals.
- Compile a list of resources to call when needed.
- Remain free from substance abuse.
- Secure a safe place to live in.

SUGGESTED NOC OUTCOMES

Coping; Distorted Thought Self-Control; Impulse Self-Control; Self-Esteem; Risk Control

INTERVENTIONS AND RATIONALES

<u>Determine:</u> Assess for suicidal/homicidal ideation, self-induced cuts or burns. Assess for self-induced vomiting or restricting of food. Thorough mental status examination. *Individuals struggling with identified issues are at an increased safety risk.*

Monitor mental status daily to be able to intervene if necessary.

Monitor weight weekly *to be able to detect changes that may require further intervention.*

<u>Perform:</u> Contract with patient for safety. Schedule meetings with patient to process feelings and experiences. *Demonstrating care and compassion for the patient allows him or her to feel safe and promotes healing.*

<u>Inform:</u> Instruct patient to journal feelings and list coping strategies. *Journaling can help a patient maintain self-control and may increase insight.*

<u>Attend:</u> Accept patient in his or her struggle. Reinforce taking healthy risks and appropriate expression of feelings. *Appropriate expression of feelings enhances self-esteem and promotes resiliency.*

<u>Manage:</u> Refer patients to mental health services for medication and symptom management. *Disturbed personal identity may require ongoing mental health care.*

SUGGESTED NIC INTERVENTIONS

Coping Enhancement; Environmental Management: Safety; Role Enhancement; Self-Esteem Enhancement; Journaling

REFERENCE

Jørgensen, C. R., et al. (2012, July). Identity-related autobiographical memories and cultural life scripts in patients with Borderline Personality Disorder. *Conscious Cognition, 21*(2), 788–798.

DEFINITION

Accentuated risk of accidental exposure to or ingestion of drugs or dangerous products in doses sufficient to cause poisoning

RISK FACTORS

Internal

- Cognitive or emotional difficulties
- Insufficient resources
- Lack of drug education
- Lack of safety precautions
- Occupational setting without adequate safeguards
- Reduced vision

External

- Dangerous products or drugs stored within reach of children or confused people or in unlocked cabinets
- Storing of large amounts of drugs in home
- Availability of illegal drugs contaminated with poisonous additives

ASSESSMENT FOCUS

(Refer to comprehensive assessment parameters.)

- Coping
- Neurocognition
- Risk management
- Tissue integrity

EXPECTED OUTCOMES

The patient/family will

- Not ingest or be exposed to dangerous products.
- Communicate understanding of need for self-protection.
- Explain method for safekeeping of dangerous products.

SUGGESTED NOC OUTCOMES

Risk Control: Drug Use; Risk Detection; Safe Home Environment; Knowledge: Substance Use Control

INTERVENTIONS AND RATIONALES

<u>Determine:</u> Observe, record, and report falls, seizures, and unsafe practices *to ensure implementation of appropriate interventions. Overdose of certain medications can cause such neurologic problems as seizures.*

Monitor and record patient's respiratory status *because certain poisons can cause respiratory depression.*

Monitor and record neurologic status *because excessive toxic exposure can cause coma. Patient may have pinpointed or dilated pupils, depending on the type of drug ingested and the length of time patient has been hypoxic.*

Monitor vital signs, intake and output, and level of consciousness. Record and report changes. *Severe hypotension may develop following overdose. It may be related to central nervous system defect, direct myocardial depression, or vasodilation. Marked hyperthermia can occur with salicylate overdose, which affects metabolic rate. Dehydration may develop in some patients from an increased respiratory rate, sweating, vomiting, and urine losses.*

Perform: Remove dangerous or potentially dangerous products from the environment *to avoid injury.*

Check the settings on oxygen flow meters every hour on patients known to retain carbon dioxide (e.g., some patients with chronic obstructive pulmonary disease). *This avoids carbon dioxide narcosis from excessive oxygen therapy in poorly ventilated patients; if unchecked, patient may stop breathing.*

Inform: Provide patient and family members with information about such specific products as medications, oxygen, and total parenteral nutrition. Tailor instructions to a specific product and patient's ability to learn self-care. *This enables patient and family members to identify and alter environmental or lifestyle factors to achieve optimum health level.*

Attend: Encourage patient to report safety hazards and to incorporate safe behaviors in the home and work environment *to decrease the chance of poisoning.*

Manage: Refer patient to appropriate community resources (police, fire, and home health agency) for more information *to enhance safety measures.*

SUGGESTED NIC INTERVENTIONS

Home Maintenance Assistance; Medication Management; Risk Identification; Surveillance: Safety; Environmental Management: Safety; Environmental Risk Protection; Health Education

REFERENCES

Oerther, S. E. (2011, January). Plant poisonings: Common plants that contain cardiac glycosides. *Journal of Emergency Nursing, 37*(1), 102–103.

Ruth-Sahd, L. A., Zulkosky, K., & Fettr, M. E. (2011, November–December). Carbon monoxide poisoning: Case study and review. *Dimensions of Critical Care Nursing, 30*(6), 303–314.

Wieland, D. M., Halter, M. J., & Levine, C. (2012, February). Bath salts: They are not what you think. *Journal of Pyschosocial Nursing and Mental Health Services, 50*(2), 17–21.

DEFINITION

Sustained maladaptive response to a traumatic, overwhelming event

DEFINING CHARACTERISTICS

- Aggression, anxiety, anger, rage
- Avoidance, alienation, altered moods
- Compulsive behavior
- Denial, grief, fear, depression
- Detachment
- Exaggerated startle response, flashbacks
- Guilt
- Headaches
- Hypervigilance
- Intrusive dreams, nightmares, or thoughts; difficulty concentrating
- Irritability
- Numbness
- Panic attacks
- Psychogenic amnesia
- Repression
- Shame
- Substance abuse

RELATED FACTORS

- Abuse (physical or psychological)
- Disasters
- Epidemics
- Serious accident, injury, or threat to self or loved one
- Sudden destruction of home and/or community
- Torture; held prisoner of war
- Wars
- Witnessing mutilation or violent death

ASSESSMENT FOCUS

(Refer to comprehensive assessment parameters.)

- Behavior
- Coping
- Emotional
- Neurocognition
- Risk management
- Self-perception

EXPECTED OUTCOMES

The patient will

- Recover or be rehabilitated from physical injuries to the extent possible.
- State feelings and fears related to traumatic event.
- Express feelings of safety.
- Use available support systems.
- Use effective coping mechanisms to reduce fear.
- Maintain or reestablish adaptive social interactions with family members.

SUGGESTED NOC OUTCOMES

Anxiety Self-Control; Body Image; Coping; Depression Level; Fear Self-Control; Hope; Impulse Self-Control; Quality of Life; Self-Esteem; Stress Level; Abuse Protection; Abuse Recovery: Physical, Emotional, and Financial

INTERVENTIONS AND RATIONALES

<u>Determine:</u> Assess factors in patient's culture that may affect his or her response to trauma; remain supportive and nonjudgmental *to show patient that you support and accept his or her response to trauma.*

<u>Perform:</u> Follow medical regimen to manage physical injuries. *Attention to physical needs remains primary, according to Maslow's hierarchy.*

<u>Inform:</u> Instruct patient in at least one fear-reducing behavior such as seeking support from others when frightened. *As patient learns to reduce fears, coping skills will increase.*

<u>Attend:</u> Provide emotional support:

- Visit patient frequently to reduce his or her fear of being alone.
- Be available to listen *to respond empathetically to patient's feelings.*
- Accept and encourage the statement of patient's feelings *to reassure patient that feelings are appropriate and valid.*
- Assure patient of his or her safety, and take the measures needed to ensure it. *Frequent nightmares or flashbacks may cause patient to question the safety of his or her environment.*
- Avoid care-related activities or environmental stimuli that may intensify symptoms associated with trauma (loud noises, bright lights, abrupt entrances to patient's room, or painful procedures or treatment). *Environmental stimuli can easily intensify flashbacks to a traumatic event.*

Reorient patient to surroundings and reality as frequently as necessary. *Posttrauma psychic numbing impairs orientation, memory, and reality perception.*

Support patient's family members by providing time for them to express feelings and helping them understand patient's reactions. *This reduces their anxiety and gives them a chance to help patient.*

<u>Manage:</u> Offer referrals to other support persons or groups, including clergy, mental health professionals, and trauma support groups. *Referrals help patient regain a sense of universality, reduce isolation, share fears, and deal constructively with feelings.*

SUGGESTED NIC INTERVENTIONS

Active Listening; Anxiety Reduction; Coping Enhancement; Counseling; Forgiveness Facilitation; Mood Management; Security Enhancement; Socialization Enhancement; Support Group; Referral; Culture Brokerage; Support System Enhancement

REFERENCE

Seng, J. S. (2011, November–December). Integrating care for posttraumatic stress and physical comorbidities: The road is clear. *Journal of the American Psychiatric Nurses Association, 17*(6), 376–377.

DEFINITION

At risk for sustained maladaptive response to traumatic, overwhelming event

RISK FACTORS

- Diminished ego strength
- Displacement from home
- Duration of the event
- Exaggerated sense of responsibility
- Inadequate social support
- Unsupportive environment
- Occupation
- Perception of the event
- Survivor's role in the event

ASSESSMENT FOCUS

(Refer to comprehensive assessment parameters.)

- Behavior
- Communication
- Coping
- Emotional status
- Self-perception

EXPECTED OUTCOMES

The patient will

- Be free from chronic posttrauma response, substance abuse, or other mental health disorders.
- Express understanding of posttrauma response.
- Express feelings of safety.
- Employ effective coping skills and reach out to appropriate sources of support to reduce fear.

SUGGESTED NOC OUTCOMES

Coping; Depression Level; Depression Self-Control; Risk Detection; Social Support; Spiritual Health; Stress Level; Abuse Protection

INTERVENTIONS AND RATIONALES

<u>Determine:</u> Assess nature of the trauma; losses that occurred from the traumatic event; effect of the trauma on social interactions; patient's perception of what has occurred; coping responses; mental status; use of chemicals, for example, alcohol, drugs; available support systems. *Information from assessments factors will help identify appropriate interventions.*

<u>Perform:</u> Structure time to build a trusting relationship with the patient. *The patient will likely talk about fears and be open to ideas about ways to reduce stress only from someone who is trusted.*

<u>Inform:</u> Teach self-healing techniques to both the patient and the family, such as meditation, guided imagery, yoga, and prayer, *to prevent anxiety and aid in keeping patient in a frame of mind to make positive decisions.*

Teach patient how to incorporate the use of self-healing techniques in carrying out usual daily activities *in an effort to prevent the development of posttraumatic stress disorder.*

Demonstrate procedures and encourage participation in patient's care. *Have patient participate to whatever level possible without increasing stress level.*

Provide patient with concise information about decision-making skills. *This will produce benefits that can reinforce health-seeking behaviors.*

<u>Attend:</u> Listen attentively to patient's statements about the power in caring for himself. Provide encouragement to boost self-confidence of the patient *to encourage a trusting relationship and open discussion.*

Facilitate opportunities for spiritual nourishment and growth *to address patient's holistic needs for maximal therapeutic environment.*

Reinforce the family's efforts to care for the patient. *Let them know they are doing well to ease adaptation to new caregiver roles.*

Encourage family to support patient's independence. *Family members may be inclined to make decisions and do things to protect the patient.*

Encourage patient's cooperation as you continue with healing techniques, such as therapeutic touch. *Some patients may resist being touched.*

Caution patient before you touch him or her. Avoid approaching patient from behind *to avoid actions that may be misinterpreted and trigger flash back of the traumatic event.*

Assist patient to be aware of persons, places, and things that act as triggers or reduces the traumatic response *to encourage active participation in treatment.*

Provide emotional support to the family to be available to answer questions. *Members of the family may have difficulty coping with the risks the patient faces.*

<u>Manage:</u> Schedule time to meet with family and patient *to listen to ways in which they plan to enhance their coping skills in the present situation.* Refer family to community resources and support groups available *to assist in managing patient's illness and providing emotional and financial assistance to caregivers.*

Refer to a member of the clergy or a spiritual counselor, according to the patient's preference, *to show respect for the patient's beliefs and provide spiritual care.*

SUGGESTED NIC INTERVENTIONS

Active Listening; Coping Enhancement; Hope Instillation; Mood Management; Self-Awareness Enhancement Support System Enhancement

REFERENCE

Melvin, K. C., Gross, D., Hayat, M. J., Jennings, B. M., & Campbell, J. C. (2012, April). Couple functioning and post-traumatic stress symptoms in US Army couples: The role of resilience. *Research in Nursing and Health, 35*(2), 164–177.

DEFINITION

A pattern of participating knowingly in change that is sufficient for well-being and can be strengthened

DEFINING CHARACTERISTICS

Expresses readiness to enhance:
- Awareness of possible changes to be made
- Freedom to perform changes to be made
- Identification of choices that can be made for change
- Involvement in creating change
- Knowledge for participation in change
- Participation in choices for daily living and health
- Power

ASSESSMENT FOCUS

(Refer to comprehensive assessment parameters.)
- Behavior
- Coping
- Knowledge
- Roles/responsibilities
- Values/beliefs

EXPECTED OUTCOMES

The patient will
- Express perceived control in influencing health outcomes.
- Participate in choices that enhance his or her care and well-being.
- Develop a plan for adjusting to significant life changes.

SUGGESTED NOC OUTCOMES

Family Resiliency; Health Beliefs; Perceived Control; Personal Autonomy; Psychosocial Adjustment: Life Change; Knowledge: Health Promotion; Health Promoting Behavior

INTERVENTIONS AND RATIONALES

<u>Determine:</u> Assess patient's perception of present state of power; perception of ability to enhance power; support systems; patient's ability to identify choices; readiness for change to occur; reliance on the health care system to resolve problems; level of knowledge for positive decision making. *Assessment information will help identify appropriate interventions.*

<u>Perform:</u> Work with the patient to list those areas of health-related issues in which he or she needs to take greater responsibility and control. *The patient may feel the need to be in greater control without being able to articulate the specifics himself.*

List questions in writing that a patient may want to ask his or her primary caregiver and suggest strategies at further clarifying information that seems unclear. *The patient's anxiety may cause him to forget important point he needs clarified unless he is prepared for the visit.*

Inform: Keep patient informed about what to expect and when to expect it. *Accurate information reduces anxiety.*

Teach self-healing techniques to both the patient and the family such as meditation, guided imagery, yoga, and prayer. Teach patient how to incorporate the use of self-healing techniques in carrying out usual daily activities. *Repeatedly performing these techniques throughout the day will help further reduce anxiety.*

Attend: Encourage patient to talk about personal assets and accomplishments and improvements in his or her condition, no matter how small they may seem. Give positive feedback. *Conversation assists you to evaluate the patient's self-concept and adaptive abilities.*

Direct the patient's focus beyond the present state.

Manage: Help patient involve the family, community, clergy, and friends with changes to the care plan *to increase the potential of the patient's control over self-care outcomes.*

Refer patient and family to other professional caregivers, for example, dietitian, social worker, clergy, and mental health professional. *Support groups such as Ostomy clubs, I Can Cope, and Reach for Recovery can be helpful to the patient and the family.*

Assist patient to utilize appropriate resources by contacting family and scheduling follow-up appointments. *This helps give the patient a sense of direction and control over his or her future care.*

SUGGESTED NIC INTERVENTIONS

Assertiveness Training; Coping Enhancement; Self-Modification Assistance; Self-Responsibility Facilitation; Support Group; Guided Imagery; Meditation; Religious Ritual Enhancement

REFERENCE

Gutierrez, K. M. (2012, September). Experiences and needs of families regarding prognostic communication in an intensive care unit: Supporting families at the end of life. *Critical Care Quarterly, 35*(3), 299–313.

DEFINITION

Perception that one's own action will not significantly affect an outcome; a perceived lack of control over a current situation or immediate happening

DEFINING CHARACTERISTICS

- Depression over physical deterioration
- Expressed dissatisfaction over inability to perform previous tasks
- Expressed lack of control over self-care, current situation, and outcome
- Expressed feelings of shame or doubt regarding role performance
- Nonparticipation in care
- Dependence on others

RELATED FACTORS

- Health care environment
- Illness-related regimen
- Interpersonal interaction

ASSESSMENT FOCUS

(Refer to comprehensive assessment parameters.)
- Communication
- Coping
- Knowledge
- Roles/responsibilities
- Values and beliefs

EXPECTED OUTCOMES

The patient will
- Acknowledge fears, feelings, and concerns about current situation.
- Make decisions regarding course of treatment.
- Decrease level of anxiety by changing response to stressors.
- Participate in self-care activities.
- Express feeling of regained control.
- Accept and adapt to lifestyle changes.

SUGGESTED NOC OUTCOMES

Depression Self-Control; Family Participation in Professional Care; Health Beliefs; Health Beliefs: Perceived Ability to Perform; Participation in Healthcare Decisions

INTERVENTIONS AND RATIONALES

Determine: Assess mobility; behavioral responses; coping strategies; past experiences with illness; knowledge; environment, including equipment and supplies, health care professionals and personnel, lighting, noise, privacy, number and types of stressors; social factors; spiritual beliefs. *Information gained from assessment will help identify appropriate interventions.*

<u>Perform:</u> Work with the patient to identify specific issues in which the patient feels powerless. *Understanding several areas will help the patient focus on setting goals.*

Help the patient develop focused goals. *Having goals will give the patient confidence that his and her efforts will produce results.*

<u>Inform:</u> Teach coping strategies to patient and family members. Have patient practice role-playing *to increase the confidence in his or her ability to handle difficult situation in the health care system.* Teach self-healing techniques to both the patient and the family such as meditation, guided imagery, yoga, and prayer. Teach patient how to incorporate the use of self-healing techniques in carrying out usual daily activities. *The more routine the use of these techniques becomes, the greater will be the effectiveness.*

<u>Attend:</u> Help patient identify his values, beliefs, hopes, dreams, skills, and interest. *The patient's deficits may lie in a lack of self-exploration, problem-solving methods used, or separation issues with parents.*

Promote choices with the most likeliness of success. *Specific instructions can help the patient gain problem-solving ability and maturity.*

Listen to patient's personal values and beliefs, but remain nonjudgmental, even if his or her values and beliefs differ from your own. *Remaining nonjudgmental, but attentive, shows your support. Explore personal identity issues distressing to the patient to isolate issues into small, more solvable units.*

Accept patient's feelings of powerlessness as normal. *This indicates respect for the patient and enhances feelings of self-respect.*

Encourage patient to take an active role as a health team member and in self-care. *Active participation will promote self reliance.*

<u>Manage:</u> Organize family conferences to explore potential reactions to the patient's choices, and promote support for the patient's independent decision making. *Meetings can help the patient and family members ventilate true feelings in a safe environment.*

SUGGESTED NIC INTERVENTIONS

Cognitive Restructuring; Decision-Making Support; Emotional Support; Health Education; Mood Management; Presence; Self-Assistance; Self-Responsibility Facilitation; Values Clarification; Coping Enhancement

REFERENCE

Lavoie, M., et al. (2011, January/February). The autonomy experience of patients in palliative care. *Journal of Hospice and Palliative Care, 13*(1), 47–53.

DEFINITION

At risk for perceived lack of control over a situation and/or one's ability to significantly affect an outcome

RISK FACTORS

- Anxiety
- Caregiving
- Chronic low self-esteem
- Deficient knowledge
- Economically disadvantaged
- Illness
- Ineffective coping patterns
- Lack of social support
- Pain
- Social marginalization
- Stigmatized condition or disease
- Unpredicatable course of illness
- Progressive debilitating disease process
- Situational low self-esteem

ASSESSMENT FOCUS

(Refer to comprehensive assessment parameters.)

- Health care system
- Self-perception
- Knowledge
- Coping

EXPECTED OUTCOMES

The patient will

- Make decisions regarding course of action.
- Decrease level of anxiety by changing response to stressors.
- Participate in self-care activities.
- Describe modifications or adjustments to the environment that allows feelings of control.
- Discuss factors in the illness-related regimen over which control can be maintained.
- Demonstrate ability to plan for controllable factors.
- Express feeling of maintaining control.
- Accept and adapt to lifestyle.

SUGGESTED NOC OUTCOMES

Anxiety Level; Body Image; Coping; Endurance; Information Processing; Personal Autonomy; Risk Control; Social Support

INTERVENTIONS AND RATIONALES

Determine: Assess for high-risk behaviors; health-promoting activities; coping skills; activities of daily living, including rest and sleep; sensory perception; decision-making skills; sexuality patterns. *Assessment information helps identify appropriate interventions.*

<u>Perform:</u> Modify environment when possible *to meet patient's self-care needs to promote sense of control over the environment.*

Orient patient to space by walking with patient around space and assisting him to place personal belongings.

<u>Inform:</u> Teach patient about risk factors and other aspects of the patient's medical condition *to help patient feel in control of his or her care.*

<u>Attend:</u> Be present when patient is facing situations in which the patient feels powerlessness *to help patient cope.*

Encourage patient to express concerns. Set aside time for discussions with the patient about daily events. *This helps the patient feel vaguely understood emotions into focus.* Discuss situations that provoke feelings of anxiety, anger, and powerlessness *to identify areas of patient concern and to prevent anger from being inappropriately directed at self.*

Encourage participation in self-care. Provide patient with as many decisions as possible with regard to self-care (such as positioning, choosing an injection site, and receiving visitors) *to communicate respect for patient and enhance feelings of independence.*

Provide positive environment for patient's activities. Encourage patient to take an active role as a member of his or her health care team. *This enhances patient's sense of control and reduces passive and dependent behavior.*

Encourage family members to support patient without taking control *to increase patient's feelings of self-worth.*

<u>Manage:</u> Arrange to accommodate patient's spiritual needs. *Spiritual assistance may help patient gain courage and resist despair.*

Refer to mental health professional *for additional assistance with coping.* Refer patient to community resources *that may offer assistance to the patient when needed.*

Offer written information that can be referred to when needed.

SUGGESTED NIC INTERVENTIONS
Decision-Making Support; Risk Control; Presence; Self-Assistance

REFERENCE

Nurses called upon as advocates for patient empowerment through technology. (2012, February). *Computers Informatics Nursing,* 30(2), 69–70.

DEFINITION

Decrease in the ability to guard self from internal or external threats such as illness or injury

DEFINING CHARACTERISTICS

- Altered clotting, anorexia, chilling, cough
- Deficient immunity, disorientation
- Dyspnea, fatigue, immobility, impaired healing, perspiring
- Insomnia
- Itching
- Maladaptive stress response
- Restlessness
- Weakness
- Pressure ulcers

RELATED FACTORS

- Abnormal blood files (leukopenia, thrombocytopenia, anemia, coagulation)
- Substance abuse
- Cancer
- Drug therapies (e.g., antineoplastic, corticosteroid, immune, anticoagulant, thrombolytic)
- Extremes of age
- Immune disorders
- Inadequate nutrition
- Treatment-related side effects (e.g., surgery, radiation)

ASSESSMENT FOCUS

(Refer to comprehensive assessment parameters.)

- Cardiac function
- Fluids and electrolytes
- Pharmacological function
- Physical regulation
- Respiratory function
- Risk management

EXPECTED OUTCOMES

The patient will

- Not experience chills, fever, or other signs and symptoms.
- Demonstrate use of protective measures, including conservation of energy, maintenance of balanced diet, and attainment of adequate rest.
- Demonstrate effective coping skills.
- Demonstrate personal cleanliness and maintain clean environment.
- Maintain safe environment.
- Demonstrate increased strength and resistance.
- Exhibit improved immune system as evidenced by normal WBC, CBC and differential, normal sedimentation rate, and immunoelectrophoresis.
- Express desire for additional health information.

SUGGESTED NOC OUTCOMES

Abuse Protection; Immune Status; Immunization Behavior; Knowledge: Infection Control; Energy Conservation; Sleep

INTERVENTIONS AND RATIONALES

Determine: Assess vital signs; high-risk behaviors, knowledge of present condition; coping skills, comfort level; activities of daily living; cardiac, respiratory status, neurologic status; protective mechanisms; CBC and differential, sedimentation rate, immunoelectrolytes, immunoelectro-phoresis, blood cultures, wound exudate, sputum, urine. *Assessment information helps identify appropriate interventions.*

Perform: Take vital signs every 4 hours. *This allows for early detection of complications.*

Administer medications as ordered for symptoms. *Discomfort interferes with rest, interferes with nutritional intake, and places added stress on the patient.*

Inform: Teach protective measures, including the need to conserve energy, obtain adequate rest, and eat a balanced diet. *Adequate sleep and nutrition enhance immune function. Energy conservation can help decrease the weakness caused by anemia.*

Teach coping strategies, including stress management and relaxation techniques. *Relaxation and decreased stress can increase function, thereby improving strength and resistance.*

Teach patient to guard against falls, cuts, abrasions, and other types of accidents to prevent infections. Provide written instruction for the patient so he or she has it to review when needed.

Attend: Promote personal and environmental cleanliness *to decrease threat from microorganisms.*

Manage: Order nutritious foods with supplements for the patient. Encourage him to eat *to prevent further complications.* Offer to have dietitian visit patient to assist with this.

If patient has new insights on his own condition or treatment, encourage him to share this information with his oncologist *to foster a sense of responsibility for obtaining health care.* Suggest that patient present practitioner with a summary of his or her findings in advance of his or her appointment *to allow the practitioner time to review the information.*

SUGGESTED NIC INTERVENTIONS

Coping Enhancement: Environmental; Management: Safety; Infection Control; Knowledge: Personal Safety Health

REFERENCE

Kasberg, H., et al. (2011, October/December). Aggressive disease, aggressive treatment: The adult hematopoietic stem cell transplant patient in the intensive care unit. *AACN Advanced Critical Care, 22*(4), 349–364.

DEFINITION

Sustained maladaptive response to a forced, violent sexual penetration against the victim's will and consent

DEFINING CHARACTERISTICS

- Anger, anxiety, and depression
- Agitation
- Changes in relationships
- Confusion
- Denial
- Dependence
- Disorganization
- Dissociative disorders
- Embarrassment or shame
- Fear or paranoia
- Guilt and self-blame
- Helplessness
- Humiliation
- Hyperalertness
- Impaired decision making
- Loss of self-esteem
- Mood swings
- Muscle spasms
- Muscle tension
- Nightmares, sleep disturbances, and phobias
- Physical trauma
- Powerlessness
- Revenge
- Sexual dysfunction
- Shame
- Shock
- Sleep disturbances
- Substance abuse
- Suicide attempts
- Vulnerability

RELATED FACTORS

- Rape

ASSESSMENT FOCUS

(Refer to comprehensive assessment parameters.)

- Coping
- Emotional
- Values/beliefs

EXPECTED OUTCOMES

The patient will

- Recover from physical injuries to the fullest possible extent.
- Express feelings and fears.
- Make contact with appropriate sources of support.

SUGGESTED NOC OUTCOMES

Abuse Protection; Abuse Recovery: Emotional; Coping; Abuse Recovery: Sexual

INTERVENTIONS AND RATIONALES

<u>Determine:</u> Assess history of traumatic event; physical injuries sustained at the time of the trauma; emotional reactions to the event; support systems available to the patient; coping; problem-solving strategies. *Assessment information will help establish realistic goals and identify appropriate interventions.*

<u>Perform:</u> Explain assessment procedures to the patient *to reduce the level of fear associated with data gathering following a rape.*

<u>Inform:</u> Teach patient relaxation techniques such as guided imagery, deep breathing, meditation, aromatherapy, and progressive muscle relaxation. Practice with the patient at bedtime. *Purposeful relaxation efforts usually help promote sleep.*

Educate patient about various emotional responses to trauma. *Rape-trauma syndrome is a variant of posttraumatic distress disorder. Responses such as suicidal ideation, disorientation, confusion, extreme detachment, nightmares, guilt, depression, and flashbacks are common. The patient may believe that the emotional turmoil she experiences after rape is abnormal. Pointing out that others have gone through the same experience may lessen the patient's isolation, help her talk about the symptoms, and motivate her to seek follow-up care.*

Teach a variety of techniques that will help the woman cope. *Patient may believe that the emotional turmoil one experiences after rape is abnormal.*

<u>Attend:</u> Provide emotional support. Be available to listen, and accept the patient's feelings *to let her know her feelings are valid and acceptable.*

Approach patient in a warm, caring manner *to cultivate her trust and cooperation.* Assure patient of her safety, and take all necessary measures to ensure it.

<u>Manage:</u> Offer referral to other support groups or professionals, such as clergy, a crisis center, mental health professionals, rape counselors, and Women Organized Against Rape. *This will help the patient express her feelings and develop coping skills.*

SUGGESTED NIC INTERVENTIONS

Abuse Protection Support; Active Listening; Anxiety Reduction; Crisis Intervention; Rape-Trauma Treatment; Self-Esteem Enhancement; Referral

REFERENCE

Hinton, S. T., et al. (2010, December). Domestic violence and the role of the parish nurse. *Journal of Christian Nursing, 27*(4), 302–305.

DEFINITION

A pattern of mutual partnership that is sufficient to provide each other's needs and can be strengthened

DEFINING CHARACTERISTICS

- Expresses desire to enhance communication between partners
- Expresses satisfaction with sharing of information and ideas between partners
- Expresses satisfaction with fulfilling physical and emotional needs by one's partner
- Demonstrates mutual respect between partners
- Meets developmental goals appropriate for family life-cycle stage
- Demonstrates well-balanced autonomy and collaboration between partners
- Demonstrates mutual support in daily activities between partners
- Identifies each other as a key person
- Demonstrates understanding of partner's insufficient (physical, social, and psychological) function
- Expresses satisfaction with complementary relation between partners

ASSESSMENT FOCUS

(Refer to comprehensive assessment parameters.)
- Sexuality
- Emotional
- Roles/relationships

EXPECTED OUTCOMES

The patient will
- Communicate effectively with partner and family members.
- Articulate ways to mutually meet physical and emotional needs of partner and self.
- Participate in appropriate counseling (premarital, preconceptual, sexual) as needed.
- Verbalize that relationships are characterized by well-balanced autonomy and self-efficacy.

SUGGESTED NOC OUTCOMES

Family Functioning; Role Performance; Sexual Functioning; Social Interaction Skills

INTERVENTIONS AND RATIONALES

<u>Determine:</u> Assess communication techniques and effectiveness of couple and family *to be able to counsel and/or refer appropriately as needed.*
<u>Perform:</u> Suggest that patient and partner/family members attend counseling sessions as appropriate for their life-cycle stage. *Patients may*

need permission from a health care professional to feel comfortable seeking relationship assistance.

<u>Inform:</u> Teach patient and family members normal family life-cycle stages *so that they can better understand what is normal and are able to anticipate challenges.*

<u>Attend:</u> Encourage patient and family members to share information and ideas *in order to enhance their communication.*

<u>Manage:</u> Refer as needed to colleagues in other disciplines such as social workers or counselors *to facilitate enhanced communication.*

SUGGESTED NIC INTERVENTIONS

Family Integrity Promotion; Family Support; Preconception Counseling; Sexual Counseling; Socialization Enhancement; Support System Enhancement

REFERENCE

Kovar, C. L., et al. (2012, April). Does a satisfactory relationship with her mother influence when a 16-year-old begins to have sex? *MCN. The American Journal of Maternal/Child Nursing,* 37(2), 122–129.

DEFINITION

Risk for a pattern of mutual partnership that is insufficient to provide for each other's needs.

RISK FACTORS

- Cognitive changes in one partner
- Developmental crises
- History of domestic violence
- Incarceration of one partner
- Poor communication skills
- Stressful life events
- Substance abuse
- Unrealistic expectations

ASSESSMENT FOCUS

(Refer to comprehensive assessment parameters.)
- Behavior
- Coping
- Emotional
- Knowledge
- Roles/relationships
- Sexuality

EXPECTED OUTCOMES

The patient will:
- Actively participate in activities that help build cohesion with partner/family.
- Express understanding of his/her role as an individual, a partner, and/or member of the family.
- Identify healthy coping mechanisms that will support the patient as an individual, a partner, and/or family member.
- Verbalize desire to work with partner/family in developing healthy communication skills.

SUGGESTED NOC OUTCOMES

Family Functioning; Family Integrity; Role Performance; Psychosocial Adjustment; Life Change; Social Interaction Skills; Social Support

INTERVENTIONS AND RATIONALES

<u>Determine:</u> Assess patient and partner/family *since the partner/family can provide additional information/perspectives that the patient may not be aware of.*

Assess support system and availability. *Partner may travel frequently and immediate family may not live in proximity to the patient, which can cause emotional strain.*

<u>Perform:</u> Assist the patient and partner/family to identify positive activities that they can participate in together *to help build cohesion.*

Assist patient with cognitive therapies and stress reduction techniques. *Positive coping skills can help foster self-confidence and a positive attitude and positive behaviors towards personal relationships.*

<u>Inform:</u> Educate patient and partner/family regarding the need for family treatment *as the partner/family is also affected by the status of the relationship, and only together can they begin to repair the relationship.*

<u>Attend:</u> Provide a safe environment and assist patient and partner/family in communicating openly *in order to help facilitate a positive interaction.*

<u>Manage:</u> Work with patient and partner/family to ensure that the treatment plan is sensitive to their cultural practices and developmental needs *in order to help build unity and confidence in their ability to follow through with the treatment plan.*

SUGGESTED NIC INTERVENTIONS

Anxiety Reduction; Abuse Protection Support; Complex Relationship Building; Family Support; Role Enhancement; Sexual Counseling; Substance Use Treatment; Support Group

REFERENCE

Mazanec, P., Daly, B. J., Ferrell, B. R., & Prince-Paul, M. (2011). Lack of communication and control: Experiences of distance caregivers of parents with advanced cancer. *Oncology Nursing Forum, 38*(3), 307–313.

DEFINITION
Impaired ability to exercise reliance in beliefs and/or participate in rituals of a particular faith tradition

DEFINING CHARACTERISTICS
- Difficulty adhering to prescribed religious beliefs and rituals (e.g., religious ceremonies, dietary regulations, clothing, worship, prayer, private religious behaviors/reading religious materials/media, holiday observances, meetings with religious leaders)
- Expresses emotional distress because of separation from faith community
- Expresses a need to reconnect with previous belief patterns
- Expresses a need to reconnect with previous religious customs
- Questions religious belief patterns
- Questions religious customs

RELATED FACTORS
- Aging
- End-stage life crises
- Life transitions
- Illness
- Pain
- Anxiety
- Fear of death
- Ineffective coping
- Ineffective support
- Lack of security
- Cultural barriers to practicing religion
- Spiritual crises
- Suffering

ASSESSMENT FOCUS
(Refer to comprehensive assessment parameters.)
- Values/beliefs

EXPECTED OUTCOMES
The patient will
- Describe conflicts with his or her religious beliefs and the effects of his or her illness on these beliefs.
- Accept counsel of a person trained in spirituality.
- Engage in religious practices to the extent that it is therapeutic.
- Begin differentiating between delusional thinking and reality arterial blood gas levels.

SUGGESTED NOC OUTCOMES
Hope; Motivation; Quality of Life; Spiritual Health

INTERVENTIONS AND RATIONALES

Determine: Assess spiritual or religious beliefs; religious affiliation; importance of religion in daily life; religious involvement of family; religious dietary restrictions; importance of religion in helping with usual coping. *Assessment information helps identify appropriate interventions.*

Attend: Approach patient in a nonjudgmental way when he or she is discussing religious beliefs or spiritual needs. *The nurse's beliefs may differ radically but it is a professional responsibility to assist the patient in an ethically sensitive way.*

Help patient list the religious practices most important to him or her *to determine what is possible to provide in the hospital.*

Acquire simple-to-obtain items, such as books, pictures, CD, cross, *to provide comfort to the patient.*

Confirm that patient's spiritual needs are being satisfied *so that modifications can be made in the plan.*

Involve family members in helping meet patient's spiritual needs if the patient agrees. *If family members have strong spiritual beliefs, they can be a help to one another in times of pain and difficulty.*

Encourage patient and family to express feelings associated with diagnosis, treatment, and recovery. *Expression of feelings helps patient and family cope with treatment.*

Schedule time to spend with the family. *They need time with health care providers to ask questions.*

Manage: Suggest a referral to a clergy person or faith community nurse *so that the person can discuss deeper spiritual issues.*

SUGGESTED NIC INTERVENTIONS

Acid–Base Management; Bedside Laboratory Testing; Active Listening; Spiritual Growth; Spiritual Support

REFERENCE

Smith, A. R. (2011, October–December). What if the patient doesn't want prayer? *Journal of Christian Nursing, 28(4),* 235.

DEFINITION

A pattern of reliance on religious beliefs and/or participation in rituals of a particular faith tradition that is sufficient for well-being and can be strengthened

DEFINING CHARACTERISTICS

- Expresses desire to strengthen religious belief patterns that have provided comfort in the past
- Expresses desire to strengthen religious belief patterns that have provided religion in the past
- Expresses desire to strengthen religious customs that have provided religion in the past
- Questions and/or rejects belief patterns or customs that are harmful
- Requests assistance to expand religious options
- Requests forgiveness
- Requests reconciliation
- Requests meetings with religious leaders
- Requests religious experiences and/or religious materials

ASSESSMENT FOCUS

(Refer to comprehensive assessment parameters.)

- Communication
- Coping
- Knowledge
- Roles/responsibilities
- Values/beliefs

EXPECTED OUTCOMES

The patient will

- Articulate what gives him or her strength and hope.
- Discuss important aspects of religion to work with the patient to establish a trusting relationship.
- Perform if the patient is to talk about spiritual needs, it must be in a nonjudgmental, warm, caring environment.
- List how staff can facilitate his or her participation in religious practices.
- Request or agree to talk to a religious professional.
- Express a feeling of peace with provided religious opportunities.

SUGGESTED NOC OUTCOMES

Health Beliefs; Health Promoting Behavior; Hope; Motivation; Quality of Life; Spiritual Health

INTERVENTIONS AND RATIONALES

<u>Determine:</u> Assess support system; involvement in religion; religious affiliation; religious practices and/or spiritual practices that are meaningful

to the patient; perceptions of faith, life, death, and suffering. *Information from assessment helps identify appropriate interventions.*

<u>Perform:</u> Obtain for the patient objects of religious significance that he requests, for example, a cross, a copy of the Bible or Koran, a menorah. *Patients often find comfort in having religious objects at the bedside.*

<u>Attend:</u> Listen attentively to the patient. Do not argue about the patient's beliefs or perceptions of faith. Ask for clarification when it is needed. Honest communication is important to gain the patient's trust.

Offer to provide whatever things can easily be found to support the patient's spiritual needs, such as reading material, pictures, music, and so forth. *This may promote comfort.*

Explore with the patient to what extent he wishes to incorporate his religious beliefs into his daily life. *This would introduce the idea of making a plan to enhance religiosity.*

Help patient list the religious practices that are most important to him *to comfort him while planning much more complex support.*

<u>Manage:</u> Evaluate to what extent the patient perceives that his or her spiritual needs are being met. *This way modifications can be made if indicated.*

Arrange a referral to a member of the clergy or person designated by the patient as a spiritual guide *so the patient may discuss deeper spiritual issues.*

SUGGESTED NIC OUTCOMES

Presence; Religious Ritual Enhancement; Spiritual Growth Facilitation; Spiritual Support; Values Clarification

REFERENCE

Lazenby, J. M. (2010, December). On "spirituality," "religion," and "religions": A concept analysis. *Palliative Support Care, 8*(4), 469–476.

DEFINITION

At risk for an impaired ability to exercise reliance on religious beliefs and/or participate in rituals of a particular faith tradition

RISK FACTORS

- Cultural or environmental barriers
- Illness or hospitalization
- Ineffective support/coping systems
- Lack of social interaction
- Lack of transportation
- Life transitions
- Suffering

ASSESSMENT FOCUS

(Refer to comprehensive assessment parameters.)
- Coping
- Communication
- Values/beliefs
- Knowledge

EXPECTED OUTCOMES

The patient will
- Articulate those religious practices that are important to him.
- Decide what changes to his practices are realistic and acceptable.
- Cope with the limitations placed on him by current circumstances.
- Make use of the available spiritual resources.
- Express satisfaction with ability to practice his religion.

SUGGESTED NOC OUTCOMES

Health Beliefs; Health-Promoting Behavior; Hope; Motivation; Quality of Life; Spiritual Health

INTERVENTIONS AND RATIONALES

<u>Determine:</u> Assess religious affiliation; degree of active participation in religious activities; support/coping systems; social interaction; present living circumstances. *Assessment information helps identify appropriate interventions.*

<u>Inform:</u> Teach patient about the resources that are available to him or her as a preparation for developing a realistic plan. *The plan will be more meaningful to the patient if he or she has already lined up possible resources.*

<u>Attend:</u> Encourage patient to talk about the religious practices that are important to him or her *to provide focus for appropriate interventions.*

Help patient explore modifications to his or her activities without compromising spiritual comfort. *Decision making promotes feelings of independence and control.*

Have patient list options for participation in religious activities *to promote optimism or acceptance in present situations.*

<u>Manage:</u> Involve family, friends, and clergy *to provide appropriate spiritual support.*

Check daily or weekly with the patient *to evaluate the effectiveness of the patient's plan.*

SUGGESTED NIC INTERVENTIONS

Active Listening; Emotional Support; Hope Instillation; Presence; Religious Ritual Enhancement; Spiritual Growth Facilitation; Spiritual Support; Values Clarification

REFERENCE

Sartori, P. (2010, July). Spirituality 1: Should spiritual and religious beliefs be part of patient care? *Nursing Times, 106*(28), 20–26.

DEFINITION
Physiological and/or psychosocial disturbance following transfer from one environment to another

DEFINING CHARACTERISTICS
- Alienation
- Anger
- Anxiety related to separation
- Concern over relocation
- Dependency
- Depression
- Fear
- Frustration
- Increased physical symptoms or illness
- Increased verbalized needs or unwillingness to move
- Insecurity
- Loneliness
- Loss of identity or self-worth
- Pessimism
- Sleep disturbance
- Withdrawal
- Worry

RELATED FACTORS
- Decreased health status
- Feelings of powerlessness
- Impaired psychosocial health
- Isolation from familiar locations and persons
- Lack of adequate support system or predeparture counseling or social support
- Move from one environment to another
- Language barrier
- Losses
- Passive coping
- Unpredictability of experience

ASSESSMENT FOCUS
(Refer to comprehensive assessment parameter.)
- Activity/exercise
- Coping
- Emotional
- Knowledge
- Neurocognition
- Risk management
- Roles/relationships

EXPECTED OUTCOMES

The patient will
- Request information about new environment.
- Communicate understanding of relocation.
- Take steps to prepare for relocation.
- Use available resources.
- Express satisfaction with adjustment to new environment.

SUGGESTED NOC OUTCOMES

Loneliness Severity; Psychosocial Adjustment: Life Change; Quality of Life; Stress Level

INTERVENTIONS AND RATIONALES

Determine: Assess patient's needs for additional health care services before relocation *to ensure receipt of appropriate care in the new environment.*

Perform: Assign a primary nurse to patient *to provide a consistent, caring, and accepting environment that enhances patient's adjustment and well-being.*

Help patient and family members prepare for relocation. Conduct group discussions, provide pictures of the new setting, and communicate any additional information that will ease transition *to help patient cope with a new environment.*

If possible, allow patient and family members to visit the new location, and provide introductions to the new staff. *The more familiar the environment, the less stress patient will experience during relocation.*

Inform: Educate family members about relocation stress syndrome and its potential effects *to encourage family members to provide needed emotional support throughout the transition period.*

Attend: Encourage patient to express emotions associated with relocation *to provide opportunity to correct misconceptions, answer questions, and reduce anxiety.*

Reassure patient that family members and friends know his or her new location and will continue to visit *to reduce feelings of abandonment and anxiety.*

Manage: Communicate all aspects of patient's discharge plan to appropriate staff members at the new location *to ensure continuity of care.*

SUGGESTED NIC INTERVENTIONS

Active Listening; Coping Enhancement; Self-Responsibility Facilitation

REFERENCE

Bekhet, A. K., & Zauszniewski, J. A. (2012, July 24). Resourcefulness, positive cognitions, relocation controllability and relocation adjustment among older people: A cross-sectional study of cultural differences. *International Journal of Older People Nursing.*

DEFINITION
At risk for physiological and/or psychosocial disturbance following transfer from one environment to another

RISK FACTORS
- Decreased health status
- Feelings of powerlessness
- Lack of adequate support system or group
- Lack of predeparture counseling
- Moderate to high degree of environmental change
- Moderate mental competence
- Move from one environment to another
- Passive coping
- Past, current, or recent losses
- Unpredictability of experiences

ASSESSMENT FOCUS
(Refer to comprehensive assessment parameters.)
- Activity/exercise
- Coping
- Emotional
- Knowledge
- Neurocognition
- Risk management
- Roles/relationships

EXPECTED OUTCOMES
The patient will
- Request information about the new environment.
- Participate in decision making regarding relocation.
- Communicate understanding of need for relocation.
- Express satisfaction with adjustment to new environment.
- Take steps to prepare for relocation along with family members or partner.

SUGGESTED NOC OUTCOMES
Loneliness Severity; Psychosocial Adjustment: Life Change; Quality of Life; Stress Level

INTERVENTIONS AND RATIONALES
<u>Determine:</u> Assess patient's needs for additional health care services before relocation *to ensure that patient receives appropriate care in the new environment.*
<u>Perform:</u> Assign a primary nurse to patient *to provide a consistent, caring, and accepting environment that enhances patient's adjustment and well-being.*

If possible, include patient in the decision-making process regarding potential location, dates, and circumstances of relocation *to promote a feeling of participation in choices, which will allow feeling of control.*

If possible, allow patient and family members to visit the new location, and provide introductions to the new staff. *The more familiar the environment, the less stress patient will experience during relocation.*

<u>Inform:</u> Educate family members about relocation stress syndrome and its potential effects *to encourage family members to provide needed emotional support throughout the transition period.*

<u>Attend:</u> Help patient and family members prepare for relocation. Conduct group discussions, provide pictures of setting, and communicate any information that will ease transition *to help patient with the new environment.*

Encourage patient to express emotions associated with relocation or provide an opportunity to correct misconceptions and answer questions. *This helps reduce anxiety about relocation.*

<u>Manage:</u> Communicate all aspects of patient's discharge plan to appropriate staff members at the new location *to ensure continuity of care.*

Reassure patient that family members and friends know his or her new location and will continue to visit *to reduce feelings of abandonment.*

SUGGESTED NIC INTERVENTIONS

Active Listening; Coping Enhancement; Self-Responsibility Facilitation

REFERENCE

Johnson, R., Popejoy, L. L., & Radina, M. E. (2010). Older adults participation in nursing home placement. *Clinical Nursing Research, 19*(4), 358–375.

DEFINITION

At risk for a decrease in blood circulation to the kidney that may compromise health

RISK FACTORS

- Systemic inflammatory response syndrome
- Hypoxia
- Hypovolemia
- Infection
- Treatment-related side effects
- Renal artery stenosis
- Renal disease
- Hypertension
- Diabetes mellitus

ASSESSMENT FOCUS

(Refer to comprehensive assessment parameters.)

- Cardiac function
- Elimination
- Fluid and electrolytes

EXPECTED OUTCOMES

The patient will

- Identify risk factors that contribute to risk for decreased renal perfusion.
- Make appropriate lifestyle changes to minimize risks, including careful management of chronic health conditions.
- Verbalize signs and symptoms of possible renal dysfunction related to impaired perfusion.
- Maintain fluid balance.

SUGGESTED NOC OUTCOMES

Cardiac Pump Effectiveness; Electrolyte & Acid/Base Balance; Kidney Function; Knowledge: Health Promotion

INTERVENTIONS AND RATIONALES

Determine: Assess patient current management of preexisting health conditions that increase the risk of decreased renal perfusion. *Effective management of chronic health conditions will help preserve kidney function.*

Monitor intake and output to evaluate need for fluid replacement.

Perform: Collect and evaluate laboratory and urine data that may indicate renal damage. *Serum creatinine levels and urine protein and creatinine are sensitive indicators of renal function.*

Maintain mean arterial pressure of at least 60 to 70 *to provide continuous perfusion needed for optimal renal function.*

Inform: Provide patient teaching regarding the need to control modifiable risk factors and the signs and symptoms that indicate renal dysfunction. *Prevention and early intervention are essential in maintaining renal function.*

Attend: Provide patient and family with encouragement and psychological support *to reinforce positive health behaviors.*

Manage: Collaborate with other members of the health care team to develop an individualized plan of care to reduce risk factors. *A multidisciplinary approach results in positive patient outcomes.*

SUGGESTED NIC INTERVENTIONS

Electrolyte Monitoring; Hemodynamic Regulation; Fluid Management; Urinary Elimination Management

REFERENCE

Lambers Heerspink, H. J., Perkovic, V., & de Zeeuw, D. (2011). Is doubling of serum creatinine a valid clinical "hard" endpoint in clinical nephrology trials? *Nephron Clinical Practice, 119*(3), c195–c199.

DEFINITION
Decreased ability to sustain a pattern of positive responses to an adverse situation or crisis

DEFINING CHARACTERISTICS
- Maladaptive coping responses (e.g., drug use, violence)
- Renewed elevation of distress
- Decreased interest in academic or vocational activities
- Depression
- Guilt
- Low self-esteem
- Social isolation
- Isolation

RELATED FACTORS
- Demographics that increase chance of maladjustment
- Inconsistent parenting, large family size, or low maternal education
- Gender, minority status
- Poor impulse control, substance abuse, or violence
- Psychological disorders
- Vulnerability factors which encompass indices that exacerbate the negative effects of the risk condition

ASSESSMENT FOCUS
(Refer to comprehensive assessment parameters.)
- Support systems
- Substance use
- Self-care
- Depression
- Safety
- Decision making
- Anxiety
- Spiritual needs

EXPECTED OUTCOMES
The patient will
- Remain free from harming self or others.
- Avoid abusing substances.
- Identify personal strengths.
- Engage in activities that promote health.
- Identify strategies that have been successful in previous times of stress.

SUGGESTED NOC OUTCOMES
Role Performance; Knowledge: Health Behavior; Risk Control; Stress Level; Symptom Control; Personal Resiliency

INTERVENTIONS AND RATIONALES

Determine: Explore with patients what maladaptive behaviors they are exhibiting because of impaired individual resilience. *The patient must take ownership of behaviors before change can occur.*

Monitor responses to change *to assess their effect on patient.*

Perform: Assist patient in making a list of strengths and resources with contact information and the parameters for contacting those resources. *Planning for needs decreases anxiety and increases self-care.*

Inform: Instruct patient to engage in positive health behaviors. *Adequate sleep, nutritional intake, and activity improve decision making.*

Attend: Encourage patient to wait to make life-changing decisions until the current crisis is over. *Decision making is impaired during times of crisis.*

Manage: Refer patients to mental health resources in the event of maladaptive coping or safety risk. *Individuals with impaired individual resilience face an increased risk of physical and mental illness.*

SUGGESTED NIC INTERVENTIONS

Anxiety Reduction; Coping Enhancement; Decision-Making Support; Spiritual Support; Risk Identification; Resiliency Promotion

REFERENCE

Peereboom, K. (2012, June). Goals-of-care discussions for patients with life-limiting disease. *Contemporary Nurse, 14*(1), 251–258.

DEFINITION
At risk for decreased ability to sustain a pattern of positive responses to an adverse situation or crisis

RISK FACTORS
- Chronicity of existing crises
- Multiple coexisting adverse situations
- Presence of additional new crisis (e.g., unplanned pregnancy, death of a spouse or family member, loss of job, illness, loss of housing)

ASSESSMENT FOCUS
(Refer to comprehensive assessment parameters.)
- Support systems
- Comfort
- Self-care
- Autonomic system
- Physical regulation
- Decision making
- Coping
- Spiritual needs

EXPECTED OUTCOMES
The patient will
- Identify available support systems to maintain resilience.
- Identify healthy coping strategies.
- Verbalize belief in self to withstand current situation.
- Engage in activities that promote health.
- Identify strategies that have been successful in previous times of stress.

SUGGESTED NOC OUTCOMES
Coping; Health Promoting Behavior; Role Performance; Personal Resiliency; Stress Level;Knowledge: Health Behavior

INTERVENTIONS AND RATIONALES
<u>Determine:</u> Evaluate previous mechanisms of effective coping in difficult situations. *Assimilating current situation to previous successes enhances resilience.*

<u>Perform:</u> Assist patient in making a list of strengths and resources. Be knowledgeable of cultural aspects of resilience. *Cultural relevance is critical to all aspects of patient care.*

<u>Inform:</u> Instruct patient to engage in positive self-talk: "I can handle this," "I will accomplish one thing today and celebrate it." *A positive outlook increases endorphins and enhances self-efficacy.*

<u>Attend:</u> Encourage patient to maintain activities of health promotion including adequate sleep, nutritious eating, and activity. *Maintaining adequate self-care enhances resilience.*

<u>Manage:</u> Refer patients to mental health resources in the event of maladaptive coping or safety risk. *Risk of compromised resilience may lead to actual compromised resilience.*

SUGGESTED NIC INTERVENTIONS

Anxiety Reduction; Coping Enhancement; Decision-Making Support; Spiritual Support; Culture Brokerage; Self-Awareness Enhancement; Resiliency Promotion

REFERENCE

Peters, K. (2011, December). Surviving the adversity of childlessness: Fostering resilience in couples. *Contemporary Nurse*, *40*(1), 130–140.

DEFINITION

A pattern of positive responses to an adverse situation or crisis that can be strengthened to optimize human potential

DEFINING CHARACTERISTICS

- Expressed desire to enhance resilience
- Presence of crisis
- Effective use of conflict management strategies
- Increases positive relationships with others
- Identifies support systems
- Identifies available resources
- Sets goals
- Makes progress toward goals
- Enhances personal coping skills
- Takes responsibility for actions
- Involvement in activities
- Enhanced sense of control
- Effective use of communication skills
- Demonstrates positive outlook
- Verbalizes self-esteem
- Access to resources

ASSESSMENT FOCUS

(Refer to comprehensive assessment parameters.)

- Thought process
- Perception of self
- Stability of relationships

EXPECTED OUTCOMES

The patient will

- Acknowledge readiness for increased resilience.
- Verbalize the feeling of resilience.
- Identify impact of resilience toward growth.

SUGGESTED NOC OUTCOMES

Self-Esteem; Knowledge: Health Behavior; Personal Resiliency

INTERVENTIONS AND RATIONALES

<u>Determine:</u> Explore with patients their process and growth in mastering a situation or crisis that enhanced their resilience. *Mastery of responses in crisis situations can generalize to future situations.*

Monitor attainment of goals *to assess need for further intervention.*

<u>Perform:</u> Listen therapeutically to patient's self-exploration and mastery. *Active listening is the key to the therapeutic alliance and accurate assessment.*

Demonstrate conflict resolution principles through role playing *to be able to practice in a controlled environment.*

<u>Inform:</u> Instruct the patient to journal experiences for future reflection. *Journaling is a therapeutic tool for self-exploration and expansion.*

<u>Attend:</u> Guide patient to review life goals that might now be attainable. *Personal potential is maximized in an environment of resilience.*

<u>Manage:</u> Encourage patient to assist others or get involved to enrich the lives of others. *Humans benefit from shared positive experiences.*

SUGGESTED NIC INTERVENTIONS

Coping Enhancement; Conflict Mediation; Journaling; Resiliency Promotion

REFERENCE

Gill, J. M., et al. (2010, December). Facilitating resilience using a society-to-cells framework: A theory of nursing essentials applied to research and practice. *Advances in Nursing Science, 33*(4), 329–343.

DEFINITION
Parent experience of role confusion and conflict in response to crisis

DEFINING CHARACTERISTICS
- Anxiety
- Disruption in care-taking routines
- Expressed concern about changes in parental role and family functioning, communication, and health
- Expressions of inadequacy to provide for child's needs
- Expressed loss of control over decisions relating to child
- Expressed or demonstrated feelings of guilt, anger, fear, anxiety, and frustration about the effect of the child's illness on family
- Reluctance to participate in usual care giving activities, even with support

RELATED FACTORS
- Change in marital status
- Home care of a child with special needs
- Interruptions of family life due to home care regimen
- Intimidations with invasive or restrictive modalities
- Parent–child separation due to chronic illness

ASSESSMENT FOCUS
(Refer to comprehensive assessment parameters.)
- Behavior
- Communication
- Coping
- Roles/relationships
- Self-perception

EXPECTED OUTCOMES
The parents will
- Communicate feelings about present situation.
- Participate in their child's daily care.
- Express feelings of greater control and ability to contribute more to the child's well-being.
- Express knowledge of child's developmental needs.
- Hold, touch, and convey warmth and affection to child.
- Use available support systems or agencies to assist with coping.

SUGGESTED NOC OUTCOMES
Caregiver Adaptation to Patient Institutionalization; Caregiver Performance: Direct and Indirect Care; Coping: Family

INTERVENTIONS AND RATIONALES
<u>Determine:</u> Assess the child's special needs; age and maturity of parents; roles within the family; available support systems for parents; parent–child relationship; and presence of conflict between family's lifestyle

and child's needs. *Assessment information will be useful in establishing appropriate interventions.*

Perform: Make changes in the environment with child-friendly pictures, and so forth, *to foster enhanced communication between parents and child.*

Provide family-centered care by involving the parents in the child's care. *Parents are responsible for decisions about the child's care.*

Inform: Provide information on informed consent *because parents will be making decisions for child's care.*

Teach parents about normal growth and development and advocate that they provide as much normalcy for the child with special needs as possible. *Treating them differently will retard progress in socialization.*

Teach patient and caregiver the skills necessary to manage care adequately. *Teaching will encourage compliance and adjustment to optimum wellness.*

Teach parents how to find areas in activities of living in which it is possible to maintain control *in order to avoid feelings of powerless.*

Teach parents to assist child with self-care activities in a way that maximizes the child's potential. *This enables caregivers to participate in child's care while supporting child's independence.*

Attend: Encourage visit by friends to promote socialization.

Encourage parents to pay attention to needs of siblings at home, and to discuss with siblings their feelings about having a sister or brother with special needs. *The goal is to have siblings be supportive but feel important in their own rites.*

Provide respite care *to promote emotional well-being of parents.* Encourage parents to spend time away from child *to enhance their marital relationship.*

Manage: Act as a liaison between family and multidisciplinary health care team *to provide support to the patients as they reach out for help.*

Refer parents to home care agencies and ensure that an appropriate assessment is done *to encourage long-term support.*

Refer parents to a mental health specialist *to enable support for the family members as they continue coping with the child's special needs.*

Arrange for parents to meet with parents who are coping positively with the same kinds of issues. *Peer support will help parents cope with their child's issues.*

SUGGESTED NIC INTERVENTIONS

Family Process Maintenance; Limit Setting; Mutual Goal-Setting; Parenting Promotion; Role Enhancement; Family Presence Facilitation

REFERENCE

Mikkelsen, G., & Frederikseen, K. (2011, May). Family-centered care of children in hospital-a concept analysis. *Journal of Advances in Nursing, 67*(5), 1152–1162.

DEFINITION

Patterns of behavior and self-expression that do not match the environmental context, norms, and exceptions

DEFINING CHARACTERISTICS

- Anxiety related to role performance, or altered role perceptions
- Change in capacity to resume role, perception of role (by self and others), or usual responsibilities
- Conflict among vocational, family, cultural, and social roles
- Discrimination
- Domestic violence or harassment
- Inadequate adaptation to change or transition
- Inadequate self-management, motivation, confidence, competence, or coping skills for fulfilling role
- Inappropriate developmental expectations
- Lack of external support or opportunities for enacting role
- Lack of knowledge about roles and responsibilities
- Pessimism
- Powerlessness
- Role ambivalence, denial, conflict, confusion, dissatisfaction, overload, or strain

RELATED FACTORS

- Knowledge (e.g., inadequate role model)
- Physiological (e.g., depression, cognitive deficits)
- Social (e.g., domestic violence, lack of resources)

ASSESSMENT FOCUS

(Refer to comprehensive assessment parameters.)

- Coping
- Emotional
- Knowledge
- Roles/relationships

EXPECTED OUTCOMES

The patient/family will

- Express feelings about diminished ability to perform usual roles.
- Recognize and state feelings about limitations imposed by illness.
- Make decisions about course of treatment and management of illness.
- Continue to function in usual roles as much as possible.
- Express feelings of making productive contribution to self-care, to others, or to environment.

SUGGESTED NOC OUTCOMES

Caregiver Lifestyle Disruption; Psychosocial Adjustment: Life Change; Role Performance; Coping; Psychomotor Energy

INTERVENTIONS AND RATIONALES

<u>Determine:</u> Assess patient's knowledge of illness *to establish baseline data.*

<u>Perform:</u> If possible, assign the same nurse to patient each shift *to establish rapport and foster development of a therapeutic relationship.*

Spend ample time with patient each shift to *foster a sense of safety and decrease loneliness.* If possible, assign the same nurse to patient each shift to *establish rapport and promote a therapeutic relationship.*

Encourage patient to express thoughts and feelings *to identify life affects of altered role performance.*

Express belief in ability of patient to develop coping skills *to help patient gain confidence.*

Be aware of patient's emotional vulnerability, and allow open expression of all emotions. *An accepting attitude will help patient deal with the effects of chronic illness and loss of functioning.*

Provide opportunities for patient to make decisions. *Showing respect for patient's decision-making ability enhances feelings of independence.*

<u>Inform:</u> Educate patient and family members about redefining *roles to promote optimal functioning. Through education, family members may become resources in patient's care.*

Offer patient and family members a realistic assessment of patient's illness, and communicate hope for the immediate future. *Education helps promote patient safety and security and helps family members plan for future health care requirements.*

<u>Attend:</u> Encourage patient to participate in self-care activities, keeping in mind his or her physical and emotional limitations. *Involvement in self-care promotes optimal functioning.*

Help patient recognize and use personal strengths *to maintain optimal functioning and promote a healthy self-image.*

Encourage patient to continue to fulfill life roles within the constraints posed by illness. *This will help patient maintain a sense of purpose and preserve connections with other people.*

Encourage patient to participate in his or her care as an active member of the health care team. *This will help establish mutually accepted goals between patient and his or her caregivers. Patient who participates in care is more likely to take an active role in other aspects of life.*

<u>Manage:</u> Help family members identify their feelings about patient's decreased role functioning. *Encourage participation in a support group. Relatives of patient may need social support, information, and an outlet for ventilating feelings.*

SUGGESTED NIC INTERVENTIONS

Caregiver Support; Family Process Maintenance; Role Enhancement; Family Mobilization

REFERENCE

Wong, N., Sarver, D. E., & Beidle, D. C. (2012, January). Quality of life impairments among adults with social phobia: The impact of subtype. *Journal of Anxiety Disorders, 26*(1), 50–57.

DEFINITION

A pattern of performing activities for oneself that helps to meet health-related goals and can be strengthened

DEFINING CHARACTERISTICS

- Expresses desire to enhance independence in maintaining life
- Expresses desire to enhance independence in maintaining health
- Expresses desire to enhance independence in maintaining personal development
- Expresses desire to enhance independence in maintaining well-being
- Expresses desire to enhance knowledge of responsibility and strategies for self-care

ASSESSMENT FOCUS

(Refer to comprehensive assessment parameters.)

- Behavior
- Coping
- Emotional
- Self-care

EXPECTED OUTCOMES

The patient will

- Demonstrate positive decision making toward maximizing potential for self-care.
- Express satisfaction with independence in assuming responsibility for planning self-care.
- Involve staff, family, and community in developing strategies for self-care.
- Seek out health-related information as needed.
- Monitor self-care measures taken for effectiveness and make alterations as needed.

SUGGESTED NOC OUTCOMES

Adherence Behavior; Client Satisfaction: Functional Assistance; Decision-Making; Health Beliefs: Perceived Ability to Perform

INTERVENTIONS AND RATIONALES

<u>Determine:</u> Assess patient's satisfaction with level of self-care *to support general well-being.*

Assess current ability to provide self-care *to establish a baseline.*

Assess effectiveness of self-care measures *to identify the need for adjustments.*

<u>Perform:</u> Assist patient to develop plan *to promote autonomous decision making to increase patient's responsibility for facilitating care.*

<u>Inform:</u> Provide information that supports implementation of a program to sustain health-seeking behavior *to promote patient autonomy in self-care.*

Attend: Encourage health team, family, and community efforts to participate in patient's self-care initiatives *to promote satisfactory mutual goal-setting and group efforts.*

Encourage patient and his or her family to participate in support networks that promote patient independence, where possible, *to promote patient and family resilience.*

Manage: Develop a referral list for community resources to promote patient's enhanced self-care.

SUGGESTED NIC INTERVENTIONS

Mutual Goal-Setting; Resiliency Promotion; Self-Responsibility Facilitation; Self-Efficacy Enhancement

REFERENCE

Colandrea, M., et al. Patient care heart failure model: The hospitalization to home plan of care. *Home Health Nurse, 30*(6), 337–344.

DEFINITION

Impaired ability to perform or complete bathing/hygiene activities for oneself

DEFINING CHARACTERISTICS

- Inability to dry body
- Inability to get into and out of bathroom
- Inability to obtain bath supplies
- Inability to obtain or get water source
- Inability to regulate water temperature or flow
- Inability to wash body or body parts

RELATED FACTORS

- Cognitive impairment
- Decreased motivation
- Environmental barriers
- Inability to perceive body part
- Musculoskeletal, perceptual, and/or neuromuscular impairment
- Pain
- Severe anxiety
- Weakness

ASSESSMENT FOCUS

(Refer to comprehensive assessment parameters.)

- Activity/exercise
- Coping
- Self-care
- Self-perception

EXPECTED OUTCOMES

The patient will

- Have self-care needs met.
- Have few, if any, complications.
- Communicate feelings about limitations.
- Demonstrate correct use of assistive devices.
- Carry out bathing and hygiene program daily.

SUGGESTED NOC OUTCOMES

Adaptation to Physical Disability; Energy Conservation; Self-Care: Activities of Daily Living (ADLs); Self-Care: Bathing; Self-Care: Hygiene

INTERVENTIONS AND RATIONALES

Determine: Observe patient's functional level every shift; document and report any changes. *Careful observation helps you adjust nursing actions to meet patient's needs.*

Monitor the completion of bathing and hygiene daily. Praise patient's accomplishments. *Reinforcement and rewards may encourage renewed effort.*

<u>Perform:</u> Perform the prescribed treatment for underlying musculoskeletal impairment. Monitor patient's progress, reporting favorable and adverse responses to treatment. *Applying therapy consistently aids patient's independence.*

Provide assistive devices, such as a long-handled toothbrush, for bathing and hygiene; instruct patient on use. *Appropriate assistive devices encourage independence.*

Assist with or perform bathing and hygiene daily. Assist only when patient has difficulty *to promote feeling of independence.*

<u>Inform:</u> Instruct patient and family members in bathing and hygiene techniques (you can give family members written instructions). Have patient and family members demonstrate bathing and hygiene under supervision. *Return demonstration identifies problem areas and increases patients' and family members' self-confidence.*

<u>Attend:</u> Encourage patient to voice feelings and concerns about self-care deficits *to help patient achieve the highest functional level possible.*

<u>Manage:</u> As needed, refer patient to a psychiatric liaison nurse, support group, or home health care agency. *These extra resources will reinforce activities planned to meet patient's needs.*

SUGGESTED NIC INTERVENTIONS

Behavior Modification; Discharge Planning; Bathing; Ear Care; Foot Care; Hair Care; Nail Care; Self-Care Assistance; Self-Care Assistance: Bathing/Hygiene

REFERENCE

Guler, E. K., Eşer, I., Khorshid, L., & Yücel, S. Ç. (2012, January). Nursing diagnoses in elderly residents of a nursing home: A case in Turkey. *Nursing Outlook, 60*(1), 21–28.

DEFINITION

Impaired ability to perform or complete dressing activities for self

DEFINING CHARACTERISTICS

- Inability to choose clothing
- Inability to put clothing on upper and/or lower body
- Inability to maintain appearance at a satisfactory level
- Inability to pick up clothing
- Inability to put on shoes, socks, or other items of clothing
- Inability to remove clothes
- Inability to use assistive devices

RELATED FACTORS

- Cognitive impairment
- Decreased motivation
- Environmental barriers
- Inability to perceive body part
- Musculoskeletal, perceptual, and/or neuromuscular impairment
- Pain
- Severe anxiety
- Weakness

ASSESSMENT FOCUS

(Refer to comprehensive assessment parameters.)

- Activity/exercise
- Coping
- Self-care
- Self-perception

EXPECTED OUTCOMES

The patient will

- Have self-care needs met.
- Have few, if any, complications.
- Communicate feelings about limitations.
- Demonstrate the correct use of assistive devices.
- Carry out dressing and grooming program daily.

SUGGESTED NOC OUTCOMES

Self-Care: Activities of Daily Living (ADLs); Self-Care: Dressing; Care-giver Performance: Direct Care

INTERVENTIONS AND RATIONALES

<u>Determine:</u> Observe patient's functional level every shift; document and report any changes. *Careful observation helps you adjust nursing actions to meet patient's needs.*

Monitor patient's abilities to dress and groom daily. *This identifies problem areas before they become sources of frustration.*

<u>Perform:</u> Perform the prescribed treatment for underlying musculoskeletal impairment. Monitor patient's progress, reporting favorable and adverse responses to treatment. *Applying therapy consistently aids patient's independence.*

Provide enough time for patient to perform dressing and grooming. *Rushing creates unnecessary stress and promotes failure.*

Provide necessary assistive devices, such as a long-handled shoehorn and zipper pull, as needed. Instruct patient on use. *Appropriate assistive devices encourage independence.*

Assist with or perform dressing activities: fasten clothes, comb hair, and clean nails. Provide help only when patient has difficulty *to promote feeling of independence.*

<u>Inform:</u> Instruct patient and family members in dressing techniques (you can give family members written instructions). Have patient and family members demonstrate dressing and grooming techniques under supervision. *Return demonstration reveals problem areas and increases self-confidence.*

<u>Attend:</u> Encourage patient to voice feelings and concerns about self-care deficits *to help patient achieve the highest functional level possible.*

Encourage family members to provide clothing patient can easily manage. Patient may benefit from clothing slightly larger than regular size and Velcro straps. *Such clothing makes independent dressing easier.*

<u>Manage:</u> As needed, refer patient to a psychiatric liaison nurse, support group, or home health care agency. *These extra resources will reinforce activities planned to meet patient's needs.*

SUGGESTED NIC INTERVENTIONS
Self-Care Assistance: Dressing/Grooming; Dressing

REFERENCE
Boltz, M., Resnick, B., Capezuti, E., Shabbat, N., & Secic, M. (2011, November–December). Function-focused care and changes in physical function in Chinese American and non Chinese American hospitalized older adults. *Rehabilitation Nursing, 36*(6), 233–240.

DEFINITION
Impaired ability to perform or complete self-feeding activities

DEFINING CHARACTERISTICS
Inability to perform one or more of the following:

- Bring food from receptacle to mouth
- Chew food
- Complete meals
- Get food onto utensil
- Handle a cup or glass
- Handle utensils
- Ingest food safely and in a socially acceptable manner
- Ingest sufficient food
- Open containers
- Prepare food
- Swallow food
- Use assistive devices

RELATED FACTORS
- Cognitive impairment
- Decreased motivation
- Environmental barriers
- Fatigue
- Musculoskeletal, perceptual, and/or neuromuscular impairment
- Pain
- Severe anxiety
- Weakness

ASSESSMENT FOCUS
(Refer to comprehensive assessment parameters.)

- Activity/exercise
- Coping
- Self-care
- Self-perception

EXPECTED OUTCOMES
The patient will

- Express feelings about feeding limitations.
- Maintain weight at ___ lb.
- Have no evidence of aspiration.
- Consume ___ % of diet.
- Demonstrate the correct use of assistive devices.
- Carry out feeding program daily.

SUGGESTED NOC OUTCOMES
Aspiration Prevention; Nutritional Status; Self-Care: Activities of Daily Living (ADLs); Self-Care: Eating; Swallowing Status

INTERVENTIONS AND RATIONALES
<u>Determine:</u> Observe patient's functional level every shift; document and report any changes. *Careful observation helps you adjust nursing actions to meet patient's needs.*

Monitor and record breath sounds every 4 hours *to check for aspiration of food.* Report crackles, wheezes, or rhonchi.

<u>Perform:</u> Perform the prescribed treatment of underlying musculoskeletal impairment. Monitor patient's progress, reporting favorable and

adverse responses to treatment. *Applying therapy consistently aids patient's independence.*

Weigh patient weekly and record his or her weight. Report a change of more than 1 lb/week *to ensure adequate nutrition and fluid balance.*

Initiate an ordered feeding program:

- Determine the types of food best handled by patient *to encourage patient's feelings of independence.*
- Place patient in high Fowler's position to feed *to aid swallowing and digestion.* Support weakened extremities, and wash patient's face and hands before meals *to promote a sense of well-being and safety.*
- Provide assistive devices such as plate guard, rocker knife *to allow more independence*; instruct patient on their use *to promote independence.*
- Supervise or assist at each meal, for example, cut food into small pieces. *This aids chewing, swallowing, and digestion, and reduces the risk of choking or aspiration.*
- Feed patient slowly. *Rushing causes stress, reducing digestive activity and causing intestinal spasms.*
- Keep suction equipment at the bedside *to remove aspirated foods if necessary.*
- Record the percentage of food consumed *to ensure adequate nutrition.*

Inform: Instruct patient and family members in feeding techniques and equipment. *This aids understanding and encourages compliance.*

Return demonstration reveals problem areas and increases self-confidence.

Attend: Encourage patient to express feelings and concerns about feeding deficits *to help patient achieve the highest functional level.*

Encourage patient to carry out the aspects of feeding according to his or her abilities. *This gives patient a sense of achievement and control.*

Manage: Refer patient to a psychiatric liaison nurse, support group, or community agencies such as Visiting Nurse Association and Meals on Wheels. *Additional resources reinforce activities planned to meet patient's needs.*

SUGGESTED NIC INTERVENTIONS

Aspiration Precautions; Fluid Management; Nutrition Management; Nutritional Monitoring; Self-Care Assistance: Feeding; Swallowing Therapy

REFERENCE

Chang, C. C. (2012, March). Prevalence and factors associated with feeding difficulty in institutionalized elderly with dementia in Taiwan. *Journal of Nutrition and Health in Aging, 16*(3), 258–266.

DEFINITION
Impaired ability to perform or complete toileting activities for self

DEFINING CHARACTERISTICS
- Inability to carry out proper toilet hygiene
- Inability to flush toilet or empty commode
- Inability to get to toilet or commode
- Inability to manipulate clothing for toileting
- Inability to sit on or rise from toilet or commode

RELATED FACTORS
- Cognitive impairment
- Decreased motivation
- Environmental barriers
- Fatigue
- Impaired transfer ability
- Musculoskeletal, perceptual, and/or neuromuscular impairment
- Pain
- Severe anxiety
- Weakness

ASSESSMENT FOCUS
(Refer to comprehensive assessment parameters.)
- Activity/exercise
- Coping
- Self-care
- Self-perception

EXPECTED OUTCOMES
The patient will
- Have self-care needs met.
- Have few, if any, complications.
- Communicate feelings about limitations.
- Maintain continence.
- Demonstrate the correct use of assistive devices.
- Carry out toileting program daily.

SUGGESTED NOC OUTCOMES
Urinary Continence; Bowel Continence; Self-Care: Activities of Daily Living (ADLs); Self-Care: Hygiene; Self-Care: Toileting

INTERVENTIONS AND RATIONALES
<u>Determine:</u> Observe patient's functional level every shift; document and report any changes. *Careful observation helps you adjust nursing actions to meet patient's needs.*

Monitor intake and output and skin condition; record episodes of incontinence. *Accurate intake and output records can identify potential imbalances.*

<u>Perform:</u> Perform the prescribed treatment of underlying musculoskeletal impairment. Monitor patient's progress, reporting favorable and adverse responses to treatment. *Applying therapy consistently aids patient's independence.*

Use assistive devices, as needed, such as an external catheter at night, a bedpan or urinal every 2 hours during the day, and adaptive equipment for bowel care. Instruct on use. As control improves, reduce the use of assistive devices. *Assisting at an appropriate level helps maintain patient's self-esteem.*

Assist with toileting only if needed. Allow patient to perform independently as much as possible *to promote independence.*

Perform urinary and bowel care if needed. Follow urinary or bowel elimination plans. *Monitoring success or failure of toileting plans helps identify and resolve problem areas.*

<u>Inform:</u> Instruct patient and family members in toileting routine (you can give family members written instructions). Have patient and family members demonstrate toileting routine under supervision. *Return demonstration identifies problem areas and increases patient's self-confidence.*

<u>Attend:</u> Encourage patient to voice feelings and concerns about his or her self-care deficits *to help patient achieve the highest functional level possible.*

<u>Manage:</u> As needed, refer patient to a psychiatric liaison nurse, support group, or home health care agency. *Additional resources reinforce activities planned to meet patient's needs.*

SUGGESTED NIC INTERVENTIONS

Bowel Training; Self-Care Assistance: Toileting; Urinary Elimination Management; Urinary Bladder Training; Urinary Incontinence Care; Bowel Incontinence Care

REFERENCE

Dean, E. (2012, February). Dignity in toileting. *Nursing Standard, 26*(24), 18–20.

DEFINITION

A pattern of perceptions or ideas about self that is sufficient for well-being and can be strengthened

DEFINING CHARACTERISTICS

- Accepts strengths and limitations
- Actions are congruent with expressed feelings and thoughts
- Expresses confidence in abilities
- Expresses satisfaction with thoughts about self, sense of worthiness, role performance, body image, and personal identity
- Expresses willingness to enhance self-concept

ASSESSMENT FOCUS

(Refer to comprehensive assessment parameters.)
- Coping
- Emotional
- Growth and development
- Roles/relationships
- Self-perception
- Values/beliefs

EXPECTED OUTCOMES

The patient will
- Articulate long- and short-term goals.
- Express motivation necessary to achieve goals.
- Develop realistic plan to achieve stated goals.
- Practice self-management strategies needed to be successful.
- Evaluate progress and modify behavior as needed.

SUGGESTED NOC OUTCOMES

Adherence Behavior; Health Beliefs: Perceived Ability to Perform: Health Promoting Behavior: Knowledge: Health Promotion; Motivation; Personal Well-Being; Risk Control; Body Image; Personal Autonomy; Self-Esteem

INTERVENTIONS AND RATIONALES

<u>Determine:</u> Assess patient's satisfaction with level of self-concept *to support general well-being.*

<u>Perform:</u> Provide patient with materials and resources on health-related issues that affect her attitude. *Knowledge will enhance patient's motivation or resolve.*

Have patient list one or two realistic, practical behaviors that will facilitate achieving goals. *The more positive her behaviors are, the greater the chance patient has of being successful.*

<u>Inform:</u> Answer questions related to written material *so patient is adequately prepared to establish realistic goals.*

<u>Attend:</u> Assist patient in writing long- and short-term goals. *These goals can serve as tools for self-evaluation as new behaviors are being practiced.*

Assist patient to determine positive rewards for successful behavior changes. *Reinforcers are needed for new behavior to continue.*

<u>Manage:</u> Develop a referral list for community resources *to promote patient's enhanced self-concept.*

SUGGESTED NIC INTERVENTIONS

Hope Inspiration; Journaling; Self-Awareness Enhancement; Self-Responsibility Facilitation; Self-Efficacy Enhancement; Self-Esteem Enhancement

REFERENCE

Young-Mason, J. (2012, August). Nursing and the arts: Empowering women since 1912 the Girl Scouts of America. *Clinical Nurse Specialist: The Journal for Advanced Nursing Practice, 26*(4), 227–228.

DEFINITION

At risk for behavior in which an individual demonstrates that he or she can be physically, emotionally, and/or sexually harmful to others

RISK FACTORS

- Age: 15 to 19 years; over 45 years
- Verbal or behavioral clues
- Conflictual interpersonal relationships
- Emotional problems
- Employment problems
- Engagement in autoerotic sexual acts
- Family background
- History of multiple suicide attempts
- Lack of personal resources
- Lack of social resources
- Mental or physical health problems
- Marital status
- Occupation
- Sexual orientation
- Suicidal ideation or plan

ASSESSMENT FOCUS

(Refer to comprehensive assessment parameters.)

- Behavior
- Coping
- Emotional
- Risk management
- Self-perception
- Values/belief

EXPECTED OUTCOMES

The patient will

- Maintain environment that is free from potential suicidal weapons.
- Recover from suicidal episode.
- Discuss feelings that precipitated suicide attempt.
- Consult mental health professional.
- Describe available resources for crisis prevention and management.
- Verbalized noticed improvement in self-worth.

SUGGESTED NOC OUTCOMES

Impulse Self-Control; Self-Mutilation Restraint; Suicide Self-Restraint

INTERVENTIONS AND RATIONALES

<u>Determine:</u> Assess life situation; recent stressors; available support systems; history of suicidal attempts; history of substance/alcohol abuse; history of violence against person or property; history of antisocial

behavior. *Assessment information will help identify appropriate intervention for this diagnosis.*

<u>Perform:</u> Remove all objects from the environment that the patient could use to harm himself or herself *in order to provide safety and protect potential victims of violence to self.*

Administer prescribed medications *to help patient control aggressive behavior and remain calm.* Monitor for effectiveness. *When used appropriately, medications will help reduce suicidal ideations.*

<u>Inform:</u> Explain medication program to patient *to promote compliance.* Make sure that the medication is swallowed, as prescribed, *to ensure compliance and produce calmness.*

Teach coping strategies and self-healing techniques to patient and family members, including meditation, guided imagery, and prayer.

Teach patient how to incorporate the use of self-healing techniques in carrying out usual daily activities. *These techniques help calm the mind and promote ability to cooperate with the difficulties associated with suicidal behavior.*

<u>Attend:</u> Use a warm, caring nonjudgmental manner *to show unconditional positive regard.*

Demonstrate understanding but don't reinforce denial of the present situation *because denial can mask the roots of suicidal feelings.*

Listen carefully to the patient and do not challenge him or her *to communicate caring and support.*

<u>Manage:</u> Make a short-term contract with the patient that he or she will not harm him/herself during a specific period. Continue negotiating until no evidence of suicidal ideation exists. *A contract gets the subject of suicide out in the open, places some responsibility to the patient, and conveys acceptance of the patient as a person.*

Provide patient with telephone numbers and other information about crisis centers, hotlines, and counselors. *Alternatives may ease anxiety about the perceived threat of long-term psychotherapy.*

SUGGESTED NIC INTERVENTIONS

Behavior Management: Self-Harm; Environmental Management: Violence Prevention; Impulse Control Training; Suicide Prevention; Crisis Intervention

REFERENCE

Plawecki, L. H. (2010, May). Someone to talk to. The nurse and the depressed or suicidal older patient. *Journal of Gerontology Nursing, 36*(5), 15–18.

DEFINITION

Long-standing negative self-evaluation/feelings about self or self-capabilities

DEFINING CHARACTERISTICS

- Dependent on others' opinions
- Evaluation of self as unable to deal with events
- Exaggerates negative feedback about self
- Hesitant to try new situations
- Indecisive behavior
- Lack of eye contact
- Nonassertive behavior
- Overly conforming
- Passive
- Rejects positive feedback about self
  - Reports feelings of guilt
  - Reports feelings of shame
  - Excessively seeks reassurance

RELATED FACTORS

- Lack of affection, approval, or membership in group
- Ineffective adaptation to loss
- Perceived lack of belonging or respect from others
- Repeated failures
- Repeated negative reinforcement
- Traumatic event or situation

ASSESSMENT FOCUS

(Refer to comprehensive assessment parameters.)

- Behavior
- Coping
- Emotional
- Role/responsibilities
- Self-perception

EXPECTED OUTCOMES

The patient will

- Voice feelings related to current situation and its effect on self-esteem.
- Report feeling safe in agency environment.
- Make a verbal contract not to harm self while in the facility.
- Gradually join in self-care and decision-making process.
- Decrease number of negative self-defeating comments.
- Accept positive and negative feedback without exaggeration.

SUGGESTED NOC OUTCOMES

Body Image; Depression Self-Control; Mood Equilibrium; Motivation; Personal Autonomy; Quality of Life; Self-Esteem; Risk Detection; Decision-Making; Suicide Self-Restraint

INTERVENTIONS AND RATIONALES

<u>Determine:</u> Assess reason for hospitalization; perception of self; and cognitive ability. *Information gained from the assessment will assist to identify appropriate goals and interventions.*

<u>Perform:</u> Provide for a specific amount of uninterrupted time each day to engage the patient in conversation. *This will allow the patient time for self-exploration, which promotes future change.*

When appropriate, institute suicide precaution according to protocol. *Patient needs supervision until he or she demonstrates adequate self-control to ensure his or her own safety.*

Provide the patient with a simple structured daily routine. *Structured activity limits the patient's anxious behavior.*

Encourage discussion of problems patient considers important. Have patient make a list of three most critical issues. *This creates opportunity for patient to identify problems and begin setting realistic goals to build self-confidence.*

Encourage bathing, grooming, and other hygiene functions for the patient every day, as needed. Encourage patient to do as much as possible for himself or herself. *Greater independence will help strengthen self-esteem.*

<u>Inform:</u> Teach self-healing techniques to patient and family such as meditation, guided imagery, yoga and prayer *to prevent anxiety and encourage a positive frame of mind.*

Provide patient with concise information about decision-making skills *to produce benefits that can reinforce health-seeking behaviors.*

<u>Attend.</u> Provide patient with positive feedback for verbal reports or behaviors that indicate a return to positive self-appraisal. *This gives patient feelings of significance, approval, and competence, which can help cope effectively with stressful situations.*

Encourage social interaction. *Disturbed interpersonal relationships may be an outward expression of self-hate.*

Facilitate opportunities for spiritual nourishment and growth *to address patient's holistic needs for maximal therapeutic environment.*

Be available to answer any questions patient's family may have *to provide accurate information and emotional support.*

<u>Manage:</u> Assist patient to seek assistance when discharged *in order to help replace maladaptive coping behaviors with more adaptive ones.*

Schedule time to meet with family and patient to listen to ways in which they plan to enhance their coping skills in the present situation. *This better ensures success in meeting established goals.*

Refer family to community resources and support groups available *to assist in managing patient's illness and providing emotional and financial assistance to caregivers.*

SUGGESTED NIC INTERVENTIONS

Active Listening; Body Image Enhancement; Coping Enhancement; Decision-Making Support; Hope Instillation; Self-Esteem Enhancement; Support Group; Suicide Prevention

REFERENCE

Korpershoek, C., van der Bijl, J., et al. (2011, September). Self-efficacy and its influence on recovery of patients with stroke: A systematic review. *Journal of Advanced Nursing, 67*(9), 1876–1894.

DEFINITION

At risk for longstanding negative self-evaluating/feelings about self or self-capabilities.

RISK FACTORS

- Ineffective adaptation to loss
- Lack of affection
- Lack of membership in a group
- Perceived discrepancy between self and cultural norms
- Perceived discrepancy between self and spiritual norms
- Perceived lack of belonging
- Perceived lack of respect from others
- Psychiatric disorder
- Repeated failures
- Repeated negative reinforcement
- Traumatic event
- Traumatic situation

ASSESSMENT FOCUS

(Refer to comprehensive assessment parameters.)
- Behavior
- Coping
- Emotional
- Roles/Relationships
- Self-perception

EXPECTED OUTCOMES

The patient will:
- Attend milieu therapies and interact with peers.
- Use cognitive therapies to modify negative thoughts about self.
- Maintain safety and report any thoughts of self-harm to staff.
- Report decrease in feelings of anger, fear, guilt, and self-doubt.
- Verbalize positive self characteristics and accomplishments.

SUGGESTED NOC OUTCOMES

Anxiety Control; Body Image; Coping; Depression Level; Mood Equilibrium; Risk Control; Self-Esteem; Social Interaction Skills

INTERVENTIONS AND RATIONALES

<u>Determine:</u> Assess patient's mental status per unit protocols. *Recurring assessments will aid in identifying interventions, expected outcomes, and allow for modifications based on patient's progress.*

Obtain thorough history upon admission *in order to determine if patient's past history has additional risk factors for low self-esteem.*

<u>Perform:</u> Assist patient in applying cognitive therapies and positive self-talk *in order to identify and modify negative actions and thoughts that lead to feelings of anger, fear, guilt, and self-doubt.*

Work with patient to set a daily schedule that promotes self-care and attendance at milieu therapies, and give sincere praise when patient follows through. *Independence and positive feedback from peers and staff will aid in developing self-confidence and increasing self-esteem.*

<u>Inform:</u> Educate the patient on the importance of being assertive and reinforce by having the patient state their particular needs or preferences for the day *as this will help build independence, self-confidence, and decrease fear of rejection.*

Educate patient regarding the importance of setting realistic treatment goals *in order to continue to build self-confidence and self-esteem.*

Educate patient regarding resources available in the community such as support groups and *their positive impact on building self-esteem.*

<u>Attend:</u> Dedicate quality time to patient in a therapeutic and consistent manner *in order to help patient feel safe, allow time for open expression of feelings, and allow for the development of a trusting relationship.*

<u>Manage:</u> Work together with patient to develop a treatment plan and schedule appointments. *This will help to build the patient's independence, confidence, social skills, and self-esteem.*

SUGGESTED NIC INTERVENTIONS

Anxiety Reduction; Body Image Enhancement; Cognitive Restructuring; Coping Enhancement; Self-Esteem Enhancement; Support Group

REFERENCE

Erder, A., & Magnusson, A. (2012, March). Caregivers' difficulties in activating long-term mental illness patients with low self-esteem. *Journal of Psychiatric and Mental Health Nursing, 19*(2), 140–145.

DEFINITION

Development of a negative perception of self-worth in response to a current situation

DEFINING CHARACTERISTICS

- Evaluation of self as being unable to deal with situations or events
- Expressions of helplessness or uselessness
- Indecisive or nonassertive behavior
- Self-negating verbalizations
- Verbally reports current situational challenge to self-worth

RELATED FACTORS

- Behavior inconsistent with values
- Changes in development or social role changes
- Disturbed body image
- Failures, rejections, or loss
- Functional impairment
- Lack of recognition

ASSESSMENT FOCUS

(Refer to comprehensive assessment parameters.)

- Behavior
- Coping
- Emotional
- Role/responsibilities
- Self-perception

EXPECTED OUTCOMES

The patient will

- Voice feelings related to current situation and its effect on self-esteem.
- Verbally appraise self before and during current health problems.
- Participate in decisions related to care and therapies.
- Report a sense of control over life events.
- Articulate return to previous positive feelings about self.

SUGGESTED NOC OUTCOMES

Decision-making; Psychosocial Adjustment: Life Change; Self-Esteem; Suffering Severity

INTERVENTIONS AND RATIONALES

<u>Determine:</u> Assess health history, including mental status (affect, general appearance, and mood) and cognitive ability; as well as unhealthy coping and environmental factors. *Information gained from the assessment will assist to identify appropriate interventions.*

<u>Perform:</u> Spend time alone with patient listening to the problems that are important to him or her at this time. Have patient make a list of the three most critical issues he or she has now *to help patient identify his*

or her strengths and begin setting some realistic goals to build his or her self-confidence.

Encourage bathing, grooming, and other hygiene functions for the patient every day, as needed. Encourage patient to do as much as possible for himself or herself. *Greater independence will help strengthen self-esteem.*

<u>Inform:</u> Teach self-healing techniques to both the patient and family such as meditation, guided imagery, yoga, and prayer *to prevent anxiety and aid in keeping patient in a frame of mind to make positive decisions.*

Provide patient with concise information about decision-making skills. *This will produce benefits that can reinforce health-seeking behaviors.*

<u>Attend:</u> Encourage patient to express feelings about self (past and present). *Self-exploration encourages patient to consider future change.*

Provide patient with positive feedback for verbal reports or behaviors that indicate a return to positive self-appraisal. *This gives patient feelings of significance, approval, and competence, which can help cope effectively with stressful situations.*

Provide a specific amount of noncore time to engage patient in conversation. *Such discussions help patient assume responsibility for coping responses.*

Facilitate opportunities for spiritual nourishment and growth *to address patient's holistic needs for maximal therapeutic environment.*

Reinforce the family's efforts to care for the patient and support patient's independence. Let them know they are doing well *in order to ease adaptation to new caregiver roles.* Provide emotional support to family by being available to answer questions. *Accurate information will help family cope with current situation.*

<u>Manage:</u> Schedule time to meet with family and patient to listen to ways in which they plan to enhance their coping skills in the present situation. *Helping patient and/or family develop a realistic plan will better ensure success in meeting established goals.*

Refer family to community resources and support groups available *to assist in managing patient's illness and providing emotional and financial assistance to caregivers.*

Refer to a member of the clergy or a spiritual counselor, according to the patient's preference, *to show respect for the patient's beliefs and provide spiritual care.*

SUGGESTED NIC INTERVENTIONS

Anticipatory Guidance; Decision-Making Support; Self-Esteem Enhancement; Behavior Management; Relaxation Therapy

REFERENCE

Lavoic, M., et al. (2011, January/February). The autonomy experience of patients in palliative care. *Journal of Hospice and Palliative Nursing, 13*(1), 47–53.

DEFINITION

Risk for developing negative perception of self-worth in response to a current situation

RISK FACTORS

- Behavior inconsistent with values
- Decreased control over environment
- Change in developmental or social role changes
- Disturbed body image
- Failures, rejections, or loss
- Functional impairment
- History of abandonment, abuse, neglect, or learned helplessness
- Lack of recognition
- Physical illness
- Unrealistic self-expectations

ASSESSMENT FOCUS

(Refer to comprehensive assessment parameters.)

- Behavior
- Coping
- Emotional

EXPECTED OUTCOMES

The patient will

- Participate in decisions related to care and therapy.
- Maintain eye contact and initiate conversation.
- Maintain an open and upright posture.
- Verbally assess feelings about current situation and health problems and impact on lifestyle.
- Express positive feelings about self (verbally or through behaviors), indicating acceptance of changes caused by health problems or situation.
- Perform hygiene and self-care activities indicating attention to appearance.
- Express interest in talking to others who have successfully overcome the problem of low self-esteem.

SUGGESTED NOC OUTCOMES

Self-Esteem; Life Changes; Decision Making; Perceived Control; Psychosocial Adjustment

INTERVENTIONS AND RATIONALES

Determine: Assess developmental stage; family system; role in family; sibling position; health history; mental status, including affect, general appearance, mood; cognitive ability; support systems; patient's ability to identify choices; readiness for change to occur; level of knowledge for positive decision making, coping mechanisms, environmental factors.

Information from assessment will assist the nurse to identify appropriate interventions.

<u>Perform:</u> Encourage bathing, grooming, and other hygiene functions for the patient every day, as needed. Encourage patient to do as much as possible for himself or herself. *Greater independence will help strengthen self-esteem.*

<u>Inform:</u> Keep patient informed about what to expect and when to expect it. *Accurate information reduces anxiety.*

Teach self-healing techniques to both the patient and family such as meditation, guided imagery, yoga, and prayer. Teach patient how to incorporate the use of self-healing techniques in carrying out usual daily activities. *These techniques help calm the mind and promote ability to cooperate with the difficulties associated with low self-esteem.*

<u>Attend:</u> Encourage patient to talk about personal assets and accomplishments and about improvements in condition no matter how small these may seem. Give positive feedback. *Conversation assists you to evaluate the patient's self-concept and adaptive abilities.*

Direct the patient's focus beyond the present state. *As long as a patient focuses only on the present state, he or she will have difficulty planning activities that will move him or her forward.*

<u>Manage:</u> Help patient involve the family, community, clergy, and friends with changes to the care plan *to increase the potential of the patient's control over self-care outcomes.*

Refer patient and family to other professional caregivers, for example, dietitian, social worker, clergy, and mental health professional. *Support groups such as Ostomy clubs, I Can Cope, and Reach for Recovery can provide physical, material, financial, and emotional resources to patient and the family during the recovery period.*

Assist patient to utilize appropriate resources by contacting family and scheduling follow-up appointments. *This helps give the patient a sense of direction and control over his or her future care.*

SUGGESTED NIC INTERVENTIONS

Assertiveness Training; Coping Enhancement; Self-Modification Assistance; Self-Responsibility Facilitation; Referral

REFERENCE

Rouse, S. V. (2012, January). Universal worth: Construct and scale development. *Journal of Personal Assessment,* 94(1), 62–72.

DEFINITION

Pattern of regulating and integrating into daily living a therapeutic regimen for treatment of illness and its sequelae that is unsatisfactory for meeting specific health goals

DEFINING CHARACTERISTICS

- Failure to include treatment regimens in daily living
- Failure to take action to reduce risk factors
- Makes choices in daily living ineffective for meeting health goals
- Verbalizes desire to manage the illness
- Verbalizes difficulty with prescribed regimen

RELATED FACTORS

- Complexity of health care system and therapeutic regimen
- Decisional conflicts
- Economic difficulties
- Excessive demands made (e.g., individual, family)
- Family conflict and patterns of health care
- Inadequate number of cues to action
- Knowledge deficit
- Mistrust of regimen
- Powerlessness
- Perceived: barriers, seriousness, susceptibility, and benefits
- Social support deficit

ASSESSMENT FOCUS

(Refer to comprehensive assessment parameters.)
- Self-care
- Behavior
- Knowledge

EXPECTED OUTCOMES

The patient will
- Acknowledge responsibility to manage own health condition.
- Identify any barriers to optimal self-health management and determine plan to address them.
- Refine problem-solving skills over time.
- Increase self-efficacy, the confidence that one can carry out a behavior necessary to reach a desired goal.

SUGGESTED NOC OUTCOMES

Adherence Behavior; Compliance Behavior; Decision-Making; Health Orientation; Health Promoting Behavior; Personal Health Status; Self-Direction of Care; Knowledge: Health Promotion

INTERVENTIONS AND RATIONALES

Determine: Monitor patient's self-efficacy and use of problem-solving skills as patient manages own health. *These concepts reflect a new paradigm in health management that acknowledges that patients need many skills and confidence to carry out plan of care.*

Perform: Assist patient in setting goals and making informed choices. *This patient–nurse collaborative relationship helps patient and nurse identify barriers to optimal health management and overcome them.*

Inform: Teach patients about their disease states and regimens but, more importantly, teach patients problem-solving skills *to ensure that they actively participate in their self-health management despite any setbacks that they might experience.*

Attend: Provide encouragement to help motivate patient to maximize healthy behaviors. *This highlights that behavior is best changed by internal motivation rather than by external motivation.*

Manage: Coordinate with social services and colleagues in other disciplines *to ensure that family, economic, and social barriers to optimal self-health management have been addressed.*

SUGGESTED NIC INTERVENTIONS

Behavior Modification; Complex Relationship Building; Decision-Making Support; Health Education; Learning Facilitation; Mutual Goal-Setting; Self-Awareness Enhancement

REFERENCE

Mackey, E. R., et al. (2010). Individual and family strengths: An examination of the relation to disease management and metabolic control in youth with type I diabetes. *Family Systems Health, 29*(4), 314–326.

DEFINITION

Deliberate self-injurious behavior causing tissue damage with the intent of causing nonfatal injury to attain relief of tension

DEFINING CHARACTERISTICS

- Abrading
- Biting
- Constricting a body part
- Cuts on body
- Hitting
- Ingestion of harmful substances
- Inhalation of harmful stance
- Insertion of object into body orifice
- Picking at wounds
- Scratches on body
- Self-inflicted burns
- Severing

RELATED FACTORS

- Adolescence
- Autistic individual
- Battered child
- Borderline personality disorder
- Character disorder
- Dissociation
- Disturbed body image
- History of inability to plan solutions
- Impulsivity

ASSESSMENT FOCUS

(Refer to comprehensive assessment parameters.)

- Communication
- Coping
- Emotional
- Knowledge
- Roles/responsibilities

EXPECTED OUTCOMES

The patient will

- Refrain from harming self while in the hospital.
- Express an increased sense of security.
- Report being able to cope better with disorganization, aggressive impulses, anxiety, and hallucinations.
- Verbalize absence of or fewer dissociative states.
- Participate in therapeutic milieu.
- Describe community resources that can provide assistance when she feels out of control.

SUGGESTED NOC OUTCOME

Impulse Self-Control; Risk Control; Self-Mutilation Restraint

INTERVENTIONS AND RATIONALES

<u>Determine:</u> Assess behavioral responses; coping strategies; number and types of stressors; social factors; and spiritual beliefs. *Assessment information will assist in identifying appropriate goal and interventions.*

<u>Perform:</u> Move patient to a quiet room *to reduce stimuli if he or she is in a dissociative state.* Remove all dangerous objects from patient's room *to prevent injury.* Place patient under observation *to provide protection and increase his or her sense of security.*

Administer psychotropic medications, as prescribed, *to reduce tension, impulse behavior, hallucinations, and panic.*

Inform: Teach patient's coping strategies to family members. *Family members and friends can help patient practice adaptive methods of coping with self destructive feelings.*

Have patient and family members practice role-playing *to increase the confidence in the patient's ability to handle difficult situations.*

Teach self-healing techniques to both patient and family such as meditation, guided imagery, yoga, and prayer. Teach patient how to incorporate the use of self-healing techniques in carrying out usual daily activities. *These techniques can reduce the anxiety that comes from attempting to cope with his or her disease.*

Teach additional skills that enhance coping and relaxation strategies for the patient and family (i.e., meditation, guided imagery, yoga, exercise). *Self-healing gives the patient a better sense of control over regaining independence.*

Attend: Limit the number of staff who interact with patient *to provide continuity of care and enhance a sense of security.*

If patient is participating in a therapeutic milieu, discuss his or her risk of self-harm with community members *to provide patient with enhanced protection and psychological support.*

If patient causes harm to self, provide care in a calm, nonjudgmental manner. *Encourage discussion of feelings that caused self-mutilation to help patient connect self-destructive behavior to feelings that preceded it, and provide an opportunity to explore alternative ways of dealing with negative feelings.*

Accept patient's feelings of powerlessness as normal. *This indicates respect for the patient and enhances feelings of self-respect.*

Encourage patient to take an active role in self-care *to promote a sense of control.*

Manage: Organize frequent staff meetings *to ensure patient care is consistent with current behavior.*

Organize family conferences to allow opportunities for the family to discuss their particular frustrations and hopes in relation to the patient's current situation. *Family conferences can help the patient and family members ventilate true feelings in a safe environment.*

SUGGESTED NIC INTERVENTIONS

Area Restriction; Self-Harm; Environmental Management; Impulse Control; Coping Behaviors; Guided Imagery; Meditation Facilitation

REFERENCE

Rissanen, M. L., Kylma, J., & Laukkanen, E. (2012). Helping self-mutilating adolescents: Description of Finnish nurses. *Issues in Mental Health Nursing, 33*(4), 251–262.

DEFINITION

At risk for deliberate self-injurious behavior causing tissue damage with the intent of causing nonfatal injury to attain relief of tension

RISK FACTORS

- Adolescence
- Autistic individuals
- Battered child
- Character disorders
- Disturbed body image
- Isolation from peers
- Living in a nontraditional setting
- Low self-esteem
- Loss of significant relationship
- Peers who self-mutilate
- Perfectionism
- Substance abuse
- Violence between parental figures

ASSESSMENT FOCUS

(Refer to comprehensive assessment parameters.)

- Behavior
- Coping
- Emotional
- Self-perception
- Values/beliefs

EXPECTED OUTCOMES

The patient will

- Refrain from harming self.
- Express increased feelings of security.
- Report improved ability to cope with self-destructive feelings.
- Experience no episodes of dissociation.
- Participate in therapeutic milieu.
- Report suicidal ideations to staff.

SUGGESTED NOC OUTCOMES

Abuse Recovery Status; Anxiety Level; Impulse Self-Control; Risk Control; Self-Mutilation Restraint

INTERVENTIONS AND RATIONALES

<u>Determine:</u> Assess high-risk behaviors; health-promoting activities; coping skills; activities of daily living, including rest and sleep; sensory perception; decision-making skills; and sexuality patterns. *Information from the assessment will help establish outcomes to be developed.*

<u>Perform:</u> Administer psychotropic medications, as prescribed, *to reduce tension, impulsive behavior, hallucinations, and panic.*

Remove all dangerous objects from the environment *to enhance security.*

Move patient to a quiet room *to reduce stimuli if he or she is in a dissociative state.*

Place patient under observation *to provide protection and increase patient's sense of security.*

<u>Inform:</u> Teach patient about risk factors and other aspects of patient's medical condition *to help patient feel in control of his or her care.*

Teach patient's coping strategies to family members *so they can help patient practice adaptive methods of coping with self-destructive feelings.*

Have patient and family members practice role-playing *to increase the confidence in the patient's ability to handle difficult situations.*

Teach self-healing techniques to both the patient and family such as meditation, guided imagery, yoga, and prayer. *These techniques can reduce the anxiety that comes from attempting to cope with his or her disease.*

<u>Attend:</u> Make short-term verbal contracts with patient in which the patient states he will not harm himself. *This makes patient aware that he is ultimately responsible for his own safety and he can guarantee it.*

Ask patient directly whether he is thinking about suicide and if so, what plan he has. *A self-destructive patient may become suicidal and may require additional precautions.*

If patient harms himself or herself, care for him or her in a calm, nonjudgmental manner. Encourage patient to talk about feelings that prompted the self-mutilation. *Discussion of the event may help the patient connect self-destructive behavior to feelings that preceded it. Discussion may also provide him or her with an opportunity to explore alternative ways of dealing with negative thoughts and feelings.*

<u>Manage:</u> Organize frequent staff meetings to ensure consistency in managing the patient's care that is consistent with his current behavior.

Organize family conferences to allow opportunities for the family to discuss their particular frustrations and hopes in relation to the patient's current situation. *Family conferences can help the patient and family members ventilate true feelings in a safe environment.*

SUGGESTED NIC INTERVENTIONS

Area Restriction; Behavior Management: Self-Harm; Environmental Management: Violence Prevention; Impulse Control Training; Coping Enhancement

REFERENCE

Cromwell, S. E., et al. (2012, January). Differentiating adolescent self-injury from adolescent depression: Possible implications for borderline personality development. *Journal of Abnormal Psychiatry, 40*(1), 45–57.

DEFINITION
A constellation of culturally framed behaviors involving one or more self-care activities in which there is a failure to maintain a socially accepted standard of health and well-being

DEFINING CHARACTERISTICS
- Inadequate personal hygiene
- Inadequate environmental hygiene
- Nonadherence to health activities

RELATED FACTORS
- Cognitive impairment
- Depression
- Learning disability
- Fear of institutionalization
- Frontal lobe dysfunction and/or executive processing ability
- Functional impairment
- Lifestyle/choice
- Malingering
- Substance abuse
- Major life stressor (e.g., coping difficulty)
- Capgras syndrome

ASSESSMENT FOCUS
(Refer to comprehensive assessment parameters.)
- Activity/exercise
- Self-care
- Neurocognition
- Behavior

EXPECTED OUTCOMES
The patient will
- Demonstrate improved cognitive, functional, and mental health status.
- Adhere to prescribed health activities.
- Experience increased safety.
- Demonstrate improved coping with complex health circumstances including personal and environmental hygiene, nutrition, and fitness.
- Have fewer acute hospitalizations and emergency room visits.

SUGGESTED NOC OUTCOMES
Adherence Behavior; Compliance Behavior; Coping; Decision-Making; Health Orientation; Motivation; Personal Well-Being; Risk Control; Self-Care Status

INTERVENTIONS AND RATIONALES

Determine: Assess patient with complex health issues for adequate coping abilities *because poor coping skills may lead to unintentional self-neglect.*

Assess patient with failing self-care for changes in cognitive function *because neglected self-care may be the first noticeable sign of diminishing cognitive function.*

Perform: Involve patient's family in care activities as appropriate *to improve the chance that the patient will incorporate recommended regimens into lifestyle as long-term choice.*

Inform: Teach strategies to enhance adherence to medication and other health regimens. *Some instances of self-neglect occur because the patient has not been able to incorporate recommended regimens into his or her lifestyle.*

Attend: Encourage patient to identify internally motivating factors for adhering to health regimens. *Persons who intentionally neglect self-care as a lifestyle choice (i.e., fail to comply with medication and treatment regimens) will fare better if the decision to improve self-care is theirs.*

Manage: Refer patient demonstrating a significant decline in self-care abilities (i.e., posing a threat to self and/or community) for competency evaluation *because unintentional self-neglect may indicate diminished competency.*

SUGGESTED NIC INTERVENTIONS

Behavior Management; Counseling; Exercise Promotion; Limit Setting; Mutual Goal Setting; Self-Care Assistance; Self-Efficacy Enhancement; Self-Responsibility Facilitation

REFERENCES

Dong, X., Simon, M. A., & Evans, D. A. (2012). Prevalence of self-neglect across gender, race, and socioeconomic status: Findings from the Chicago Health and Aging Project. *Gerontology, 58*(3), 258–268.

Mauk, K. L. (2011, March–April). Ethical perspectives on self-neglect among older adults. *Rehabilitation Nursing, 36*(2), 60–65.

DEFINITION

The state in which an individual experiences a change in sexual function during the sexual response phases of desire, excitation, and/or orgasm, which is viewed as unsatisfying, unrewarding or inadequate

DEFINING CHARACTERISTICS

- Alterations in achieving sexual satisfaction
- Actual or perceived limitation imposed by disease or therapy
- Change in achieving perceived sex role
- Change in relationship with spouse or significant other
- Change of interest in self and others
- Conflicts involving values
- Inability or change in ability to achieve sexual satisfaction
- Need for confirmation of sexual desirability
- Verbal expression of problem

RELATED FACTORS

- Absent role models
- Altered body function
- Altered body structure
- Biopsychosocial alteration of sexuality
- Ineffectual role models
- Lack of privacy
- Lack of significant other
- Physical or psychosocial abuse
- Deficient knowledge or misinformation

ASSESSMENT FOCUS

(Refer to comprehensive assessment parameters.)

- Coping
- Emotional
- Knowledge
- Pharmacological function
- Self-perception

EXPECTED OUTCOMES

The patient will

- Acknowledge problems or potential problems in sexual function.
- Voice feelings about changes in sexual identity.
- Express understanding of reason for sexual dysfunction.
- Express willingness to obtain counseling.
- Reestablish sexual activity at pre-illness level.

SUGGESTED NOC OUTCOMES

Adaptation to Physical Disability; Body Image; Fear Level; Physical Aging; Role Performance; Sexual Functioning; Sexual Identity; Stress Level

INTERVENTIONS AND RATIONALES

Determine: Access marital status, sexual patterns, living arrangements, usual sexual patterns, attitudes toward modifying sexual patterns, and knowledge about appropriate options available, anxiety, and loss. *In combination with a general assessment, these factors will help establish realistic outcomes for a plan.*

Perform: Arrange for patient and partner to have periods of privacy for sexual expression by closing the door, using a privacy sign, and arranging with the staff to refrain from entering the room for a predetermined period of time. *Hospital routines allow too few opportunities for a patient to have private time. Sexual expression will not occur where privacy does not exist.*

Inform: Teach patient and partner about alternative methods of intimacy and expression of affection. *This can raise patient's self-esteem until impotence is evaluated.*

Teach coping strategies, including stress management and relaxation techniques. *Relaxation and decreased stress can increase function, thereby improving strength and resistance.*

Attend: Encourage patient to ask questions about personal sexuality. *A nonthreatening atmosphere encourages patients to ask questions specifically related to the particular situation.*

Provide support for the partner. *Supportive interventions (such as active listening) communicate concern, interest, and acceptance.*

Suggest patient discuss concerns with partner. *Open discussion fosters sharing of concerns and strengthens relationship.*

Manage: Suggest referral to a sex counselor or other appropriate professional for future guidance *to provide patient with a resource for postdischarge support.*

SUGGESTED NIC INTERVENTIONS

Anxiety Reduction; Emotional Support; Role Enhancement; Sexual Counseling; Coping Enhancement; Environmental Management; Self-Awareness Enhancement; Self-Esteem Enhancement

REFERENCE

Rees, M., et al. (2012, December). Sex and support model for stroke survivors. *Journal of Australian Nursing, 19*(6), 41.

DEFINITION

Expressions of concern regarding own sexuality

DEFINING CHARACTERISTICS

- Alterations in achieving perceived sex role
- Alteration in relationship with significant other
- Conflicts involving values
- Reported changes in sexual behaviors
- Reported changes in sexual activities
- Reported difficulties in sexual behaviors
- Reported difficulties in sexual activities
- Reported limitations in sexual behaviors
- Reported limitations in sexual activities

RELATED FACTORS

- Absent role model
- Conflicts with sexual orientation or variant preferences
- Fear of acquiring a sexually transmitted disease
- Fear of pregnancy
- Impaired relationship with a significant other
- Ineffective role model
- Knowledge/skill deficit about alternative responses to health-related issues
- Lack of privacy
- Lack of significant other

ASSESSMENT FOCUS

(Refer to comprehensive assessment parameters.)

- Coping
- Emotional
- Knowledge
- Values/beliefs

EXPECTED OUTCOMES

The patient will

- Voice feelings about reported changes in sexual activity.
- Express concern about self-concept, self-esteem, and body image.
- State at least one effect of illness or treatment on sexual behavior.

The patient and partner will

- Resume effective communication patterns.
- Use available counseling referrals or support.

SUGGESTED NOC OUTCOMES

Anxiety Level; Body Image; Role Performance; Sexual Identity; Stress Level Sexual Functioning

INTERVENTIONS AND RATIONALES

<u>Determine:</u> Assess for current treatment/medication regimen, marital status and family members, perception of sexual identity and role, and perception of changes in sexual activities resulting from illness or treatment. *Assessment information may help discover reasons for the problem and will assist to identify desirable outcomes and interventions.*

<u>Perform:</u> Arrange to spend time each shift with the patient to develop a trusting relationship. *The patient may need to discuss his or her difficulty but is more inclined to do that with a person he or she trusts.*

<u>Inform:</u> Teach patient relaxation techniques such as guided imagery, deep breathing, meditation, aromatherapy, and progressive muscle relaxation. Practice with the patient at bedtime. *Purposeful relaxation efforts usually help reduce anxiety.*

Educate patient and partner about the illness and treatment. Answer questions that might clarify any misconceptions they may have. *This may help them focus on specific concerns, encourage questions, and avoid misunderstandings.*

<u>Attend:</u> Provide time for privacy *to allow the patient and his or her partner to discuss feelings about sexuality and to engage in alternatives for intimacy while the patient is in the hospital.*

Be available to listen; accept patient's feelings to let him or her know that the feelings are valid and acceptable. *A nonjudgmental approach demonstrates unconditional positive regard for the patient and his or her feelings.*

<u>Manage:</u> Offer referral to counselors or support persons such as mental health professional, sex counselor, and illness-related support group *to provide postdischarge support.*

SUGGESTED NIC INTERVENTIONS

Anticipatory Guidance; Body Image Enhancement; Coping Enhancement; Sexual Counseling; Emotional Support; Self-Awareness Enhancement; Support Group; Guided Imagery; Teaching: Sexuality; Teaching: Disease Process

REFERENCE

Bates, J. (2011, December). Broaching sexual health issues with patients. *Nursing Times, 107*(48), 20–22.

DEFINITION
At risk for an inadequate blood flow to the body's tissues which may lead to life-threatening cellular dysfunction

RISK FACTORS
- Systemic inflammatory response syndrome
- Hypoxia
- Hypoxemia
- Sepsis
- Hypovolemia
- Infection
- Hypotension

ASSESSMENT FOCUS
(Refer to comprehensive assessment parameters.)
- Cardiac function
- Physical regulation

EXPECTED OUTCOMES
The patient will
- Maintain adequate blood pressure to provide tissue perfusion.
- Not experience hemodynamic complications from underlying medical condition.
- Understand the need for aggressive management of underlying medical condition in an effort to prevent shock.
- Verbalize reportable signs and symptoms of possible hypotension and hypoperfusion.

SUGGESTED NOC OUTCOMES
Tissue Perfusion: Cerebral; Hydration; Fluid Balance; Vital Signs; Circulation Status; Electrolyte & Acid/Base Balance

INTERVENTIONS AND RATIONALES
<u>Determine:</u> Monitor hemodynamic status frequently, including blood pressure, heart rate, and oxygen saturation. *Trending of vital signs will provide database for early intervention and treatment.*

Assess level of consciousness (LOC) with each vital sign check. *Change in LOC is an early indicator of cerebral hypoperfusion.*

<u>Perform:</u> Administer intravenous fluids, oxygen, and medications as prescribed *to maintain fluid volume and organ perfusion.*

Collect and evaluate serum laboratory specimens *to provide data to effectively treat underlying medical condition and avoid complication of shock.*

<u>Inform:</u> Educate patient and family of reportable signs and symptoms of inadequate perfusion, for example, dizziness, confusion, restlessness, and dyspnea. *Early intervention and treatment is essential in preventing permanent organ damage.*

<u>Attend:</u> Encourage patient and family to express concerns and fears *to reduce anxiety*.

<u>Manage:</u> Collaborate with other members of the health care team *to effectively manage underlying medical condition and prevent complications*.

SUGGESTED NIC INTERVENTIONS

Acid–Base Management; Acid–Base Monitoring; Fluid/Electrolyte Management; Hypovolemia Management; Shock Management; Laboratory Data Interpretation

REFERENCE

Moore, K. (2011, November). Managing hemorrhagic shock in trauma: Are we still drowning patients in the field? *Journal of Emergency Nursing, 37*(6), 594–596.

DEFINITION
Altered epidermis and/or dermis

DEFINING CHARACTERISTICS
- Destruction of skin layers
- Disruption of skin surface
- Invasion of body structures

RELATED FACTORS
- External: chemical substances, extremes in age, humidity, hyper- or hypothermia, mechanical factors—shearing forces, pressure, restraint, medications, moisture, physical immobilization, and radiation
- Internal: changes in fluid status, pigmentation, or turgor; developmental factors; imbalanced nutritional state—obesity, emaciation; immunological deficit; impaired circulation, metabolic state, or sensation; skeletal prominence

ASSESSMENT FOCUS
(Refer to comprehensive assessment parameters.)
- Activity/exercise
- Knowledge
- Nutrition
- Tissue integrity

EXPECTED OUTCOMES
The patient will
- Show no evidence of skin breakdown.
- Show normal skin turgor.
- Regain skin integrity (specify); for example, pressure ulcer will decrease in size.
- Have a healed surgical wound.
- Communicate understanding of skin protection measures.
- Demonstrate skill in care of wound, burn, or incision.
- Demonstrate skin inspection technique.
- Perform skin care routine.
- Communicate feelings about change in body image.

SUGGESTED NOC OUTCOMES
Immobility Consequences: Physiological; Tissue Integrity: Skin & Mucous Membranes; Tissue Perfusion: Peripheral; Wound Healing: Primary Intention; Wound Healing: Secondary Intention; Body Image

INTERVENTIONS AND RATIONALES
Determine: Inspect skin every shift. Describe and document skin condition, and report changes. *These measures provide evidence of the effectiveness of the skin care regimen.*

Monitor frequency of turning and skin condition *to reduce pressure, promote circulation, and minimize skin breakdown.*

Perform: Perform prescribed treatment regimen for the skin condition involved and monitor progress. Report responses to the treatment regimen *to maintain or modify current therapy.*

Provide supportive measures, as indicated:

- Assist with general hygiene and comfort measures *to promote comfort and sense of well-being.*
- Administer pain medication and monitor its effectiveness. *Patient needs pain relief to maintain health.*
- Maintain proper environmental conditions *to promote patient's sense of well-being.*
- Use a foam mattress, bed cradle, or other devices *to minimize skin breakdown.*
- Warn against tampering with the wound or dressings *to reduce potential for infection.*
- Maintain infection control standards *to reduce the risk of spreading disease.*

Position patient for comfort and minimal pressure on bony prominences. Change his or her position at least every 2 hours. *These measures reduce pressure, promote circulation, and minimize skin breakdown.*

Inform: Explain the therapy to patient and family members *to encourage compliance.*

Instruct patient and family members in a skin care regimen *to encourage compliance.* Supervise patient and family members in skin care management. Provide feedback *to improve skill in managing skin care.*

Attend: Allow patient to express his or her feelings about skin problem. *Verbalization of feelings helps allay anxiety and develops coping skills.*

Manage: Provide a referral to a psychiatric liaison nurse, social service, or support group, as appropriate, *to provide additional support for patient and his or her family.*

SUGGESTED NIC INTERVENTIONS

Fluid Management; Infection Protection; Positioning; Pressure Management; Pressure Ulcer Care; Pressure Ulcer Prevention; Skin Surveillance; Wound Care; Body Image Enhancement

REFERENCE

Kinnunen, U. M., et al. (2012, July–August). Developing the standardized wound care documentation model: A Delphi study to improve the quality of patient care documentation. *Journal of Wound Ostomy Continence Nursing, 39*(4), 397–407.

DEFINITION
At risk for alteration in epidermis and/or dermis

RISK FACTORS
- External: chemical substances, extremes in age, humidity, hyper- or hypothermia, mechanical factors—shearing forces, pressure, restraint, medications, moisture, physical immobilization, radiation
- Internal: changes in fluid status, pigmentation, or turgor; developmental factors; imbalanced nutritional state—obesity, emaciation; immunological deficit; impaired circulation, metabolic state, or sensation; skeletal prominence

ASSESSMENT FOCUS
(Refer to comprehensive assessment parameters.)
- Activity/exercise
- Knowledge
- Nutrition
- Tissue integrity

EXPECTED OUTCOMES
The patient will
- Experience no skin breakdown.
- Maintain muscle strength and joint range of motion (ROM).
- Sustain adequate food and fluid intake.
- Have intact mucous membranes.
- Maintain adequate skin circulation.
- Communicate understanding of preventive skin care measures.
- Demonstrate preventive skin care measures.
- Correlate risk factors and preventive measures.

SUGGESTED NOC OUTCOMES
Immobility Consequences: Physiological; Nutritional Status; Physical Aging; Risk Control; Risk Detection; Tissue Integrity: Skin & Mucous Membranes; Joint Movement

INTERVENTIONS AND RATIONALES
<u>Determine:</u> Inspect skin every shift. Describe and document skin condition and report changes. *These measures provide evidence of the effectiveness of the skin care regimen.*

Monitor nutritional intake and maintain adequate hydration. *Anemia (<10 mg hemoglobin) and low serum albumin concentrations (<2 mg) are associated with the development of pressure ulcers. Hydration helps maintain skin integrity.*

<u>Perform:</u> Change patient's position at least every 2 hours following turning schedule posted at bedside. Monitor frequency of turning. *These measures reduce pressure on tissues, promote circulation, and help prevent skin breakdown.*

Use preventive skin care devices, as needed, such as a foam mattress, alternating pressure mattress, sheepskin, pillows, and padding, *to avoid discomfort and skin breakdown.*

Keep patient's skin clean and dry and lubricate as needed. Avoid the use of irritating soap, and rinse skin well. *These measures alleviate skin dryness, promote comfort, and reduce the risk of irritation and skin breakdown.*

Protect bony prominences with foam padding. *Prominences have little subcutaneous fat and are prone to breakdown; using foam padding may help promote skin integrity.*

Lift patient's body when moving him or her, using a lifting sheet, if needed. Avoid shearing force. *Shearing force results when tissues slide against each other; a lifting sheet reduces sliding.*

Keep linen dry, clean, and free from wrinkles or crumbs. Change wet bed linens and incontinence pads immediately. *Dry, smooth linens help prevent excoriation and skin breakdown.*

Inform: Educate patient and family in preventive skin care ways to maintain good personal hygiene including use of nonirritating (nonalkaline) soap, patting rather than rubbing skin dry; inspecting skin regularly; avoiding prolonged exposure to water, sun, cold, and wind; avoiding rubber rings, recognizing the beginning of skin breakdown (redness, blisters, and discoloration); and reporting signs and symptoms. *These measures explain the importance of practicing preventive skin care measures to encourage compliance with skin care regimen.*

Supervise patient and family in preventive skin care measures and provide constructive feedback. Practice helps improve skill in managing the skin care regimen and encourages compliance.

Attend: Encourage ambulation or perform or assist with active ROM exercises at least every 4 hours while patient is awake. *Exercises prevent muscle atrophy and contracture. Ambulation promotes circulation and relieves pressure.*

Manage: Indicate the risk factor potential on patient's chart and care plan and reevaluate weekly, using an accepted form such as the Braden Scale. *The risk factor score helps evaluate treatment progress.*

SUGGESTED NIC INTERVENTIONS

Circulatory Precautions; Infection Prevention; Positioning; Pressure Management; Pressure Ulcer Prevention; Skin Surveillance; Splinting

REFERENCE

Rush, A., & Muir, M. (2012, April). Maintaining skin integrity in bariatric patients. *British Journal of Community Nursing, 17*(4), 154, 156–159.

DEFINITION

Prolonged periods of time without sleep (sustained natural, periodic suspension of relative consciousness)

DEFINING CHARACTERISTICS

- Acute confusion
- Agitation
- Anxiety
- Apathy
- Combativeness
- Daytime drowsiness
- Decreased ability to function
- Fatigue
- Fleeting nystagmus
- Hallucinations
- Hand tremors
- Heightened sensitivity to pain
- Irritability
- Malaise
- Restlessness
- Slowed reaction
- Transient paranoia

RELATED FACTORS

- Aging-related sleep stage shifts
- Dementia
- Familial sleep paralysis
- Idiopathic central nervous system hypersomnolence
- Narcolepsy
- Nightmares
- Periodic limb movement
- Sleep apnea
- Sundowner's syndrome
- Sustained uncomfortable sleep environment or circadian asynchrony
- Prolonged discomfort, use of antisoporifics, or pharmaceutical agents

ASSESSMENT FOCUS

(Refer to comprehensive assessment parameters.)

- Comfort
- Coping
- Emotional
- Knowledge
- Pharmacologic function
- Sleep/rest

EXPECTED OUTCOMES

The patient will

- Identify factors that prevent or disrupt sleep.
- Achieve uninterrupted sleep for ____ hour(s).
- Express feelings of being well rested.
- Show no signs of physical sleep deprivation.
- Alter diet and habits to promote sleep.
- Not exhibit sleep-related behavioral symptoms, such as irritability, lethargy, listlessness, restlessness, anxiety, worry, or depression.
- Perform relaxation exercises at bedtime.

SUGGESTED NOC OUTCOMES

Concentration; Endurance; Energy Conservation; Mood Equilibrium; Rest; Sleep; Stress Level; Symptom Severity

INTERVENTIONS AND RATIONALES

Determine: Assess usual sleep patterns, daytime activity and work patterns, recent life changes, sleep environment, activities that promote sleep, and dietary and drug history. *Information gained during the assessment will assist in identifying outcomes and interventions.*

Perform: Offer interventions to promote sleep, such as a warm bath, back rub, comfortable positioning, additional pillows, and food or drink. *Personal hygiene routine precedes sleep for many individuals. Milk and some high-protein snacks like cheese or nuts contain L-tryptophan and are sleep promoters.*

Inform: Teach patient relaxation techniques such as guided imagery, meditation, and progressive muscle relaxation. Practice them with patient at bedtime. *Purposeful relaxation efforts commonly promote sleep.*

Instruct patient to limit alcohol and caffeine intake. Avoid foods and beverages with caffeine 4 to 5 hours before bedtime. *Dietary changes may help promote restful sleep.*

Advise patient to avoid daytime naps *to promote restful nocturnal sleep.*

Attend: Encourage patient to discuss factors in the environment that make sleeping difficult. *A strange or new environment may affect rapid-eye-movement and non-rapid-eye-movement sleep.*

Ask patient what changes would help promote sleep (such as reducing noise, changing medication or treatment schedule, or changing lighting) *to encourage patient to play an active role in care.* Make immediate changes to accommodate patient.

Avoid quick, unanticipated movements when turning and positioning patients with neuromuscular dysfunction *to prevent spasticity, which may interrupt sleep.*

Manage: Suggest a referral to sleep disorder center especially if daily activities are affected or sleep apnea occurs. *A specialist may be required to assist in treatment.*

Help patients with chronic illnesses or disabilities find resources for addressing psychosocial issues. *Fears and concerns about future prevent restful sleep.*

SUGGESTED NIC INTERVENTIONS

Anxiety Reduction; Energy Management; Comfort; Progressive Muscle Relaxation; Sleep Enhancement; Guided Imagery; Meditation Facilitation; Relaxation Therapy

REFERENCE

Stuck, A., Clark, M. J., & Connelly, C. D. (2011, November–December). Preventing intensive care delirium: A patient-care centered approach to reducing sleep disruption. *Dimensions in Critical Care Nursing, 30*(6), 315–320.

DEFINITION

A pattern of natural, periodic suspension of consciousness that provides adequate rest, sustains a desired lifestyle, and can be strengthened

DEFINING CHARACTERISTICS

- Amount of sleep is congruent with developmental needs
- Expresses a feeling of rest after sleep
- Expresses willingness to enhance sleep
- Follows sleep routines that promote sleep habits
- Occasional use of medications to induce sleep

ASSESSMENT FOCUS

(Refer to comprehensive assessment parameters.)

- Activities
- Knowledge
- Pharmacologic function
- Sleep/rest

EXPECTED OUTCOMES

The patient will
- Identify factors that enhance readiness for sleep.
- Demonstrate readiness for enhanced sleep through the use of appropriate sleep hygiene measures.
- Express feeling rested after sleep.
- Have an appropriate amount of sleep and rapid-eye-movement sleep that is congruent with developmental needs.

SUGGESTED NOC OUTCOMES

Anxiety Level; Rest; Sleep

INTERVENTIONS AND RATIONALES

Determine: Assess daytime activity and work patterns; cognitive status; daytime consequences of sleeplessness; sleep environment; quality and duration of sleep; recent changes in health status or lifestyle; and dietary and drug history, including ingestion of caffeine or other stimulants.

Assessment information will help identify appropriate outcomes and interventions.

Perform: Give warm, light snacks containing protein at bedtime and small amounts of liquid *to promote a sense of comfort.*

Provide a cup of water close to bedtime *to avoid dry mouth and help return to sleep after awakening.*

Inform: Educate patient about normal age-related changes to sleep and strategies that are specific to the patient's health status, lifestyle, and environment *to decrease anxiety about sleeplessness.*

Teach patient to relax before going to bed, using music, reading, meditation, or other soothing or comforting activities *to enhance ability to sleep.*

Instruct patient to avoid dietary substances and drugs that may influence sleep, including ingestion of caffeine or other stimulants, nicotine, alcohol, sedatives, hypnotics, and fluid intake, *to enhance the ability to sleep.*

Attend· Encourage patient to make a log of sleep and wake times, number of awakenings, total time asleep, quality of sleep, and any precipitating factors that may influence sleep *to determine sleep efficiency.*

Manage: If patient begins having difficulties in sleeping, recommend a behavior modification plan based on assessment of condition, patient's history, and precipitating factors *to enhance compliance.*

SUGGESTED NIC INTERVENTIONS

Comfort; Sleep Enhancement; Environmental Management: Comfort; Progressive Muscle Relaxation; Journaling

REFERENCE

Donnelly, G. F., et al. (2012, August). From the editor: Biological rhythms: The color of light and the quality of sleep. *Holistic Nursing Practice, 26*(4), 181.

DEFINITION

Time limited interruptions of sleep amount and quality due to external factors

DEFINING CHARACTERISTICS

- Change in normal sleep pattern
- Dissatisfaction with sleep
- Decreased ability to function
- Reports being awakened
- Reports no difficulty falling asleep
- Reports not feeling well rested

RELATED FACTORS

- Ambient humidity or temperature
- Caregiving responsibilities
- Change in daylight-darkness exposure
- Interruptions (e.g., monitoring, lab tests)
- Lack of sleep control and/or privacy
- Lighting, noise, noxious odors, physical restraint
- Sleep partner
- Unfamiliar sleep furnishings

ASSESSMENT FOCUS

(Refer to comprehensive assessment parameters.)

- Comfort
- Coping
- Emotional
- Knowledge
- Pharmacologic function
- Sleep/rest

EXPECTED OUTCOMES

The patient will

- Identify factors that changed usual sleep pattern.
- Achieve uninterrupted sleep for _____ hour(s).
- Express feelings of being well rested.
- Alter diet and habits to promote sleep.
- Incorporate sleep preparation measures into evening routine.
- Perform relaxation exercise.

SUGGESTED NOC OUTCOMES

Rest; Sleep; Well-Being; Symptom Control

INTERVENTIONS AND RATIONALES

<u>Determine:</u> Complete a sleep history and help patient identify factors that may impair sleep. *Review of patterns may elicit insights that can be used to correct the problem.*

Assist patient to identify environmental factors that make sleeping difficult. Suggest the use of "white noise" machines to mask unwanted noise. *A strange or new environment may affect rapid-eye-movement and non-rapid-eye-movement sleep.*

Ask patient what changes would help promote sleep *to encourage patient to play an active role in care.*

Ask patient to evaluate the quality of sleep the night before *to help detect sleep-related behavioral symptoms.*

Assess the daytime schedule to ensure adequate time for rest. *Excessive fatigue can result in insomnia.*

Perform: Offer interventions to promote sleep, such as a warm bath, back rub, comfortable positioning, additional pillows, and food or drink. *Personal hygiene routine precedes sleep for many individuals. Milk and some high-protein snacks like cheese or nuts contain* L-tryptophan *and are sleep promoters.*

Inform: Teach patient relaxation techniques such as guided imagery, meditation, and progressive muscle relaxation. *Purposeful relaxation efforts commonly promote sleep.*

Instruct patient to limit alcohol and caffeine intake. Avoid foods and beverages with caffeine 4 to 5 hours before bedtime. *Dietary changes may help promote restful sleep.*

Advise patient to avoid daytime naps *to promote restful nocturnal sleep.*

Attend: Encourage regular evening routines that promote sleep, such as taking a warm bath or eating a small snack. *Personal hygiene routine precedes sleep for many individuals. Milk and some high-protein snacks, such as cheese or nuts, contain L-tryptophan, a sleep promoter.*

Manage: Refer patient experiencing extended sleep changes to a sleep disorder center especially if activities of daily living are affected or sleep apnea occurs. *A specialist may be required to assist in treatment.*

SUGGESTED NIC INTERVENTIONS

Anxiety Reduction; Simple Guided Imagery; Energy Management; Environmental Management: Comfort; Progressive Muscle Relaxation; Sleep Enhancement; Anticipatory Guidance; Calming Technique; Simple Relaxation Therapy

REFERENCE

Gregory, P., Morgan, K., & Lynall, A. (2012, January). Improving sleep management in people with Parkinson's. *British Journal of Community Nursing, 17*(1), 14–8, 20.

DEFINITION
Insufficient or excessive quantity or ineffective quality of social exchange

DEFINING CHARACTERISTICS
- Discomfort in social situations
- Dysfunctional interaction with others
- Family report of change in style of interaction
- Inability to receive or communicate satisfying sense of belonging, caring, interest, or shared history
- Use of unsuccessful social interaction

RELATED FACTORS
- Absence of significant others
- Communication barriers
- Deficit about ways to enhance mutuality
- Environmental barriers
- Limited physical mobility
- Disturbed thought processes
- Self-concept disturbance
- Sociocultural dissonance
- Therapeutic isolation

ASSESSMENT FOCUS
(Refer to comprehensive assessment parameters.)
- Behavior
- Communication
- Coping
- Knowledge
- Self-perception

EXPECTED OUTCOMES
The patient will
- Provide information concerning cultural background.
- Identify needs and communicate (verbally or through behavior) whether needs are met.
- Express understanding of care-related instructions.
- Participate in planning care.
- Identify effective coping techniques to deal with sociocultural differences.
- Express feelings of comfort and trust in interacting with caregivers.
- Use resources outside normal sociocultural group, as necessary.

SUGGESTED NOC OUTCOMES
Communication; Social Interaction Skills; Social Involvement; Stress Levels; Client Satisfaction: Cultural Needs Fulfillment

INTERVENTIONS AND RATIONALES

<u>Determine:</u> Assess sociocultural background; usual pattern of social interaction; dominant language; position in family; support systems, including clergy, family members, and friends; and education and level of intelligence. *Assessment information will help identify appropriate outcomes and interventions.*

<u>Perform:</u> Assist patient with self-care activities of bathing, grooming, eating, and toileting. Encourage patient to do as much as possible *in order to reduce feelings of helplessness and to build a sense of control over current situation.*

Explain care-related activities clearly and answer questions as accurately as possible *to enhance the patient's understanding of procedures and facility routines.*

<u>Inform:</u> Teach patient to use effective social interaction behaviors, such as increased eye contact, calling people by name, and asking questions. *Teaching patient effective communication skills helps him or her function more effectively in a social environment.*

<u>Attend:</u> Provide a specific time to talk to the patient and family about their sociocultural background. *In many cultural groups, trust develops slowly and may be hampered by lengthy interviews.*

Involve patient and family members in planning care and in encouraging patient's participation in self care *to increase their sense of control over the present situation.*

Demonstrate respect for the patient's privacy, personal belongings, cultural norms, and religious beliefs and practices to demonstrate sensitivity to patients from varied cultural backgrounds.

<u>Manage:</u> Use an interpreter when necessary to ensure effective communication with non-English-speaking patients. *The primary reasons to use an interpreter to communicate with a patient are legal and financial and to provide quality care.*

Involve family, friends, and clergy *to provide appropriate spiritual support.*

SUGGESTED NIC INTERVENTIONS

Behavior Modification: Social Skills; Active Listening; Anxiety Reduction; Coping Enhancement; Family Support; Normalization Promotion Spiritual Support; Family Integrity Promotion; Cultural Brokerage

REFERENCE

Smith, S., Dewar, B., et al. (2010, June). Relationship centered outcomes focused on compassionate care for older people within inpatient settings. *International Journal of Older People Nursing, 5*(2), 128–136.

DEFINITION
Aloneness experienced by the individual and perceived as imposed by others and as a negative or threatening state

DEFINING CHARACTERISTICS
- Culturally unacceptable behavior
- Description of lifestyle as solitary or circumscribed by membership in subculture
- Evidence of physical or mental disability or altered state of wellness
- Expressed feelings of being different from others
- Expressed feelings of rejection or aloneness
- Expressed frustration over inability to meet expectations of others
- Inappropriate or immature interests or activities
- Insecurity in public
- Lack of family, friends, and social groups
- Lack of purpose in life
- Preoccupation with own thoughts
- Projection of hostility in voice and behavior
- Repetitive, meaningless actions
- Sad, dull affect
- Uncommunicative and withdrawn behavior (with poor eye contact)

RELATED FACTORS
- Alterations in mental status
- Alterations in physical appearance
- Altered state of wellness
- Immature interests
- Inability to engage in satisfying personal relationships
- Inadequate personal resources
- Unaccepted social values
- Unaccepted social behavior

ASSESSMENT FOCUS
(Refer to comprehensive assessment parameters.)
- Behavior
- Coping
- Emotional
- Self-perception

EXPECTED OUTCOMES
The patient will
- Express feelings associated with social isolation.
- Identify possible causes of social isolation and participate in developing plan for increasing social activity.
- Interact with family members, friends, and caregivers.
- Perform self-care activities independently.
- Participate daily in meaningful diversional activity.
- Indicate that social relationships have improved and negative feelings have diminished.
- Achieve expected state of wellness.

SUGGESTED NOC OUTCOMES
Leisure Participation; Loneliness Severity; Personal Well-Being; Social Interaction Skills; Social Involvement; Social Support

INTERVENTIONS AND RATIONALES

<u>Determine:</u> Assess reason for hospitalization, family support systems available, functional ability, financial resources, occupation, educational level, and coping and problem-solving ability. *Assessment information will assist in identifying appropriate outcomes and interventions.*

<u>Perform:</u> Assist patient with daily self-care activities, such as bathing, grooming, dressing, eating, and ambulating. Encourage patient to take on more of this responsibility for self, as he or she is able. *This will reduce feelings of helplessness.*

<u>Inform:</u> Teach self-healing techniques to both the patient and the family such as meditation, guided imagery, yoga, and prayer *to prevent anxiety and aid in keeping patient in a frame of mind to make positive decisions.*

Teach patient coping techniques *to help increase ability to deal with especially challenging situations.*

Provide patient with concise information about decision-making skills *to produce benefits that can reinforce health-seeking behaviors.*

<u>Attend:</u> Encourage patient to express feelings about herself (past and present). *Self-exploration encourages patient to consider future change.*

Encourage patient to identify the causes of social isolation *to help her to develop a plan to reduce the isolation she is experiencing.*

Provide private time for patient to spend with family, including specific amount of noncore time to engage patient in conversation. *Such discussions help patient assume responsibility for coping responses.*

Provide patient with positive feedback for verbal reports or behaviors that indicate a return to positive self-appraisal. *This gives patient feelings of significance, approval, and competence, which can help her cope effectively with stressful situations.*

Provide emotional support to family by being available to answer questions. *Accurate information will help family cope with current situation.*

<u>Manage:</u> Arrange with patient specific periods for appropriate diversional activity *to provide pleasure, increase feelings of self-worth, and decrease negative self-absorption.*

Schedule time to meet with family and patient to listen to ways in which they plan to enhance their coping skills in the present situation.

Refer family to community resources and support groups available *to assist in managing patient's illness and providing emotional and financial assistance to caregivers.*

SUGGESTED NIC INTERVENTIONS

Behavior Modification: Social Skills; Activity Therapy; Family Integrity Promotion; Mood Management; Socialization Enhancement; Support System Enhancement; Therapy Group

REFERENCE

Viner, R. M., et al. (2012, April). Adolescence and the social determinants of health. *Lancet, 379*(9826), 1641–1652.

DEFINITION

Cyclical, recurring, and potentially progressive pattern of pervasive sadness experienced (by a parent, a caregiver, and an individual with chronic illness or disability) in response to continual loss, throughout the trajectory of an illness or disability

DEFINING CHARACTERISTICS

- Expressed feelings that vary in intensity, are periodic, may progress and intensify over time, and may interfere with patient's ability to reach highest level of personal and social well-being
- Expressions of one or more of the following: anger, being misunderstood, confusion, depression, disappointment, emptiness, fear, frustration, guilt or self-blame, helplessness, hopelessness, loneliness, low self-esteem, recurring loss, and being overwhelmed
- Expressions of periodic, recurrent feeling of sadness

RELATED FACTORS

- Crisis in management of the disability or illness
- Crisis related to developmental stages
- Death of a loved one
- Experiences chronic disability or illness (e.g., physical or mental)
- Missed opportunities
- Missed milestones
- Unending caregiving

ASSESSMENT FOCUS

(Refer to comprehensive assessment parameters.)

- Behavior
- Communication
- Coping
- Emotional
- Nutrition
- Sleep patterns
- Values/beliefs

EXPECTED OUTCOMES

The patient will

- Identify losses associated with changes in health status.
- Express feelings about changes in health status.
- Seek assistance in dealing with emotions related to loss.
- Develop healthy coping mechanisms such as open expression of grief.
- Seek out support from family, friends, clergy, or others when necessary.
- Begin to plan for discharge and the future.
- Express realistic expectations with regard to health.

SUGGESTED NOC OUTCOMES

Acceptance: Health Status; Depression; Self-Control; Hope; Mood Equilibrium

INTERVENTIONS AND RATIONALES

<u>Determine:</u> Assess history of recent loss; usual pattern of coping; behavioral manifestation of grief and loss; sleep problems; lifestyle changes related to the situation; appetite; change in weight; religious beliefs and practices; and sources of support. *Assessment information will help identify appropriate outcomes and interventions.*

<u>Perform:</u> For patient who has lost weight, weigh daily at the same time *to evaluate improvements in nutrition.*

Provide bathing, grooming, and other hygiene functions for patient every day, as needed. Encourage patient to do as much as possible for himself or herself. *Greater independence will help build self-esteem.*

<u>Inform:</u> Teach skills that enhance coping strategies and relaxation strategies such as meditation, guided imagery, yoga, and exercise. *These mechanisms help reduce the level of anxiety that prevents the patient from coping with grief and loss.*

<u>Attend:</u> Let patient know that expressions of anger are acceptable, but place limits on destructive behavior. *Inability to identify anger as a normal response to loss may cause patient to express aggression inappropriately.*

Encourage patient to reach out to people who can offer emotional support in order to increase emotional support. *Sensitive listening provides emotional support that can allow the patient to broaden his or her focus beyond the cause of the sorrow.*

Encourage patient and family to reminisce. *Engaging in life review promotes a peaceful atmosphere and helps understanding the meaning of loss in relation to health and life.*

Encourage patient to take an active part in setting goals for health care *to facilitate independence and enhance self-esteem.*

<u>Manage:</u> Help patient involve the family, community, clergy, and friends with changes to the care plan *to increase the potential of the patient's control over self-care outcomes.*

Refer patient and family to other professional caregivers (e.g., dietitian, social worker, clergy, mental health professional). *Support groups can be helpful to the patient and the family.*

SUGGESTED NIC INTERVENTIONS

Coping Enhancement; Decision-Making Support; Emotional Support; Hope Installation; Mood Management; Spiritual Support; Guided Imagery; Reminiscence Therapy

REFERENCE

Whittingham, K., Wee, D., Sanders, M. R., & Boyd, R. (2012, June 8). Predictors of psychological adjustment, experienced parenting burden and chronic sorrow symptoms in parents of children with cerebral palsy. *Child Care Health Development.*

DEFINITION

Impaired ability to experience and integrate meaning and purpose in life through connectedness with self, others, art, music, literature, nature, and/or a power greater than oneself

DEFINING CHARACTERISTICS

- Connections to self: anger; expressed lack of acceptance, courage, hope, love, meaning or purpose in life, self-forgiveness, serenity; guilt, ineffective coping
- Connections with others: expresses alienation, refuses interactions with significant others or spiritual leaders, verbalizes separation from support system
- Connections with art, music, literature, and nature: disinterest in nature or in reading spiritual literature, inability to express previous state of creativity
- Connections with power greater than self: expresses anger toward power greater than self, feeling abandoned, hopelessness, suffering; inability for introspection, to experience the transcendent, to participate in religious activities, to pray; requests to see a spiritual leader; sudden changes in spiritual practices

RELATED FACTORS

- Active dying
- Anxiety
- Chronic illness
- Death
- Life change
- Loneliness
- Pain
- Self-alienation
- Social alienation
- Sociocultural deprivation

ASSESSMENT FOCUS

(Refer to comprehensive assessment parameters.)

- Communication
- Coping
- Emotional
- Values/beliefs

EXPECTED OUTCOMES

The patient will

- Communicate conflicts about beliefs.
- Identify understanding of source of spiritual conflict.
- Specify whatever spiritual assistance is perceived as needed.
- Discuss beliefs about religious practices.
- Identify coping techniques to deal with spiritual discomfort and not harm self while in the hospital.

SUGGESTED NOC OUTCOME

Suffering Severity; Hope; Quality of Life; Spiritual Health

INTERVENTIONS AND RATIONALES

Determine: Assess behavioral responses; coping strategies; experiences with illness; knowledge; environment, social factors; spiritual beliefs and practices; and spiritual support system. *Assessment information will help the nurse identify appropriate interventions.*

Perform: Assist the patient to list those aspects of spiritual care he or she would like the hospital to provide. *Having documentation from the patient is useful to communicate the patient's spiritual needs with the staff.*

Spend time with the patient developing goals for skill development that will help the patient deal with his or her current diagnosis. *Without the necessary skills, the patient will continue to feel distressed and anxious.*

Inform: Teach patient's coping strategies to family members and friends so *they can help patient practice adaptive methods of coping with self-destructive feelings.*

Have patient and family members practice role-playing *to increase the confidence in the patient's ability to handle difficult situations.*

Teach self-healing techniques and relaxation strategies to both the patient and family such as meditation, aromatherapy, guided imagery, yoga, and prayer. *These techniques can reduce the anxiety that comes from attempting to cope with his or her disease.* Teach patient how to incorporate the use of self-healing techniques in carrying out usual daily activities.

Self-healing gives the patient a better sense of control over regaining independence.

Attend: Acknowledge patient's spiritual concerns and encourage expression of thoughts and feelings *to help build a therapeutic relationship.*

For the patient whose spiritual comfort is derived from music, art, or nature, attempt to find such items (e.g., CD's, posters, or picture books) that will provide spiritual nourishment. *Not everyone finds spiritual comfort in organized religion. Each person is entitled to find spiritual hope and consolation in whatever way his or her needs are met.*

Encourage patient to continue religious practices while in the hospital; do whatever you must to facilitate this. *These measures demonstrate support and convey caring and acceptance.*

Manage: Communicate and collaborate with patient's clergy person or with the hospital chaplain, as appropriate. *This ensures consistent care and provides a more complete database.*

SUGGESTED NIC INTERVENTIONS

Active Listening; Hope Instillation; Referral; Spiritual Growth Facilitation; Spiritual Support; Guided Imagery; Aromatherapy; Religious Ritual Enhancement

REFERENCE

Lin, W. C., et al. (2011, March). Spiritual well-being in patients with rheumatoid arthritis. *The Journal of Nursing Research, 19*(1), 1–12.

DEFINITION

At risk for an impaired ability to experience and integrate meaning and purpose in life through connectedness with self, others, art, music, literature, nature, and/or a power greater than oneself

RISK FACTORS

Physical
- Physical illness, including chronic illness
- Substance abuse, excessive drinking

Psychosocial
- Low self-esteem
- Depression, anxiety, and stress
- Poor relationships
- Separation from support systems
- Blocks to experiencing love
- Inability to forgive
- Loss
- Racial or cultural conflict
- Change in religious rituals and practices

Developmental
- Life change
- Developmental life changes

Environmental
- Environmental changes
- Natural disasters

ASSESSMENT FOCUS

(Refer to comprehensive assessment parameters.)
- Behavior
- Coping
- Emotional
- Self-perception
- Values/beliefs

EXPECTED OUTCOMES

The patient will
- Discuss current beliefs and concerns.
- Discuss effects of illness, injury, or disability on beliefs and spiritual practices.
- Express feelings of spiritual well-being.
- Use healthy coping techniques to maintain spiritual well-being.
- Refrain from causing harm to self.
- Be supported in efforts to pursue spirituality in coping with illness or disability.
- Reach out to family members, clergy, or friends for assistance.

SUGGESTED NOC OUTCOMES

Coping; Grief Resolution; Hope; Spiritual Health

INTERVENTIONS AND RATIONALES

<u>Determine:</u> Assess health history; impact of the current illness on lifestyle; spiritual status; religious affiliation; relationship with spiritual leaders; importance of spirituality in the patient's life; desire for help in coping with spiritual concerns; family status; and socioeconomic status. *Assessment information will assist in identifying appropriate interventions.*

<u>Inform:</u> Teach coping strategies that appeal to the patient such as meditation, relaxation, guided imagery. *This will help the patient focus on what he or she would like to achieve in his or her spiritual life.*

<u>Attend:</u> Express your willingness to discuss spirituality if the patient desires. *This helps reduce isolation and bring spiritual realities into the open.*

Be certain about understanding your own beliefs and accept the patient's beliefs even if they are different from your own. *It is essential to understand what you believe in order to listen and be nonjudgmental when listening to the patient. It is unacceptable for the nurse to argue with the patient about spiritual beliefs.*

Communicate to the patient that you accept his or her expression of spiritual concerns, even if his or her feelings are angry and negative to reassure him or her that his feelings are valid. *The feeling of acceptance will facilitate the patient's ability to express his or her spiritual issues more freely.*

Listen attentively to patient's discussion of spiritual concerns. *Thoughtful listening fosters open discussion.*

Encourage patient to discuss recent life-threatening experience *to help him or her clarify and cope with his or her feelings.*

Provide for continuation of the patient's religious practices. For example, help patient obtain ritual items and respect dietary restrictions, if possible, *to demonstrate support and convey caring and acceptance to patient.*

<u>Manage:</u> Collaborate with patient's clergy person or hospital chaplain *to develop a plan to integrate spiritual interventions into patient's care to ensure continuity of care.*

SUGGESTED NIC INTERVENTIONS

Active Listening; Anticipatory Guidance; Anxiety Reduction; Caregiver Support; Hope Instillation; Spiritual Growth Facilitation; Spiritual Support; Religious Ritual Enhancement

REFERENCE

Carson, V. B. (2011, September). What is the essence of spiritual care? *Journal of Spiritual Care Nursing, 28*(3), 173.

DEFINITION

A pattern of reliance on religious beliefs and/or participation in rituals of a particular faith tradition that is sufficient for well-being and can be strengthened

DEFINING CHARACTERISTICS

- Expresses desire to strengthen belief patterns that have provided religion, comfort, or customs in the past
- Questions belief patterns or customs that are harmful
- Rejects belief patterns or customs that are harmful
- Requests assistance to expand religious options; participation in prescribed religious beliefs; forgiveness; meeting with religious leader/facilitators; reconciliation; religious experiences or materials

ASSESSMENT FOCUS

(Refer to comprehensive assessment parameters.)

- Coping
- Emotional
- Knowledge
- Self-perception
- Values/beliefs

EXPECTED OUTCOMES

The patient will

- Discuss spiritual conflicts.
- Have opportunity to meet with chosen religious figure.
- Receive support in his efforts to pursue enhanced spiritual well-being.
- Pursue religious or spiritual practices to the extent he or she feels comfortable.
- Openly discuss effects of illness on his beliefs and other spiritual issues.
- Describe plan to continue to enhance spiritual well-being.
- Receive referrals for continued support.

SUGGESTED NOC OUTCOMES

Hope; Quality of Life; Spiritual Health; Comfort Status: Psychospiritual; Knowledge: Health Resources; Motivation; Personal Well-Being

INTERVENTIONS AND RATIONALES

<u>Determine:</u> Assess personal religion and church affiliation; perceptions of faith, life, death, suffering; support networks; beliefs opposed by family, friends, and health care providers. *Assessment of spiritual status will provide information that will assist in identifying expected outcomes and interventions for this diagnosis.*

<u>Perform:</u> Monitor the patient for signs of spiritual distress that might harm the patient's well-being (altered self-care, sleep pattern disturbance, and

change in eating and exercise habits). *This information will provide insight into changes in goals and interventions.*

Assess the significance of spirituality in the patient's life and in coping with illness. *Before the nurse can intervene in spiritual matters, she must determine whether spirituality is significant for the patient.*

<u>Inform:</u> Provide the patient with resources for coping with spiritual distress (such as referrals to religious or spiritual organizations or books on prayer or meditation) *to enhance the opportunity to attend to spiritual beliefs.*

If the nurse lacks knowledge about the patient's beliefs or practices, consult an authority on the patient's particular religion *to have accurate information when endeavoring to meet his or her individual needs.*

Discuss importance of maintaining a healthy diet, regular exercise, adequate sleep, and healthy interaction with family members and friends. *A patient who is predisposed to spiritual distress may neglect day-to-day well-being.*

<u>Attend:</u> Demonstrate to the patient that you are willing to discuss issues related to spirituality, such as the patient's view of God, how illness has affected his life, or how the hospital stay has affected his or her spiritual practices *to bring spiritual issues into the open.*

Praise patient's efforts to attend to his or her spiritual needs and encourage him or her to continue to develop spirituality after he or she leaves the health care setting *to reinforce the progress the patient has already made.*

<u>Manage:</u> Provide patient with referrals to appropriate religious groups, spiritually centered organizations, and social service organizations *to help provide additional support and to ensure continuity of care.*

Consider resources such as faith community nurses, home visiting services, and computer networks *to help provide continued opportunity for spiritual development and ensure continuity of care.*

SUGGESTED NIC INTERVENTIONS

Active Listening; Emotional Support; Hope Instillation; Presence; Spiritual Growth Facilitation; Spiritual Support; Referral

REFERENCE

Chase, S. K., et al. (2012, August). Sustaining health in faith community nursing practice: Emerging processes that support the development of a middle-range theory. *Holistic Nursing Practice, 26*(4), 221–227.

DEFINITION

Decreased energy reserves resulting in an individual's inability to maintain independent breathing adequate to support life

DEFINING CHARACTERISTICS

- Apprehension
- Decreased cooperation
- Decreased pO_2
- Decreased $SatO_2$
- Decreased tidal volume
- Dyspnea
- Increased heart rate
- Increased metabolic rate
- Increased pCO_2
- Increased restlessness
- Increased use of accessory muscles

RELATED FACTORS

- Metabolic factors
- Respiratory muscle fatigue

ASSESSMENT FOCUS

(Refer to comprehensive assessment parameters.)

- Cardiac function
- Coping
- Fluid and electrolytes
- Neurocognition
- Physical regulation
- Respiratory function

EXPECTED OUTCOMES

The patient will

- Maintain respiratory rate at 5 breaths/minutes within baseline.
- Demonstrate arterial blood gas (ABG) levels normal for that patient.
- Indicate feelings of comfort without pain or dyspnea.
- Have breathing pattern return to baseline.
- Demonstrate PaO_2 within normal limits as activity level increases.
- Breathe spontaneously after ventilation support is withdrawn.

SUGGESTED NOC OUTCOMES

Anxiety Level; Endurance; Energy Conservation; Respiratory Status: Gas Exchange; Ventilation; Vital Signs

INTERVENTIONS AND RATIONALES

<u>Determine:</u> Assess vital signs; respiratory status, including rate, rhythm and depth of respiration. Look for nasal flaring, effectiveness of cough; suctioning demands; sputum characteristics, including color, consistency, amount; ABGs; hemoglobin and hematocrit. *Assessment information will help identify appropriate outcomes and interventions.*

<u>Perform:</u> Check vital signs every 15 minutes to 1 hour *to detect tachypnea and tachycardia, both of which are early indicators of respiratory distress.*

Begin oxygen support using the smallest concentration needed *to make patient comfortable.* Monitor closely *to avoid oxygen toxicity.*

Place patient in Fowler's position *to increase comfort and facilitate adequate chest expansion and diaphragmatic excursion, thereby decreasing the work of breathing.*

Assist patient to progress gradually from bed rest to increased activity *to improve sense of well-being.*

Monitor vital signs and ABGs closely. If respiratory status is compromised, return to bed rest *to decrease metabolic rate and lower oxygen demands.*

<u>Inform:</u> Explain procedures to the patient, and describe specific sensations he or she may feel during each procedure. *Keeping patient informed about what to expect and when to expect it reduces anxiety.*

Teach self-healing techniques to both the patient and the family such as meditation, guided imagery, yoga, and prayer. Teach patient how to incorporate the use of self-healing techniques in carrying out usual daily activities. *These techniques help calm the mind, reduce anxiety, and promote ability to cooperate with treatment regimen.*

<u>Attend:</u> Avoid respiratory depressants such as opiates, sedatives, and paralytics because *these drugs will further depress the patient's ability to breathe adequately on his or her own and have the potential to cause respiratory arrest.*

Anticipate possible complications. Keep in mind that if the patient decompensates while on 100% fraction of inspired oxygen mask, she may require intubation. *Anticipating complications facilitates prompt intervention.*

<u>Manage:</u> If patient requires intubation, monitor him or her for spontaneous breathing and gradually wean him or her from ventilator. *Progressive weaning helps patient to adjust physiologically and emotionally to increased work of breathing.*

Refer patient and family to other professional caregivers, for example, dietitian, social worker, clergy, and mental health professional. Assist patient to utilize appropriate resources by contacting family and scheduling follow-up appointments. *These measures help give patient and family a sense of direction and control over future care.*

SUGGESTED NIC INTERVENTIONS

Acid–Base Management; Airway Suctioning; Artificial Airway Management; Coping Enhancement; Mechanical Ventilation; Oxygen Therapy; Positioning; Respiratory Monitoring; Self-Care Assistance; Guided Imagery

REFERENCE

Campbell, G. B. (2010, January/March). Symptom identification in the chronically critically ill. *AACN Advanced Critical Care, 21*(1), 64–79.

DEFINITION
Excessive amounts and types of demands that require action

DEFINING CHARACTERISTICS
- Demonstrates increased feelings of anger or impatience
- Reports feelings of pressure, tension, difficulty in functioning, excessive situational stress (e.g., rates stress level as 7 or above on a 10-point scale), anger, impatience, problems with decision-making
- Reports negative physical and psychological impact from stress such as "feeling of being sick or going to get sick"

RELATED FACTORS
- Inadequate resources (financial, social, educational)
- Intense, repeated stressors (family violence, chronic or terminal illness)
- Multiple coexisting stressors (environmental threats, physical threats)

ASSESSMENT FOCUS
(Refer to comprehensive assessment parameters.)

- Behavior
- Coping
- Emotional
- Pharmacological
- Self-perception
- Sleep/rest

EXPECTED OUTCOMES
The patient will
- Experience reduced signs of stress overload as evidenced by subjective report and observations of reduced stress, such as less facial tension and less restlessness.
- Connect environmental stressors with manifestations of stress such as insomnia, tearful outbursts, irritability, or headache.
- Set limits on activities assumed by saying "no" without expressions of guilt.
- Develop more effective coping strategies to manage stress such as guided imagery, exercise, healthy diet, and recreation and leisure activities.
- Develop strategies to reframe distorted thinking patterns relating to internal and environmental demands, such as talking about feelings and asking for help.

SUGGESTED NOC OUTCOMES
Abusive Behavior Self-Restraint; Aggression Self-Control; Anxiety Self-Control; Coping; Stress Level; Risk Control

INTERVENTIONS AND RATIONALES
<u>Determine:</u> Establish and promote a trusting relationship before asking patient to make any changes. *A trusting relationship can facilitate*

patient's attempts to make changes, whereas too many demands early in relationship can foster resistance.

<u>Perform:</u> Explore support systems with patient, such as appropriate Internet chat rooms, support groups, or hobbies and outings with partner or family and friends. *Often patient is caretaker who perceives there is little time for self and is at risk for caregiver burden. Promoting verbalization of feelings with support persons can reduce feeling of stress overload.*

Explore the lack of exercise and excessive intake of caffeine, alcohol, nicotine, and carbohydrates during periods of stress overload and adoption of healthier alternatives. *Inappropriate food choices, inactivity, and substance abuse can occur when patient feels stress overload.*

<u>Inform:</u> Teach prioritization of responsibilities and deadlines *to facilitate patient's sense of control over stressors. Stressors may seem overwhelming, and nurse can promote increased self-esteem when a plan is made cooperatively with nurse and patient as partners.*

Teach patient about positive self-talk *Positive self-talk helps change and, ultimately, reverse negative emotions of guilt, fear, and worry.*

Teach coping strategies such as reframing thoughts or using music, guided imagery, yoga, deep-breathing exercises, progressive neuromuscular relaxation, or pet therapy. *Strategies that reduce tense muscles and feelings can promote deeper relaxation and reduce heart rate, respirations, and blood pressure by promoting the parasympathetic response.*

Teach assertiveness training techniques with role-play exercises. *Assertiveness training can provide a concrete way to manage stressors and enhance feeling of being empowered, such as in communicating with demanding individuals.*

<u>Attend:</u> Provide opportunities for patient to ventilate feelings about stressors. *Promoting a time to talk can help the patient share his or her feelings of mounting stress before irritability and tension worsen.*

<u>Manage:</u> As needed, refer patient to a psychiatric liaison nurse, support group, or other mental health provider. *Stress may be an indicator of other more serious mental health problems.*

SUGGESTED NIC INTERVENTIONS

Anger Control Assistance; Assertiveness Training; Behavior Management; Behavior Modification; Calming Techniques; Cognitive Restructuring; Coping Enhancement; Impulse Control Training; Stress Management Assistance; Guided Imagery

REFERENCE

Taylor, S. G., & Kluemper, D. H. (2012, July). Linking perceptions of role and stress and incivility to workplace aggression: The moderating role of personality. *Journal of Occupational Health and Psychology, 17*(3), 316–329.

DEFINITION

Presence of risk factors for an infant under 1 year of age

RISK FACTORS

Modifiable

- Delayed prenatal care
- Infant overheating
- Infant over wrapping
- Infants placed to sleep in a prone position
- Infants placed to sleep in side-lying position
- Lack of prenatal care
- Prenatal or postnatal infant smoke exposure
- Soft underlayment (loose articles in the sleep environment)

Partially Modifiable

- Low birth weight
- Prematurity
- Young maternal age

Nonmodifiable

- Ethnicity (e.g., African American or Native American)
- Male gender
- Seasonality of sudden infant death syndrome (SIDS) (winter and fall)
- Infant age of 2 to 4 months

ASSESSMENT FOCUS

(Refer to comprehensive assessment parameters.)

- Sleep/rest
- Roles/responsibilities
- Values/beliefs

EXPECTED OUTCOMES

The parents will

- Be receptive to teaching and guidance.
- Verbalize understanding of risk factors and provide all precautions possible to prevent disorder.
- Verbalize feelings of preparedness and ability to handle emergencies utilizing cardiopulmonary resuscitation (CPR) techniques and services.
- Exhibit appropriate coping skills in dealing with high-risk infant.

The infant will

- Sleep alone in a crib on a firm sleep surface.
- Infant will be placed in proper position on back with head of crib slightly elevated.
- Maintain normal body temperature
- Monitored with an apnea monitor worn during sleep.

SUGGESTED NOC OUTCOMES

Knowledge: Infant Care; Knowledge: Parenting; Parent Performance; Risk Control; Risk Detection

INTERVENTIONS AND RATIONALES

<u>Determine:</u> Assess prenatal history; maternal history; parental experience; monitor heart rate, blood pressure; respiratory rate, quality, depth of

respirations, breath sounds; reflexes, response to touch. *The assessment information will assist in identifying appropriate interventions.*

Perform: Position infant on back when placed in the crib. *Incidence of SIDS is higher when infant is placed in a prone position.*

Elevate infant's head slightly when placed in the crib *to decrease abdominal pressure on diaphragm and allow better expansion of lungs.*

Place infant on a firm sleep surface *to prevent him or her from sinking into the mattress cover or blanket.*

Maintain room at appropriate temperature and avoid wrapping the infant in heavy blankets. *Excessive heat has been identified as a possible risk factor.*

Inform: Educate parents about risk factors of SIDS *because modification of current practices can reduce risk and prevent occurrence.* Instruct caregivers on ways to maintain a safe environment in the home. Provide written information to caregivers on all important aspects of the infant's care.

Teach parents to avoid having loose blankets, toys, or other articles in the crib *to decrease risk of accidental suffocation.*

Encourage mother to breastfeed *because there is a lower incidence of SIDS in babies who are breastfed.*

Teach parents how to correctly apply leads and set alarms of the apnea monitor. *The benefit of the monitor can be achieved only if it is used correctly.*

Instruct parents in CPR *to reduce anxiety and promote confidence in performing correct technique.* Allow time for return demonstrations *to prepare parents to cope with infant when he or she returns home.*

Attend: Encourage parents in their efforts to care for the infant. Provide suggestions for coping mechanisms *to help reduce the anxieties associated with caring for a high-risk infant.* Be aware that parents may be sensitive to your unspoken feelings about the situation.

Encourage parents to interact with other parents managing high-risk infants well. *Peer support may help to reduce fear in the parents.*

Involve parents in planning and decision making for their infant. *Investment in decision making will promote compliance with the plan.*

Manage: Refer to case manager/social worker/home health agency *to ensure that parents receive adequate support in caring for the infant.*

Refer parents to support group if one is available.

SUGGESTED NIC INTERVENTIONS

Family Support; Infant Care; Risk Control; Teaching: Infant Safety; Environmental Management; Safety

REFERENCE

Miller, L. C. (2011, August). Consequences of the "back to sleep" program on infants. *Journal of Pediatric Nursing, 269*(4), 364–328.

DEFINITION
Accentuated risk of accidental suffocation (inadequate air available for inhalation)

RISK FACTORS
- Access to unattended bathtub or pool (children)
- Consumption of large mouthfuls of food
- Discarded refrigerators or freezers with doors still in place
- Fuel-burning heater used in area without ventilation
- Habit of smoking in bed
- Household gas leaks
- Inserting small objects in airway
- Low-strung clotheslines
- Pacifier hung around neck (infant)
- Pillow in infant's crib
- Plastic bags or small objects within reach of children
- Propped bottle or pillow in infant's crib
- Vehicle left running in closed garage

ASSESSMENT FOCUS
(Refer to comprehensive assessment parameters.)
- Self-care
- Knowledge
- Values/beliefs

EXPECTED OUTCOMES
The patient will
- Demonstrate a patent airway at all times.
- Maintain vital signs within normal parameters.
- Demonstrate along with family knowledge of safety measures to prevent suffocation.

SUGGESTED NOC OUTCOMES
Aspiration Prevention; Personal Safety Behavior; Respiratory Status: Ventilation; Risk Control; Risk Detection; Knowledge: Personal Safety; Safe Home Environment

INTERVENTIONS AND RATIONALES
<u>Determine:</u> Assess vital signs; history of current situation; neurologic status; and hemoglobin, hematocrit, clotting factors, platelet count, and WBC; mental illness; history of abuse. *Assessment information will assist in formulating goals and interventions.*
<u>Perform:</u> Position patient on side or position head and neck *to prevent relaxed neck muscles from obstructing airway to allow maximal chest expansion and prevent aspiration and airway obstruction.*

Check all ventilator connections and alarms every 30 minutes if patient is on mechanical ventilation *to ensure that patient receives the proper amount of oxygen at appropriate volume and rate.*

Suction airway, as needed, *to prevent accumulation of* secretions. Suction only as needed *to prevent tracheal irritation.*

Position patient on his or her side or position his or her head and neck to prevent relaxed neck muscles from obstructing the airway. *This allows maximal chest expansion and prevents aspiration and airway obstruction.*

Obtain suction equipment, assemble, and keep at bedside *to ensure equipment readiness in case it is needed.*

Inform: Educate patient's family about safety measures in the home, for example, proper positioning, suction procedure, fall prevention *to enable them to take an active role in the patient's care and ensure performance of safety measures.*

Attend: Be attentive to the fears of both patient and family. Listen with sensitivity and reinforce safety measures to prevent injury *To achieve a level of comfort, the family may need to ask the same questions multiple times and have the information repeated frequently.*

Manage: Offer referral to counselors or support persons, as needed. *Many families will need additional support after hospitalization.*

SUGGESTED NIC INTERVENTIONS

Airway Management; Aspiration Precautions; Energy Management; Vital Signs Monitoring; Respiratory Monitoring; Security Enhancement; Surveillance

REFERENCE

Bayard, R. W., & Gilbert, J. D. (2011, November). Sleeping accidents in the elderly. *Journal of Forensic Services, 56*(6), 1645–1647.

DEFINITION

At risk for self-inflicted, life-threatening injury

RISK FACTORS

- Behavioral: Buying a gun, changing a will or creating a will, giving away possessions, history of prior attempts, marked changes in attitude or behavior, stockpiling medicines, or sudden euphoric recovery from depression
- Demographic: Age (e.g., elderly, young adult males, adolescents), divorced or widowed, gender (male), and race (e.g., Caucasian, Native American)
- Physical: Chronic pain, physical illness, or terminal illness
- Psychological: Childhood abuse, family history of suicide, gay or lesbian youth, guilt, psychiatric illness or disorder (e.g., depression, schizophrenia, bipolar disorder), or substance abuse
- Situational: Adolescents living in nontraditional settings (e.g., juvenile detention center, prison, half-way house, group home), economic instability, loss of autonomy or independence, relocation
- Social: Cluster suicides, disrupted family life, disciplinary problems, grief, helplessness, hopelessness, legal problems, loneliness, loss of important relationship, poor support systems, social isolation
- Verbal: States desire to die or makes threats of killing oneself

ASSESSMENT FOCUS

(Refer to comprehensive assessment parameters.)

- Behavior
- Coping
- Emotional
- Pharmacological function
- Self-perception

EXPECTED OUTCOMES

The patient will

- Discuss feelings that precipitate suicide attempts.
- Refrain from harming self.
- Recover from suicidal episode.
- Consult with mental health professional.
- Describe available resources for crisis prevention and management.
- Voice improvement in feelings of self-worth.

SUGGESTED NOC OUTCOMES

Impulse Self-Control; Self-Mutilation Restraint; Suicide Self-Restraint

INTERVENTIONS AND RATIONALES

<u>Determine:</u> Assess medical history, life situation, recent stressors, coping skills, history of suicidal attempts, history of substance abuse, safety hazards, and medications. *Assessment results will provide*

information that will assist in identifying goals and selecting appropriate interventions.

<u>Perform:</u> Initiate suicidal precaution protocol, including checks every 15 minutes *to ensure that the patient is protected and is in a safe environment.*

Make a short-term contract with the patient that he won't harm himself during a specific period. Continue negotiating until no evidence of suicidal ideation exists. *A contract gets the subject of suicide out in the open, places some responsibility for safety on the patient, and conveys acceptance of the patient as a worthwhile person.*

Remove anything from the patient's environment that could be used to inflict injury to self such as razor blades, belts, glass objects, knives, pills, cans, and mirrors. *This helps ensure the patient's safety.*

<u>Inform:</u> Provide the patient with telephone numbers and other information about crisis centers, hot lines, and counselors. *Alternatives may ease anxiety about the perceived threat of long-term psychotherapy.*

<u>Attend:</u> Use nonjudgmental manner *to show unconditional positive regard.*

Listen carefully to patient and avoid challenging him or her *in order to communicate caring and support.*

Demonstrate caring but do not reinforce denial of current situation *because roots of suicidal feelings can be masked by denial.*

Encourage patient to participate in group activities, especially those he or she enjoys *to help build self-esteem.* Assist patient to recognize inappropriate coping mechanisms and help identify those that enhance personal well-being *to use strengths and skills in preventing self-destructive behavior.*

<u>Manage:</u> Make a referral to mental health professional *to help patient through suicidal ideations and develop healthier alternatives.*

SUGGESTED NIC INTERVENTIONS
Impulse Control Training; Behavior Management: Self-Harm; Environmental Management: Violence Prevention, Suicide Prevention

REFERENCE
Herting, J. R. (2012, September). Promoting CARE: Including parents in youth suicide prevention. *Family & Community Health, 35*(3), 225–235.

DEFINITION
Extension of the number of postoperative days required to initiate and perform activities that maintain life, health, and well-being

DEFINING CHARACTERISTICS
- Difficulty in moving about
- Evidence of interrupted healing of surgical area
- Fatigue
- Evidence of interrupted healing of surgical area
- Loss of appetite with or without nausea
- Perception that more time is needed to recover
- Postpones resumption of work or employment activities
- Requires help to move about and/or complete self-care

RELATED FACTORS
- Extensive surgical procedure
- Infection of postoperative surgical site
- Obesity
- Pain
- Preoperative expectations
- Prolonged surgical procedure

ASSESSMENT FOCUS
(Refer to comprehensive assessment parameters.)
- Activity/exercise
- Cardiac function
- Neurocognition
- Physical regulation
- Respiratory function
- Risk management

EXPECTED OUTCOMES
The patient will
- Have vital signs and laboratory values within normal limits.
- Have evidence of wound healing; incision site will appear free from signs and symptoms of infection.
- Have resolution of any postoperative complications.
- Resume normal mobility status.
- Seek and obtain emotional support from family and friends.
- Resume normal eating, bowel, and bladder habits.
- Use community resources that are available to assist after discharge.

SUGGESTED NOC OUTCOMES
Ambulation; Endurance; Health Beliefs; Immobility Consequences: Physiological; Nutritional Status; Pain Level; Wound Healing: Primary Intention

INTERVENTIONS AND RATIONALES
<u>Determine:</u> Assess all body systems *to detect signs and symptoms of postoperative complications that delay surgical recovery.*

Assess surgical site for signs of infection, such as erythema, edema, pain, drainage, odor, incision approximation, and intact sutures. Monitor wound healing. Document and report assessment findings *to facilitate the development of an individualized care plan.*

Monitor nutritional status *optimal nutritional status promotes wound healing and provides energy for recovery.*

Monitor bowel and bladder activity. Report urine retention and absent or decreased bowel sounds. *Abnormal bowel and bladder patterns slow surgical recovery.*

Following postoperative bleeding, monitor hemoglobin level and hematocrit. *Bleeding can lead to a low hemoglobin level and hematocrit, reducing the ability of red blood cells to carry oxygen, which can hinder wound healing and diminish patient's energy level.*

Perform: Follow proper pulmonary regimen *to facilitate resolution of respiratory complications, if present, which lead to decreased oxygen levels, slow wound healing and delayed mobility.*

If patient suffers from psychosis, continue to reorient during postoperative recovery period *to prevent delay in recovery* and report psychological reaction (e.g., depression-like symptoms).

Administer pain medication, as prescribed. *A patient in pain won't move, cough, and deep-breathe as needed for timely recovery.*

As appropriate, make sure that someone is available to walk with patient or assistive devices (walkers or canes) are available. Don't allow patient to ambulate alone until steady. *Assistance enhances safety and encourages patient to improve mobility without fear of falling. Mobility facilitates improved strength, helps prevent such complications as deep vein thrombosis, and, ultimately, enhances recovery.*

Enforce use of support stockings or a sequential compression device *to facilitate venous return and prevent deep vein thrombosis.*

Inform: Educate patient and family regarding appropriate care after discharge *to promote compliance with medication and treatment regimens.*

Attend: Make sure patient and family members have access to community resources *to assist with recovery when patient returns home to ensure ongoing recovery.*

Manage: Initiate an interdisciplinary care conference for patient to *help develop a plan that will put the patient on a faster track to recovery.*

SUGGESTED NIC INTERVENTIONS

Bed Rest Care; Case Management; Discharge Planning; Energy Management; Exercise Therapy: Ambulation; Incision Site Care; Multidisciplinary Care Conference; Nutrition Management; Pain Management; Sleep Enhancement

REFERENCE

Cherry, C., & Moss, J. (2011, March). Best practices for preventing hospital-acquired pressure injuries in surgical patients. *Canadian Operating Room Nursing Journal, 29*(1), 6–8, 22–26.

DEFINITION

Abnormal functioning of the swallowing mechanism associated with deficits in oral, pharyngeal, or esophageal structure or function

DEFINING CHARACTERISTICS

- Esophageal phase impairment (observed evidence of difficulty in swallowing, heartburn or epigastric pain, food refusal, complaints of "something stuck")
- Oral phase impairment (choking or coughing before a swallow, drooling, gagging, inability to clear oral cavity, food falls from mouth)
- Pharyngeal phase impairment (delayed swallow, choking or coughing, multiple swallows, recurrent pulmonary infections, food refusal)

RELATED FACTORS

- Congenital defects (e.g., congenital heart disease, neuromuscular impairment, protein energy malnutrition, hypotonia, upper airway anomalies)
- Neurological problems (e.g., achalasia, cerebral palsy, gastroesophageal reflux, laryngeal or nasal defects, prematurity, trauma)

ASSESSMENT FOCUS

(Refer to comprehensive assessment parameters.)

- Cardiac function
- Neurocognition
- Nutrition
- Respiratory function

EXPECTED OUTCOMES

The patient will

- Show no evidence of aspiration pneumonia.
- Achieve adequate nutritional intake.
- Maintain weight.
- Maintain oral hygiene.
- Demonstrate correct feeding techniques to maximize swallowing.
- List strategies to prevent aspiration.

SUGGESTED NOC OUTCOMES

Appetite; Aspiration Prevention; Cognition; Nutritional Status: Food & Fluid Intake; Swallowing Status; Swallowing Status: Esophageal Phase; Swallowing Status: Oral Phase; Swallowing Status: Pharyngeal Phase

INTERVENTIONS AND RATIONALES

<u>Determine:</u> Monitor intake and output and weight daily until stabilized. Establish an intake goal (specify), "Patient consumes ____ mL of fluid and ____ % of solid food." Record and report any deviation from this. *Evaluating calorie and protein intake daily allows any necessary modifications to begin quickly.*

<u>Perform:</u> Elevate head of the bed 90° during mealtimes and for 30 minutes after the completion of a meal. Position patient on his or her side when recumbent. *These measures decrease the risk of aspiration.*

Keep suction apparatus at the bedside to be prepared for episodes of aspiration that require immediate suctioning. Observe and report instances of cyanosis, dyspnea, or choking. *Symptoms indicate the presence of material in the lungs.*

Provide mouth care three times daily. Keep oral mucous membrane moist by frequent rinses; use a bulb syringe or suction if necessary. *These measures promote comfort and enhance appetite.* Lubricate patient's lips *to prevent cracking and blisters.*

<u>Inform:</u> Teach patient and family about positioning, dietary requirements, and specific feeding techniques *to allow patient to take an active role in maintaining health.* These include facial exercises (such as whistling) *to promote muscle activity,* using a short straw *to provide sensory stimulation to the lips,* tipping the head forward *to decrease aspiration,* applying pressure above the lip *to stimulate mouth closure and the swallowing reflex,* and checking the oral cavity frequently *to determine presence of food particles* (remove if present).

<u>Attend:</u> Encourage patient to wear properly fitted dentures *to enhance chewing ability.*

Serve food in attractive surroundings. Encourage patient to smell and look at food. Remove soiled equipment, control smells, and provide a quiet atmosphere for eating. *A pleasant atmosphere stimulates appetite. Food aroma stimulates salivation.*

<u>Manage:</u> Consult with a dietitian to modify patient's diet, and conduct a calorie count, as needed, *to establish nutritional requirements.*

Consult with a dysphagia rehabilitation team, if available, *to obtain expert advice.*

SUGGESTED NIC INTERVENTIONS

Airway Suctioning; Aspiration Precautions; Feeding; Positioning; Referral; Risk Identification; Swallowing Therapy

REFERENCE

Mandysova, P., Skvňáková, J., Ehler, E., & Cerný, M. (2011, December). Development of the brief bedside dysphagia screening test in the Czech Republic. *Nursing in Health and Science, 13*(4), 388–395.

DEFINITION

A pattern of regulating and integrating into family processes a program for the treatment of illness and its sequelae that is unsatisfactory for meeting specific health goals

DEFINING CHARACTERISTICS

- Acceleration of illness symptoms of a family member
- Inappropriate family activities for meeting health goals
- Failure to take action to reduce risk factors
- Lack of attention to illness
- Verbalizes desire to manage illness
- Verbalizes difficulty with therapeutic regimen

RELATED FACTORS

- Complexity of health care system
- Complexity of therapeutic regimen
- Decisional conflicts
- Economic difficulties
- Excessive demands
- Family conflicts

ASSESSMENT FOCUS

(Refer to comprehensive assessment parameters.)
- Communication
- Knowledge
- Roles/responsibilities
- Risk management

EXPECTED OUTCOMES

The family members will
- Identify behaviors that lead to conflict.
- Participate in family therapy sessions and openly express feelings about illness of family member.
- Express desire to receive help to resolve conflicts.
- Describe understanding of coping mechanisms that resolve conflicts.
- Cooperate in finding ways to incorporate therapeutic regimen.
- Express desire to carry out therapeutic regimen.
- Plan for future course of illness.

SUGGESTED NOC OUTCOMES

Compliance Behavior; Family Coping; Family Functioning; Family Normalization; Family Participation in Professional Care; Knowledge

INTERVENTIONS AND RATIONALES

Determine: Assess level of education; occupation; values and beliefs; attitudes about health and illness; coping patterns; family status, including marital status, family composition, communication patterns, coping skills, drug or alcohol degree of trust in others; beliefs and attitudes about health; socioeconomic factors; spiritual status, including religious affiliation and description of faith and religious practices; perceptions about life, death, and suffering. *Assessment information will assist in identifying appropriate outcomes and interventions for this diagnosis.*

Perform: Work directly with the family to establish a daily routine for managing the therapeutic regimen that fits with their lifestyle. *Collaboration with patient and family members makes it possible to combine scientific knowledge of the illness with lifestyle factors such as culture, family dynamics, and finances.*

Inform: Provide books and videos that will help the patient's quest for enhanced knowledge. *Supplying some materials directly may be a motivation for the parents to continue searching for information.*

Direct patient to use other sources such as libraries, Internet, or professional organizations. *An independent search results in the parents developing confidence in their own ability to find answers to their questions about health and wellness.*

Select teaching strategies *that will enhance teaching/learning effectiveness,* such as discussion, demonstration, role-playing, and visual materials.

Teach those skills that the patient must incorporate into ability *to go further pursue the area of interest.*

Attend: Assist patient to set goals and develop a plan to provide concrete direction to the patient's desire *to enhance the effective management of the therapeutic regimen.*

Promote verbal reminders to reinforce health-promoting behaviors. For example, remind patient with heart disease to stop smoking. *Verbal cues may stimulate the patient to take action, if not immediately, then at a later time.*

Encourage family members to plan for future course of illness. For example, family may need to make structural changes at home to accommodate a wheelchair or hospital beds. *Planning enhances ability of patient and family to develop appropriate management strategies.*

Encourage patient and family to verbalize feelings and concerns related to the knowledge and skills that parents need. *This promotes greater ease in managing challenging situations.*

Manage: Refer family to social and community resources for ongoing assistance with parenting. *Parents can contact these sources for additional information as needed.*

SUGGESTED NIC INTERVENTIONS

Case Management; Coping Enhancement; Decision-Making Support; Family Involvement; Family Process Maintenance; Family Support; Family Therapy

REFERENCE

Albert, N., et al. (2012). Complexities of care for patients and families living with advanced cardiovascular diseases: Overview. *Journal of Cardiovascular Nursing, 27*(2), 103–113.

DEFINITION

At risk for damage to skin and mucous membranes due to extreme temperatures

RISK FACTORS

- Cognitive impairment (e.g., dementia, psychoses)
- Developmental level (e.g., infants, ages)
- Exposure to extreme temperatures
- Fatigue
- Inadequate supervision
- Inattentiveness
- Intoxication (e.g., alcohol, drugs)
- Lack of knowledge (e.g., patient, caregiver)
- Lack of protective clothing (e.g., flame-retardant sleepwear, gloves, ear covering)
- Neuromuscular impairment (e.g., stroke, amyotrophic lateral sclerosis, multiple sclerosis)
- Neuropathy
- Smoking
- Treatment-related side effects (e.g., pharmaceutical agents)
- Unsafe environment

ASSESSMENT FOCUS

(Refer to comprehensive assessment parameters.)

- Risk management
- Knowledge
- Self-care
- Sensation/perception

EXPECTED OUTCOMES

The patient will:

- Not experience thermal injury.
- Acknowledge presence of environmental hazards in home.
- Take safety precautions to prevent injury.

SUGGESTED NOC OUTCOMES

Risk Control; Risk Detection; Safe Home Environment; Knowledge: Personal Safety

INTERVENTIONS AND RATIONALES

Determine: Assess environment for potential risks for thermal injury *to prevent accidents.*

Assess patient for any cognitive impairment *that would increase risk for thermal injury.*

Assess knowledge of fire safety and emergency response *to ensure rapid notification of emergency personnel.*

<u>Perform:</u> Remove dangerous or potentially dangerous items from the environment *to avoid injury.*

Suggest a decrease in the maximum water temperature *to decrease potential scalding.*

Ensure proper functioning of all fire /smoke alarms *to provide quick intervention in case of fire.*

<u>Inform:</u> Encourage adults/family member to discuss fire safety measures with children and elderly family members *to promote household safety.*

Encourage use of flame retardant sleepware *to minimize injury in the event of a fire.*

<u>Attend:</u> Encourage patient/family to report any potential safety hazards *to decrease chance of thermal accident.*

<u>Manage:</u> Refer patient/family to community resources for fire safety *to ensure all possible precautions have been identified and implemented.*

Refer at risk patients who are living alone to home health services *for follow up home safety evaluation.*

SUGGESTED NIC INTERVENTIONS

Environmental Management: Safety; Fire Setting Precautions; Risk Identification; Surveillance: Safety

REFERENCE

Leahy, N. E., et al. (2012). Engaging older adults in burn prevention education: Results of a community-based urban initiative. *Journal of Burn Care & Research, 33*(3), 141–146.

DEFINITION
Temperature fluctuation between hypothermia and hyperthermia

DEFINING CHARACTERISTICS
- Cyanotic nail beds
- Fluctuations in body temperature above or below normal range
- Flushed skin
- Hypertension
- Increased capillary refill time
- Increased respiratory/heart rate
- Mild shivering
- Moderate pallor
- Piloerection
- Seizures
- Warm or cool skin

RELATED FACTORS
- Extremes of age
- Fluctuating environmental temperature
- Illness
- Trauma

ASSESSMENT FOCUS
(Refer to comprehensive assessment parameters.)
- Cardiac function
- Fluid and electrolytes
- Neurocognition
- Physical regulation
- Respiratory function
- Tissue integrity

EXPECTED OUTCOMES
The patient will
- Maintain body temperature at normothermic levels.
- Have no episodes of shivering.
- Express feelings of comfort.
- Exhibit skin that is warm and dry.
- Maintain heart rate and blood pressure within normal range.
- Show no signs of compromised neurologic status.
- Voice an understanding of health problem.

SUGGESTED NOC OUTCOMES
Hydration; Thermoregulation; Vital Signs

INTERVENTIONS AND RATIONALES
<u>Determine:</u> Monitor patient's body temperature every 4 hours or more often as indicated *to determine effectiveness of therapy or if intervention is needed.* Record temperature and route *(baseline data depends on route).*

Monitor and record patient's neurologic status every 8 hours. Report any changes to the physician. *Hyperthermia increases cerebral edema and thus intracranial pressure; hypothermia depresses metabolic rate.*

Monitor and record patient's heart rate and rhythm, blood pressure, and respiratory rate every 4 hours. *Hyperthermia may create hypoxia by increasing oxygen demand, which results from increased tissue metabolism (metabolism increases 7% with each increase of 1° F [0.6° C]). This, in turn, results in faster breathing and a rising pulse rate.*

<u>Perform:</u> Administer analgesics, antipyretics, and medications that prevent shivering, as indicated. Monitor and record their effectiveness. *Antipyretics help reduce fever. Shivering tends to retard the lowering of body temperature.*

If patient develops excessive fever, take the following steps:
- Reduce excessive fever.
- Remove blankets; place a loincloth over patient.
- Apply ice bags to the axilla and groin.
- Initiate a tepid water sponge bath.
- Use a hypothermia blanket if temperature rises above ____. Cool patient to ____.
- Maintain hydration.
- Monitor intake and output.
- Administer parenteral fluids, as ordered.
- Maintain the environmental temperature at a comfortable setting.
- Ensure that all metal and plastic surfaces that come into contact with patient's body are covered.
- Make sure that linens and clothing are clean and dry.

These measures aid in reducing core temperature.

<u>Inform:</u> Instruct patient and family members about
- signs and symptoms of altered body temperature.
- precautionary measures to avoid hypothermia or hyperthermia.
- adherence to other aspects of health care management to help normalize patient's temperature (such as dietary habits and measures to prevent increased intracranial pressure).
- rationale for treatment.

These measures allow patient to take an active role in health maintenance.

<u>Attend:</u> Acknowledge patient's fluid preference. Keep oral fluids at the bedside and encourage patient to drink. *These measures help maintain fluid balance and encourage patient to actively participate in the prescribed treatment.*

<u>Manage:</u> Make referral to community health agency, if needed, *to obtain adequate heating or cooling in home.*

SUGGESTED NIC INTERVENTIONS

Bathing; Environmental Management; Fever Treatment; Fluid Management; Fluid Monitoring; Temperature Regulation; Vital Signs Monitoring

REFERENCE

Block, J., Lilienthal, M., Cullen, L., & White, A. (2012, January–March). Evidence-based thermoregulation for adult trauma patients. *Critical Care Nursing Quarterly, 35*(1), 50–63.

DEFINITION
Damage to mucous membrane or to corneal, integumentary, or subcutaneous tissues

DEFINING CHARACTERISTICS
- Damaged tissue (cornea, mucous membrane, integumentary, subcutaneous)
- Destroyed tissue

RELATED FACTORS
- Altered circulation
- Chemical irritants
- Fluid deficit or excess
- Impaired physical mobility
- Knowledge deficit
- Mechanical factors (e.g., pressure, shear, friction)
- Nutritional deficit or excess
- Radiation
- Temperature extremes

ASSESSMENT FOCUS
(Refer to comprehensive assessment parameters.)
- Cardiac function
- Neurocognition
- Nutrition
- Tissue integrity

EXPECTED OUTCOMES
The patient will
- Experience relief from immediate signs and symptoms (pain, ulcers, color changes, and edema).
- Maintain collateral circulation.
- Voice intent to stop smoking.
- Voice intent to follow specific management routines after discharge.

SUGGESTED NOC OUTCOMES
Knowledge: Treatment Regimen; Self-Care Hygiene; Tissue Integrity: Skin & Mucous Membranes; Tissue Perfusion: Peripheral; Wound Healing: Secondary Intention; Smoking Cessation Behavior

INTERVENTIONS AND RATIONALES
<u>Determine:</u> Monitor intake and output and record daily weight *to detect* imbalances. Maintain adequate hydration. *Adequate hydration reduces blood viscosity and decreases the risk of clot formation.*
<u>Perform:</u> Provide scrupulous foot care *to prevent fungal infections and ingrown toenails, stimulate circulation, and promote detection of signs and symptoms to decrease tissue perfusion.*

Administer and monitor treatments according to institutional protocols. Immediately report abnormal findings to the physician.

For patient with venous insufficiency, apply antiembolism stockings or intermittent pneumatic compression stockings, removing them for 1 hour every 8 hours or according to institutional protocol. Elevate patient's feet while sitting, and elevate foot of bed 69° to 89° (15 to 20.5 cm) while lying down. *These measures promote venous return and decrease venous congestion in lower extremities.*

For patient with arterial insufficiency, elevate the head of the bed 69° to 89° while patient is lying down *to increase arterial blood supply to extremities.*

Inform: Instruct patient to avoid pressure on popliteal space. For example, say "Don't cross your legs or wear constrictive clothing" *to avoid reducing arterial blood supply and increasing venous congestion.*

Educate patient about risk factors and prevention of injury. *Teaching about factors influencing peripheral vascular disease and prevention of tissue damage helps prevent complications.*

Attend: Encourage adherence to an exercise regimen, as tolerated. *Exercise improves arterial circulation and venous return by promoting muscle contraction and relaxation.*

Manage: Refer patient to a smoking cessation program. *Smoking constricts vessels and contributes to reduced circulation.*

SUGGESTED NIC INTERVENTIONS

Circulatory Care: Arterial Insufficiency; Circulatory Precautions; Nutrition Management; Oral Health Maintenance; Positioning; Pressure Management; Pressure Ulcer Prevention; Skin Surveillance; Teaching: Foot Care; Smoking Cessation Assistance

REFERENCE

Sampaio Santos, F. A., de Melo, R. P., & Lopes, M. V. (2010, March). Characterization of health status with regard to tissue integrity and tissue perfusion in patients with venous ulcers according to the nursing outcomes classification. *Journal of Vascular Nursing, 28*(1), 14–20.

DEFINITION

At risk for a decrease in cardiac (coronary) circulation that may compromise health

RISK FACTORS

- Cardiac surgery or tamponade; coronary artery spasm
- Diabetes mellitus
- Family history of coronary artery disease
- Hyperlipidemia
- Hypertension
- Hypovolemia
- Hypoxemia
- Hypoxia
- Substance abuse
- Elevated C-reactive protein
- Birth control pills
- Lack of knowledge of modifiable risk factors (e.g., smoking, sedentary lifestyle, obesity)

ASSESSMENT FOCUS

(Refer to comprehensive assessment parameters.)
- Cardiac function
- Physical regulation

EXPECTED OUTCOMES

The patient will
- Remain hemodynamically stable.
- Not experience any signs or symptoms of decreased cardiac tissue perfusion.
- Verbalize modifiable risk factors for decreased cardiac perfusion.
- Identify reportable symptoms of possible decreased cardiac perfusion.

SUGGESTED NOC OUTCOMES

Knowledge: Cardiac Disease Management, Cardiac Pump Effectiveness, Circulation Status; Tissue Perfusion: Cardiac; Vital Signs

INTERVENTIONS AND RATIONALES

Determine: Assess hemodynamic status, including blood pressure, heart rate, oxygen saturation, and respiratory rate for any abnormalities *that may be early indicators of altered perfusion.*

Monitor cardiac rhythm for any irregularities *that may indicate cardiac irritability.*

Perform: Assist with the preparation and completion of diagnostic tests and the postprocedural patient care. *Safe completion of diagnostic test will result in improved patient outcomes.*

Treat episodes of tachycardia promptly. *Cardiac tissue is perfused during diastole and perfusion time is decreased if tachycardia is not treated.*

Inform: Provide patient with information regarding modifiable risk factors and interventions to minimize risks. *Knowledge of risk factors will contribute to informed decisions about lifestyle changes.*

Attend: Encourage patient and family to share concerns regarding outcomes of tests *to reduce anxiety.*

Manage: Collaborate with other members of health care team to ensure that all underlying medical conditions are being managed effectively. *This will minimize the possibility of cardiac perfusion complications.*

SUGGESTED NIC INTERVENTIONS

Risk Identification; Teaching: Disease Process; Cardiac Care; Hemodynamic Regulation; Vital Signs Monitoring

REFERENCE

Pereira de Melo, R., et al. (2011, November–December). Risk for decreased cardiac output: Validation of a proposal for nursing diagnosis. *Nursing and Critical Care, 16*(6):287–294.

DEFINITION

At risk for a decrease in cerebral circulation that may compromise health

RISK FACTORS

- Abnormal prothrombin and partial thromboplastin times
- Atrial fibrillation or myxoma
- Carotid stenosis
- Cerebral aneurysm, trauma, neoplasm, or tumor
- Coagulopathy
- Thrombolytic therapy
- Hypertension
- Cardiomyopathy (arterial dissection, akinetic ventricular segment, atherosclerosis, infective endocarditis, mitral stenosis, myocardial infarction, sick sinus syndrome)
- Substance abuse
- Disseminated intravascular coagulation
- Substance abuse
- Treatment side effects (cardiopulmonary bypass, medications)

ASSESSMENT FOCUS

(Refer to comprehensive assessment parameters.)
- Neurocognition
- Sensation/perception

EXPECTED OUTCOMES

The patient will
- Understand the need for frequent neurological assessments to assess for any changes.
- Experience adequate cerebral perfusion evidenced by normal neurological checks.
- Remain hemodynamically stable.
- Participate in diagnostic testing when necessary.
- Verbalize strategies to minimize or decrease modifiable risk factors.

SUGGESTED NOC OUTCOMES

Tissue Perfusion: Cerebral; Neurological Status; Circulation Status; Knowledge: Illness Care; Knowledge: Treatment Procedure

INTERVENTIONS AND RATIONALES

<u>Determine:</u> Assess patient for positive risk factors for decrease in cerebral perfusion, including carotid stenosis, hypertension, coagulopathies, atrial fibrillation, and smoking. *Risk factor reduction will result in positive patient outcomes.*

<u>Perform:</u> Facilitate completion of diagnostic tests and provide postprocedure care to prevent complications *to ensure accurate safe and timely diagnosis and treatment.*

Maintain adequate oxygenation *to ensure cerebral perfusion.*

<u>Inform:</u> Educate at-risk patients of the signs of decreased cerebral perfusion about the importance of timely medical intervention for positive symptoms. *Change in mental status is a sensitive indicator for decreased cerebral perfusion.*

Educate patients about need for prompt intervention if signs of stroke have occurred. *Early intervention can prevent or minimize stroke severity.*

<u>Attend:</u> Encourage at-risk patient and family to ask questions and share concerns *to increase their confidence and ability to recognize and respond to warning signs of decreased cerebral perfusion.*

<u>Manage:</u> Collaborate with community organizations to educate public on risk factors for and symptoms of decreased cerebral perfusion and the appropriate response. *Increased community awareness may result in a more timely intervention for decreased cerebral perfusion conditions.*

SUGGESTED NIC INTERVENTIONS

Cerebral Perfusion Promotion; Neurologic Monitoring

REFERENCE

Boly, M. (2011, August). Measuring the fading consciousness in the human brain. *Current Opinions in Neurology, 24*(4), 394–400.

DEFINITION

Decrease in blood circulation to the periphery that may compromise health

DEFINING CHARACTERISTICS

- Altered skin characteristics (e.g., hair, nails, moisture, sensation, temperature, color, elasticity)
- Blood pressure changes in extremities
- Claudication
- Color does not return to leg on lowering the leg
- Delayed peripheral wound healing
- Diminished pulses; capillary refill time >3 seconds
- Edema
- Extremity pain
- Paresthesia
- Skin color pale on elevation

RELATED FACTORS

- Lack of knowledge of disease process (e.g., diabetes, hypertension, hyperlipidemia)
- Lack of knowledge of aggravating factors (e.g., smoking, sedentary lifestyle, trauma, obesity, salt intake, immobility)

ASSESSMENT FOCUS

(Refer to comprehensive assessment parameters.)

- Activity/exercise
- Comfort
- Self-care
- Cardiac function
- Physical regulation
- Sensation/perception
- Tissue integrity

EXPECTED OUTCOMES

The patient will

- Understand the need to maintain moderate activity level to promote circulation.
- Articulate the need and rationale for smoking cessation.
- Not experience ischemic damage to involved extremity.
- Experience adequate perfusion to promote prompt wound healing.
- Acknowledge the importance of protecting involved extremity from injury.
- Recognize reportable changes in skin characteristics to the involved extremity that indicate decreased perfusion.

SUGGESTED NOC OUTCOMES

Activity Tolerance; Tissue Integrity: Skin and Mucous Membranes; Tissue Perfusion: Peripheral; Smoking Cessation Behavior

INTERVENTIONS AND RATIONALES

<u>Determine:</u> Evaluate involved extremity for clinical signs (pain, decreased temperature, pallor, delayed capillary refill, weak or absent pulse, decreased sensation, and decreased pulse oximetry) *that are indicators of ineffective peripheral perfusion.*

<u>Perform:</u> Protect the extremity from injury using sheepskin or bed cradle and position extremity at or lower than level of heart *to promote collateral blood flow.*

<u>Inform:</u> Instruct patient to increase walking activity *to promote collateral circulation and improve blood supply to extremity.*

Teach patient to avoid crossing legs or keeping legs in a dependent position *to avoid constriction of veins.*

<u>Attend:</u> Encourage patient to protect extremity from injury or extreme hot or cold temperatures. *Infection or ulcer formation may develop more easily because of decreased blood supply.*

<u>Manage:</u> Refer patients who smoke to smoking cessation program *because continued smoking will significantly increase risks for further damage.*

SUGGESTED NIC INTERVENTIONS

Circulatory Care: Arterial Insufficiency, Exercise Promotion, Positioning, Skin Surveillance; Smoking Cessation Assistance

REFERENCE

West, A. M., et al. (2011, August 30). Low-density lipoprotein lowering does not improve calf muscle perfusion, energetic, or exercise performance in peripheral arterial disease. *Journal of the American College of Cardiology, 58*(10), 1068–1076.

DEFINITION

At risk for a decrease in blood circulation to periphery that may compromise health

RISK FACTORS

- Age >60 years
- Deficient knowledge of aggravating factors (e.g., smoking, sedentary lifestyle, trauma, obesity, salt intake, immobility
- Deficient knowledge of disease process (e.g., diabetes, hyperlipidemia)
- Diabetes mellitus
- Endovascular procedures
- Hypertension
- Sedentary lifestyle
- Smoking

ASSESSMENT FOCUS

(Refer to comprehensive assessment parameters.)
- Risk Management
- Knowledge
- Self care
- Sensation/perception

EXPECTED OUTCOMES

The patient will
- Remain free of tissue injury due to decreased peripheral perfusion.
- Understand the need for smoking cessation.
- State reportable changes that indicate decreased peripheral perfusion.
- Understand the need for moderate activity to promote circulation.

SUGGESTED NOC OUTCOMES

Activity Tolerance; Tissue Integrity: Skin and Mucous Membranes; Tissue Perfusion: Peripheral; Smoking Cessation Behavior

INTERVENTIONS AND RATIONALES

<u>Determine:</u> Assess lower extremities for early signs of ineffective peripheral perfusion. *Early identification and intervention will improve patient outcomes.*

Assess patient's history for presence of heart disease, hyperlipidemia, diabetes, and smoking *which are significant risk factors for impaired peripheral tissue perfusion.*

Evaluate patient's understanding of lifestyle modifications *to enable patient participation in risk factor reduction.*

<u>Perform:</u> Administer and evaluate effectiveness of medications to treat underlying medical conditions that place patient at risk for decreased peripheral perfusion. *Control of risk factors will prevent or delay onset of tissue hypoperfusion.*

Position extremity at or lower than level of the heart *to promote peripheral perfusion.*

Inform: Instruct patient to initiate a regular walking program *to promote collateral circulation* and improve perfusion.

Teach patient to avoid crossing of the legs *to avoid constriction.*

Attend: Encourage patient to carefully follow treatment regimens for existing medical conditions *that are risk factors for decreased peripheral tissue perfusion.*

Manage: Refer patients who smoke to smoking cessation program *because continued smoking will significantly increase risks for development of peripheral tissue damage.*

SUGGESTED NIC INTERVENTIONS

Circulatory Care: Arterial Insufficiency, Exercise Promotion, Positioning, Skin Surveillance; Smoking Cessation Assistance

REFERENCE

Muir, R. (2009). Peripheral arterial disease: Pathophysiology, risk factors, diagnosis, treatment, and prevention. *Journal of Vascular Nursing, 27*(2), 26–30.

DEFINITION
Limitation of independent movement between two nearby surfaces

DEFINING CHARACTERISTICS
Impaired ability to transfer:
- Between uneven levels
- From bed to chair
- From chair to car or from car to chair
- From chair to floor or from floor to chair
- From standing to floor or from floor to standing
- In and out of tub or shower
- On or off a toilet or commode

RELATED FACTORS
- Cognitive impairment
- Deconditioning
- Environmental constraints
- Impaired balance
- Impaired vision
- Insufficient muscle strength
- Lack of knowledge
- Musculoskeletal impairment
- Neuromuscular impairment
- Obesity
- Pain

ASSESSMENT FOCUS
(Refer to comprehensive assessment parameters.)
- Activity/exercise
- Knowledge
- Physical regulation
- Pharmacological function

EXPECTED OUTCOMES
The patient will
- Have no evidence of complications associated with impaired transfer mobility, such as depression, altered health maintenance, and falls.
- Maintain or improve muscle strength and joint range of motion (ROM).
- Achieve the highest level of mobility possible (independence with regard to need for assistive device, verbalization of needs regarding transfer).
- Maintain safety during transfer.
- Adapt to alteration in ability to perform transfer.
- Demonstrate understanding of transfer techniques.
- Participate in social and occupational activities to the greatest extent possible.

SUGGESTED NOC OUTCOMES
Balance; Body Positioning: Self-Initiated; Joint Movement: Hip, Knee, Spine; Knowledge: Body Mechanics; Mobility; Transfer Performance; Coordinated Movement

INTERVENTIONS AND RATIONALES

Determine: Identify patient's level of independence using the functional mobility scale. Report findings to the staff *to provide continuity and preserve the documented level of independence.*

Monitor and record daily evidence of complications related to altered mobility or decreased ability to perform transfer with assistive device (contractures, venous stasis, skin breakdown, thrombus formation, depression, altered health maintenance, or self-care deficit). *Patients with neuromuscular dysfunction are at risk for complications.*

Assess patient's skin upon her return to bed. If patient is using a wheelchair, request a seat cushion, if necessary, *to maintain skin integrity.*

Perform: Perform ROM exercises to the joints of affected limbs, unless contraindicated, at least once per shift. Progress from passive to active ROM, as tolerated, *to prevent joint contractures and muscle atrophy.*

Inform: Teach patient transfer techniques, such as performing a standing or sitting transfer, *to maintain muscle tone, prevent complications of immobility, and promote independence.*

Adapt teaching to the limits imposed by patient's condition *to prevent injury.* As part of teaching plan, demonstrate transfer techniques to family members *to ensure that necessary adaptations are made by family.* Have patient's family perform a return demonstration *to ensure the use of proper technique and to promote continuity of care.*

Attend: Encourage patient to attend physical therapy. Request a written copy of instructions for assistive device to use as a reference *to maintain continuity of care and foster safety.*

Manage: Refer patient to a physical therapist for the development of a mobility program related to assistive device *to assist with rehabilitation of musculoskeletal deficits.*

Identify resources (stroke program, sports association for disabled, National Multiple Sclerosis Society) *to promote patient's reintegration into the community.*

SUGGESTED NIC INTERVENTIONS

Body Mechanics Promotion; Energy Management; Exercise Promotion: Strength Training; Exercise Therapy: Balance; Fall Prevention; Self-Care Assistance: Transfer; Health System Guidance

REFERENCE

Cheng, S. P., In Tang, F., Yu, S., Chen, I. J., & Wu, L.L. (2012, March–April). Factors influencing physical activity in institutionalized elderly patients with leprosy. *Rehabilitation Nursing, 37*(2), 88–93.

DEFINITION
Accentuated risk of accidental tissue injury (e.g., wound, burn, fracture)

RISK FACTORS
- Accessibility of guns
- Children playing with very dangerous objects
- Children riding in the front seat of a car
- Inadequately stored corrosives
- Contact with cold
- Contact with rapidly moving machinery
- Delayed lighting of gas appliances
- Driving at excessive speeds or a mechanically unsafe vehicle
- Driving while intoxicated
- Entering unlighted rooms
- Faulty electric plugs
- Knives stored uncovered
- Misuse of necessary headgear
- Misuse of seat restraints
- Use of cracked dishware
- Lack of safety precautions
- Unsafe home environment
  - Pot handles facing toward front of stove
  - Obstructed passageways
  - Overloaded fuse boxes
  - Litter or liquid spills in a passageway
  - Defective appliances
  - Bathing in very hot water
  - Bathtub without hand grip or antislip equipment
  - Entering unlighted rooms
  - Unsturdy or absent stair rails
  - Use of unsteady chairs or ladders
  - Slippery floors
  - Unanchored rugs

ASSESSMENT FOCUS
(Refer to comprehensive assessment parameters.)
- Behavior
- Coping
- Emotional
- Knowledge
- Risk management

EXPECTED OUTCOMES
The patient will
- Avoid injury.
- Voice need for understanding safety precautions.
- Demonstrate correct use of safety devices (i.e., walker or cane).

SUGGESTED NOC OUTCOMES
Falls Occurrence; Personal Safety Behavior; Physical Injury Severity; Risk Control; Safe Home Environment; Tissue Integrity: Skin & Mucous Membranes

INTERVENTIONS AND RATIONALES
<u>Determine:</u> Observe, record, and report falls, seizures, and unsafe practices. *Accurate assessment promotes appropriate interventions; documentation ensures continuity of care.*

Monitor and record patient's respiratory status. *Trauma increases respiratory rate; other respiratory effects depend on the nature of the trauma.*

Monitor and record patient's neurologic status *to detect changes and to report deteriorated status.*

Perform: If patient has a seizure, remain with him, loosen restrictive clothing, and protect him from environmental hazards. Don't restrain him or pry his mouth open. Keep an oral airway at the bedside and maintain a patent airway. Turn patient to his side after the seizure stops and suction if secretions occlude the airway. Record seizure characteristics, including onset, duration, and body movements. Reorient patient to his surroundings and allow a rest period. *Remaining with patient provides safety and information for accurate documentation of the event. Loosening clothing and proper positioning may prevent further harm.*

Keep bedrails raised *to ensure safety.* Maintain position of the bed as low as possible *to prevent the patient from falling and sustaining further injury.* Help debilitated, weak, or unsteady patient to get out of bed. Ensure that the floor is dry and that furniture and litter don't block patient's way *to help prevent falls.*

Inform: Instruct patient and family members on safety practices such as correct use of a walker, crutches, or cane. *These enable patient and family members to take an active role in health care and maintain a safe environment.*

Provide patient and family with information about necessary safety precautions *to enable them to take an active role in health care and maintain a safe environment.*

Instruct patient in the use of assistive devices *to ensure their proper use and provide the patient with a feeling of security.*

Attend: Encourage patient and family to express feelings and concerns related to trauma. *Discussing feelings can be therapeutic. Active listening conveys respect for the patient.*

Facilitate opportunities for spiritual nourishment and growth *to address patient's holistic needs for maximal therapeutic environment.*

Schedule time to meet with family and patient to listen to ways in which they plan to enhance their coping skills in the present situation.

Manage: Refer family to community resources and support groups available *to assist in managing patient's illness and providing emotional and financial assistance to caregivers.*

SUGGESTED NIC INTERVENTIONS

Environmental Management: Safety; Fall Prevention; Health Education; Pressure Ulcer Prevention; Seizure Precautions; Surveillance: Safety; Teaching: Disease Process

REFERENCE

Wilczweski, P., et al. (2012, January/March). Risk factors associated with pressure ulcer development in critically ill traumatic spinal cord injury patients. *Journal of Trauma Nursing, 19*(1), 5–10.

DEFINITION

Impairment in sensory and motor response, mental representation, and spatial attention of the body and the corresponding environment characterized by inattention to one side and overattention to the opposite side. Left side neglect is more severe and persistent than right side neglect

DEFINING CHARACTERISTICS

- Appears unaware of positioning of neglected limb
- Difficulty remembering details of internally represented familiar scenes that are on the neglected side
- Displacement of sounds to the nonneglected side
- Distortion of drawing on the half of the page on the neglected side
- Failure to cancel lines on the half of the page on the neglected side
- Failure to dress or groom the neglected side
- Failure to eat food from the neglected side
- Failure to move eyes, head, limbs, and trunk in the neglected hemisphere
- Failure to notice people approaching from the neglected side
- Marked deviation of the eyes, head, trunk to the non-neglected side

RELATED FACTORS

- Brain injury from tumor, or cerebrovascular, neurological, or traumatic causes
- Left hemiplegia from stroke of right hemisphere
- Hemianopsia

ASSESSMENT FOCUS

(Refer to comprehensive assessment parameters.)

- Activity/exercise
- Coping
- Neurocognition
- Self-care
- Sensation/perception
- Tissue integrity

EXPECTED OUTCOMES

The patient/family will

- Avoid injury, skin breakdown, and contractures on affected body part.
- Recognize the neglected body part.
- Demonstrate exercises for the affected body part.
- Demonstrate measures for maximum functioning and arrange environment to protect the affected body part.
- Express feelings about altered state of health and neurologic deficits.
- Identify community resources and support groups to help cope with the effects of illness.

SUGGESTED NOC OUTCOMES

Adaptation to Physical Disability; Body Image; Body Mechanics Performance; Body Positioning: Self-Initiated; Self-Care: Activities of Daily Living (ADLs); Heedfulness of Affected Side

INTERVENTIONS AND RATIONALES

<u>Determine:</u> Observe the position of the affected body part frequently *to prevent injury.*

<u>Perform:</u> Place a sling on the affected arm *to prevent dangling or injury.*

Support affected leg and foot and perform other measures, as appropriate, *to keep patient's limbs in functional position and avoid contractures.* Use a drawsheet to move patient up in bed *to avoid skin abrasions.*

Touch and rub the affected limb, and describe the limb in conversation with patient. *This reminds the patient of the neglected body part.*

Use safety belts or protective devices *to remind patient of limitations and prevent falls.* Use devices according to facility policy.

Remove splints and other devices at least every 2 hours. Inspect the skin for pressure areas. Reapply the splint. *Proper use of splints and other devices prevents deformities and maintains skin integrity.*

Perform range of motion (ROM) exercises on the affected side at least once every shift, unless medically contraindicated, *to maintain joint flexibility and prevent contractures.* Establish and follow a regular turning schedule *to maintain skin integrity.*

Arrange environment for maximum functioning; for example, place water, television controls, and the call bell within reach. *These measures enhance orientation and encourage independence.*

Assist patient with ADLs or provide supervision, as appropriate, *to protect patient's affected side.*

<u>Inform:</u> Encourage patient to perform activities that require use of the affected limb *to more easily integrate paretic or paralyzed limb into body image.*

Instruct family and nursing personnel to observe the position of the affected body part frequently; to remove food or drainage from the face if unnoticed by patient; and to place the arm or leg in the proper position as often as necessary. *These measures help avoid injury and maintain dignity.*

<u>Attend:</u> Encourage patient to check the position of the affected body part with each repositioning or transfer *to reestablish awareness of the body part.*

Encourage patient and family members to express their feelings regarding patient's condition and level of functioning *to release tension and enhance coping.*

<u>Manage:</u> Request consultations with occupational and physical therapists about adaptive equipment and exercise programs *to promote use of the affected limb.*

Refer patient and family members to appropriate support groups and other community resources *to assist in adjusting to patient's altered state of health.*

SUGGESTED NIC INTERVENTIONS

Anticipatory Guidance; Body Image Enhancement; Coping Enhancement; Exercise Therapy: Joint Mobility; Mutual Goal-Setting; Self-Care Assistance; Unilateral Neglect Management

REFERENCE

Medin, J., Windahl, J., von Arbin, M., Tham, K., & Wredling, R. (2012, March). Eating difficulties among patients 3 months after stroke in relation to the acute phase. *Journal of Advanced Nursing, 68*(3), 580–589.

DEFINITION

Dysfunction in urine elimination

DEFINING CHARACTERISTICS

- Dysuria
- Frequency
- Hesitancy
- Incontinence
- Nocturia
- Retention
- Urgency

RELATED FACTORS

- Anatomical obstruction
- Multiple causality
- Sensory motor impairment
- Urinary tract infection

ASSESSMENT FOCUS

(Refer to comprehensive assessment parameters.)
- Coping
- Elimination
- Fluid and electrolytes
- Nutrition
- Reproduction

EXPECTED OUTCOMES

The patient will
- Maintain fluid balance; intake will equal output.
- Voice increased comfort.
- Voice understanding of treatment.
- Have few, if any, complications.
- Discuss impact of urologic disorder on self and family members.
- Demonstrate skill in managing urinary elimination problem.
- Maintain urinary continence.

SUGGESTED NOC OUTCOMES

Urinary Continence; Urinary Elimination

INTERVENTIONS AND RATIONALES

<u>Determine:</u> Observe patient's voiding pattern. Document intake and output, urine color and characteristics, and patient's daily weight. Report any changes. *Accurate intake and output measurements are essential for correct fluid replacement therapy. Urine characteristics help verify diagnosis.*

Observe bowel habits; check for constipation; check for fecal impaction; if present, disimpact and institute a bowel regimen. *These measures promote comfort and prevent loss of rectal muscle tone from prolonged distention.*

<u>Perform:</u> Administer appropriate care for the urologic condition and monitor progress (e.g., strain urine). Report favorable and adverse responses to the treatment regimen. *Appropriate care helps patient recover from*

the underlying disorder. Reporting responses to treatment allows modification of the treatment, as needed.

If patient requires surgery, give appropriate preoperative and postoperative instructions and care. *Accurate information allows patient to understand the procedure and builds trust in caregivers.*

Provide supportive measures, as indicated.

- Administer pain medication and monitor patient *to reduce pain and assess the effects of medication.*
- Encourage fluids, as ordered, *to moisten mucous membranes and dilute chemical materials within the body.*
- Assist with general hygiene and comfort measures, as needed. *Cleanliness prevents bacterial growth and promotes comfort.*
- Maintain patency of catheters, drainage bags, and other urinary elimination equipment *to avoid reflux and risk of infection and ensure the effectiveness of therapy.*
- Provide mental care according to facility policy *to promote cleanliness and comfort and reduce the risk of infection.*

<u>Inform:</u> Explain reasons for therapy and intended effects to patient and family members *to increase patient's understanding and build trust in caregivers.*

If patient needs urinary diversion, prepare him or her for a change in body appearance (instruct patient and family members how to care for the ostomy site postoperatively). *Preparation and appropriate information help patient and family members cope with changes.*

Explain the urologic condition to patient and family members, including instructions on preventive measures, if appropriate. Prepare for discharge according to individual needs. *Accurate health knowledge increases patient's ability to maintain health. Involving family members assures patient that he'll be cared for.*

Assist with bladder elimination procedure, as indicated.

- For bladder training, place patient on the commode or toilet every 2 hours while awake and once during the night. Maintain regular fluid intake while patient is awake. Provide privacy. Teach patient how to perform Kegel exercises to strengthen sphincter control. *These measures aid adaptation to routine physiologic function. Women with good muscle tone can improve levator muscle action significantly if they perform Kegel exercises regularly.*
- For intermittent catheterization, catheterize patient using clean or sterile technique every 2 hours. Record amount voided spontaneously and amount obtained with catheterization (e.g., 7 a.m., spontaneous void of 200 mL; catheter void of 150 mL). Record bladder balance daily. *These measures promote normal voiding, prevent infection, and help maintain integrity of ureterovesical function. Catheterization schedule is based on flow sheet data and can provide a baseline chart.*

- Bladder balance for amount of residual urine/amount of voided urine.
- For external catheterization (in a male patient), monitor patency. Apply a condom catheter according to the established policy. *Applying a foam strip in a spiral fashion increases the adhesive surface and reduces the risk of impairing circulation.* Avoid constriction. Observe the skin condition of the penis, and clean with soap and water at least twice daily. *These measures prevent infection and ensure therapeutic effectiveness.*
- For an indwelling urinary catheter, monitor patency. Keep the tubing free from kinks and keep the drainage bag below the level of the bladder *to avoid urine reflux.* Clean the urinary meatus according to the established policy, and maintain a closed drainage system *to prevent skin irritation and bacteriuria.* Secure the catheter to patient's leg (female) or abdomen (male); avoid tension on the sphincter. *Anchoring the catheter avoids straining the trigone muscle of the bladder and prevents friction leading to inflammation.*
- For a suprapubic catheter, monitor patency. Change the dressing and clean the catheter site according to policy. Keep the tubing free from kinks; keep the drainage bag below bladder level. Maintain a closed drainage system. *Suprapubic drainage allows increased patient mobility and reduces the risk of bladder infection.*

Attend: Encourage patient to ventilate feelings and concerns related to his or her urologic problem. *Active listening conveys respect for patient; ventilation helps pinpoint patient's fears.*

Manage: Refer patient to a dietitian for instructions on diet. *Dietary changes may decrease urinary infections.*

Refer patient and family members to a psychiatric liaison nurse, sex counselor, or support group, when appropriate. *These resources help patient gain knowledge of himself or herself and the situation, reduce anxiety, and promote personal growth. Community resources usually provide support and care not available in other health care agencies.*

SUGGESTED NIC INTERVENTIONS

Anxiety Reduction; Fluid Management; Urinary Elimination Management; Urinary Retention Care; Weight Management; Urinary Bladder Training; Urinary Catheterization

REFERENCE

Tilley, C. (2012). Caring for the patient with a fecal or urinary diversion in palliative and hospice settings: A literature review. *Ostomy and Wound Management, 58*(1), 24–34.

DEFINITION

A pattern of urinary functions sufficient for meeting eliminatory needs and can be strengthened

DEFINING CHARACTERISTICS

- Amount of urine output within normal limits for age
- Expresses willingness to enhance urinary elimination
- Fluid intake adequate for daily needs
- Positions self for emptying of bladder
- Specific gravity within normal limits
- Urine straw colored with no odor

ASSESSMENT FOCUS

(Refer to comprehensive assessment parameters.)

- Coping
- Elimination
- Fluid and electrolytes
- Nutrition
- Reproduction

EXPECTED OUTCOMES

The patient will

- Maintain urine output that is clear and straw colored with no odor.
- Drink 64 oz of noncaffeinated, nonalcoholic beverages per day (unless contraindicated).
- Maintain blood pressure in normal range.
- Avoid use of nonsteroidal anti-inflammatory drugs (NSAIDs), analgesics, and anticholinergics.
- Express understanding of health promotion activities to enhance urinary elimination.

SUGGESTED NOC OUTCOMES

Urinary Continence; Urinary Elimination; Fluid Balance

INTERVENTIONS AND RATIONALES

<u>Determine:</u> Assess that weight is within established norms *to prevent pressure on bladder which contributes to incontinence.*

Assess that blood pressure is within norms; *elevated ranges contribute to renal failure.*

<u>Perform:</u> Discuss voiding and fluid intake patterns to *provide a baseline for introducing new activities.*

Discuss foods that increase acidity in the urine (cranberries, meats, eggs, whole grains, and prunes) and foods that are low in sodium. *Increased acidity in the urine impedes bacterial growth. Foods high in sodium cause fluid retention and decreased urine output.*

Discuss hygiene practices, including hand hygiene, wiping and cleaning from front to back, and taking showers rather than baths (females). *Cleaning from front to back prevents transferring microorganisms from the bowel to the urinary meatus. Showering flushes microorganisms away from the urinary meatus, preventing urinary tract infections (UTIs).*

<u>Inform:</u> Teach female patient to perform Kegel exercises *to strengthen pelvic muscles and prevent development of incontinence (which occurs in 20% to 40% of elderly women).*

Teach stress management techniques. *Stress stimulates release of antidiuretic hormones and interferes with sphincter relaxation, which causes urine retention.*

Explain reasons for activities that enhance urinary elimination *to patient to promote understanding and compliance.*

<u>Attend:</u> Encourage patient to drink six to eight glasses of noncaffeinated, nonalcoholic, noncarbonated liquid, preferably water, per day (unless contraindicated). *1,500 to 2,000 mL/day promotes optimal renal function and flushes bacteria and solutes from the urinary tract. Caffeine and alcohol promote diuresis and may contribute to excess fluid loss. Caffeine, alcohol, and carbonation are irritating to the bladder wall.*

Encourage patient to respond to the urge to void in a timely manner. *Ignoring the urge to urinate may cause incontinence.*

For female patient, encourage her to void before and after intercourse *to flush microorganisms away from the urinary meatus, preventing UTI;* to avoid bubble baths *that may cause chemical irritation to urinary meatus increasing the risk of UTI;* and to wear cotton underpants *as cotton is an absorbent fabric that prevents perineal moisture retention.*

Encourage patient to participate in regular exercise, including walking and modified sit-ups (unless contraindicated). *Weak abdominal and perineal muscles weaken bladder and sphincter control.*

Encourage patient to avoid NSAIDs, analgesics, and anticholinergics. *NSAIDs and analgesics impair renal blood flow. Anticholinergic drugs inhibit relaxation of urinary sphincter and cause urine retention.*

Encourage patient to stop smoking (if applicable) or refrain from starting. *Smoking contributes to renal and bladder cancer. Nicotine is a potent vasoconstrictor.*

Encourage patient to avoid exposure to petroleum, heavy metals, asbestos, dyes, rubber, leather, ink, and paint. *Exposure to carcinogens increases the risk of renal and bladder cancer.*

<u>Manage:</u> Advise patient to report presence of sore throat to primary care provider. *Sore throat may be indicative of streptococcal infection, which may cause renal failure.*

SUGGESTED NIC INTERVENTIONS
Urinary Elimination Management; Smoking Cessation Assistance

REFERENCE
Wang, K., & Palmer, M. H. (2011, May–June). Development and validation of an instrument to assess women's toileting behavior related to urinary elimination: Preliminary results. *Nursing Research, 60*(3), 158–164.

DEFINITION
Incomplete emptying of the bladder

DEFINING CHARACTERISTICS
- Absence of urinary output
- Dribbling
- Bladder distention
- Dysuria
- High residual urine
- Overflow incontinence (continuous dribbling)
- Sensation of bladder fullness
- Small, frequent voiding or no urine output

RELATED FACTORS
- Blockage
- High urethral pressure
- Inhibition of reflex arc
- Strong sphincter

ASSESSMENT FOCUS
(Refer to comprehensive assessment parameters.)
- Coping
- Elimination
- Fluid and electrolytes
- Nutrition
- Reproduction

EXPECTED OUTCOMES
The patient will
- Maintain fluid balance, with intake equal to output.
- Voice increased comfort with few or no complications.
- Voice understanding of treatment and demonstrate skill in managing urine retention.
- Have urinalysis within normal limits.
- Avoid bladder distention.
- Discuss impact of urologic disorder on self and family members.
- Identify resources to assist with care following discharge.

SUGGESTED NOC OUTCOMES
Urinary Continence; Urinary Elimination; Knowledge: Treatment Regimen; Symptom Control; Fluid Balance

INTERVENTIONS AND RATIONALES
<u>Determine:</u> Monitor intake and output and report if intake exceeds output *to promote adequate fluid replacement therapy.*

Monitor voiding pattern. Record data on time, place, amount, and patient's awareness of micturition *to establish a pattern of incontinence.*

Monitor therapeutic and adverse effects of prescribed medications *for early recognition and treatment of drug reactions.*

<u>Perform:</u> Assist with ordered bladder elimination procedure as follows:
- Voiding techniques. Perform Credé's or Valsalva's maneuver every 2 to 3 hours to increase bladder pressure to pass urine. Repeat until empty.
- Intermittent catheterization. Catheterize using clean or sterile technique every 2 hours. Record the amount voided spontaneously and the amount obtained with catheterization.

These measures promote normal voiding, prevent infection, and help maintain the integrity of ureterovesical function.

Perform catheter care according to established policy and maintain a closed drainage system to prevent skin irritation and bacteriuria. Secure the catheter to patient's leg (female) or abdomen (male), avoiding tension on the sphincter. *Anchoring the catheter prevents straining of the bladder's trigone muscle and prevents friction leading to inflammation.*

Use of an indwelling urinary catheter or suprapubic catheter. Monitor patency and avoid kinks in tubing. Keep the drainage bag below bladder level to avoid urine reflux. Change dressings according to facility policy. Maintain closed drainage system.

Administer pain medication, as ordered, and monitor patient *to reduce pain and assess the medication's effects.*

For fecal impaction, disimpact and institute a bowel regimen *to promote comfort and prevent the loss of rectal muscle tone from prolonged distention.*

If patient requires surgery, give appropriate preoperative and postoperative instructions and care *to increase patient's understanding.* If he undergoes urinary diversions, prepare him for a change in body image. *Preparation and appropriate information help patient and family members cope with changes.*

Inform: Instruct patient and family members on voiding techniques to be used at home. Provide for return demonstrations until they can perform the procedure well. *Knowledge of procedures and rationales reduces anxiety and promotes comfort. Demonstrations may progress through several sessions until patient can perform independently.*

Attend: Encourage high fluid intake 2000 ml (2 L)/day, unless contraindicated, *to moisten mucous membranes and dilute chemical materials in the body.* Limit fluid intake after 7 p.m. *to prevent nocturia.*

Encourage patient and family members to share feelings and concerns related to urologic problems. *Ventilation helps pinpoint patient's fears and establishes an environment of trust in which patient and family members can begin to deal with the situation.*

Manage: Refer patient and family members to a psychiatric liaison nurse, enterostomal therapist, sex counselor, support group, or home health care agency, when appropriate. *These resources help patient gain knowledge of himself and his situation, reduce anxiety, and help promote personal growth. Community resources usually provide services not available at other health care agencies.*

SUGGESTED NIC INTERVENTIONS

Perineal Care; Urinary Bladder Training; Urinary Catheterization: Intermittent; Urinary Elimination Management

REFERENCE

McKinnon, A., Higgins, A., Lopez, J., & Chaboyer, W. (2011, July–August). Predictors of acute urinary retention after transurethral resection of the prostate: A retrospective chart audit. *Urology Nursing, 31*(4), 207–212.

DEFINITION
At risk for damage to a vein and its surrounding tissues related to the presence of a catheter and/or infused solutions

RISK FACTORS
- Catheter width and type
- Impaired ability to visualize insertion site
- Inadequate catheter fixation
- Insertion site
- Length of insertion time
- Infusion rate
- Nature of solution (e.g., concentration, chemical irritant, temperature, pH)

ASSESSMENT FOCUS
(Refer to comprehensive assessment parameters.)
- Fluid and electrolytes
- Tissue integrity

EXPECTED OUTCOMES
The patient will
- Not experience vascular trauma as a result of catheter or infused solution.
- Communicate reportable signs and symptoms indicating possible catheter- or infusion-related problems.
- Maintain recommended position of extremity during treatment.

SUGGESTED NOC OUTCOMES
Tissue Integrity: Skin & Mucous Membranes; Comfort Status: Physical; Knowledge: Treatment Procedure

INTERVENTIONS AND RATIONALES
<u>Determine:</u> Assess patient for pain at insertion site. *Pain is often the first symptom of vascular trauma.*

<u>Perform:</u> Use transparent dressing over the insertion site. *This will secure the catheter and facilitate frequent assessment of the insertion site.*

Perform prescribed insertion site checks and progress of the infusion *to ensure early identification of problems and timely interventions to avoid vascular trauma.*

<u>Inform:</u> Educate patient about the purpose of the infusion and reportable symptoms indicative of trauma, for example, burning, swelling, warmth. *Prompt termination of the infusion and the catheter will minimize damage to the tissue.*

<u>Attend:</u> Support the patient throughout intravenous therapy *to decrease anxiety and promote positive patient outcomes.*

<u>Manage:</u> Collaborate with experienced team members in the management of complex intravenous therapy *to ensure that all possible steps are taken to minimize complications.*

SUGGESTED NIC INTERVENTIONS
Intravenous (IV) Therapy; Medication Administration: Intravenous (IV); Skin Surveillance; Teaching: Procedure/Treatment

REFERENCE
Johnston-Walker, E., & Hardcastle, J. (2011, July–August). Neurovascular assessment in the critically ill patient. *Nursing in Critical Care, 16*(4), 170–177.

DEFINITION

Inability to adjust to lowered levels of mechanical ventilator support that interrupts and prolongs the weaning process

DEFINING CHARACTERISTICS

Mild dysfunctional weaning response
- Breathing discomfort
- Expressed increased need for oxygen
- Fatigue
- Increased concentration on breathing
- Queries about possible machine malfunction
- Restlessness
- Slight increase in respiratory response above baseline

Moderate dysfunctional weaning response
- Apprehension
- Changes in skin color (paleness and mild cyanosis)
- Decreased air entry on auscultation
- Diaphoresis
- Hypervigilance to activities related to ventilator functioning
- Inability to cooperate
- Inability to respond to coaching
- Increase in blood pressure (no more than 20 mm Hg above baseline)
- Increase in heart rate (no more than 20 beats/minute above baseline)
- Increase in respiratory rate (no more than 5 breaths/minute above baseline)
- Slight respiratory accessory muscle use
- Wide-eyed

Severe dysfunctional weaning response
- Adventitious breath sounds
- Agitation
- Audible airway secretions
- Breathing uncoordinated with ventilator
- Cyanosis
- Decreased level of consciousness (LOC)
- Deteriorating arterial blood gas (ABG) levels
- Full use of respiratory accessory muscles
- Increased blood pressure (more than 20 mm Hg above baseline)
- Increased heart rate (more than 20 beats/minute above baseline)
- Paradoxical abdominal breathing
- Profuse diaphoresis
- Shallow, gasping breaths
- Significant increase in respiratory rate

RELATED FACTORS

- Physiological (e.g., inadequate nutrition, ineffective airway clearance, sleep pattern disturbance, uncontrolled pain)

- Psychological (e.g., anxiety, fear, decreased motivation or self-esteem, fear, hopelessness, powerlessness. Deficient knowledge of weaning process; insufficient trust in health care providers; perceived inefficacy about ability to wean)
- Situational (e.g., adverse environment, history of unsuccessful weaning attempts or ventilator dependence >4 days, inadequate social support, inappropriate pacing of diminished ventilator support, uncontrolled episodic energy demands)

ASSESSMENT FOCUS
(Refer to comprehensive assessment parameters.)
- Cardiac function
- Coping
- Communication
- Fluid and electrolytes
- Knowledge
- Neurocognition
- Physical regulation
- Respiratory function

EXPECTED OUTCOMES
The patient will
- Maintain respiratory rate at 5 breaths/minute within baseline.
- Have ABG levels normal for that patient.
- Maintain stable mental and emotional status during weaning process.
- Indicate feelings of comfort without pain or dyspnea.
- Have breathing pattern return to baseline.
- Maintain PaO_2 within normal limits as activity level increases.
- Breathe spontaneously after ventilation support is withdrawn.

SUGGESTED NOC OUTCOME
Anxiety Self-Control; Client Satisfaction; Technical Aspects of Care; Depression Self-Control; Respiratory Status; Respiratory Status: Ventilation; Risk control; Vital Signs; Electrolyte & Acid/Base Balance

INTERVENTIONS AND RATIONALES
<u>Determine:</u> Assess vital signs; respiratory status, including rate, rhythm, and depth of respiration. Look for nasal flaring, effectiveness of cough; suctioning demands; sputum characteristics, including color, consistency, amount; ABGs; hemoglobin and hematocrit; and respiratory effects of medications. *Assessment information will help identify appropriate outcomes and interventions.*

<u>Perform:</u> Check vital signs every 15 minutes to 1 hours *to detect tachypenea and tachycardia, both of which are early indicators of respiratory distress.*

Begin oxygen support by using the smallest concentration needed *to make the patient comfortable.* Monitor closely *to avoid oxygen toxicity.*

Place patient in Fowler's position *to increase comfort and facilitate adequate chest expansion and diaphragmatic excursion, thereby decreasing the work of breathing.*

Assist patient to progress gradually from bed rest to increased activity *to improve sense of well-being.*

Monitor vital signs and ABGs closely. If respiratory status is compromised, return to bed rest *to decrease metabolic rate and lower oxygen demands.*

<u>Inform:</u> Explain procedures to the patient, and describe specific sensations he or she may feel during each procedure. *Keeping patient informed about what to expect and when to expect it reduces anxiety.*

Teach self-healing techniques to both the patient and the family, such as meditation, guided imagery, yoga, and prayer. Teach patient how to incorporate the use of self-healing techniques in carrying out usual daily activities. *These measures help reduce the anxiety related to respiratory problems and will be less likely to hyperventilate and panic when he or she experiences difficulty breathing normally.*

<u>Attend:</u> Avoid respiratory depressants such as opiates, sedatives, and paralytics *because these drugs further depress respirations and have the potential to cause respiratory arrest* that if the patient decompensates while on 100% fraction of inspired oxygen mask, he or she may require intubation. *Anticipating complications facilitates prompt intervention.*

Explain in a firm, calm voice that you will help the patient maintain control. *This encourages the patient to take control of his or her behavior.*

<u>Manage:</u> Organize family conferences to explore ways in which the family can help support the ventilatory weaning process. *Meetings can help the family members ventilate fears in a safe environment.*

SUGGESTED NIC INTERVENTIONS

Acid–Base Management; Airway Management; Anxiety Reduction; Mechanical Ventilatory Weaning; Respiratory Monitoring; Support System Enhancement; Teaching: Procedure/Treatment; Vital Signs Monitoring; Guided Imagery

REFERENCE

Haas, C. F., et al. (2012, January/March). Advanced ventilator modes and techniques. *Critical Care Nursing Quarterly, 35*(1), 27–38.

DEFINITION

Decreased, delayed, or absent ability to receive, process, transmit, and/or use a system of symbols

DEFINING CHARACTERISTICS

- Disorientation to person, space, time
- Difficulty comprehending and maintaining usual communication pattern
- Difficulty expressing thoughts verbally (aphasia, dysphasia, apraxia, dyslexia)
- Difficulty forming words or sentences (aphonia, dyslalia, dysarthria)
- Difficulty using or inability to use facial expressions or body language
- Dyspnea
- Impaired articulation
- Inability or lack of desire to speak
- Inability to speak dominant language
- Inappropriate verbalizations
- Lack of eye contact or poor selective attention
- Stuttering or slurring
- Visual deficit (partial or total)

RELATED FACTORS

- Absence of significant others
- Altered perceptions
- Alteration in self-concept, self-esteem, or central nervous system
- Anatomical defect (e.g., cleft palate, alteration of the neuro-muscular visual system, phonation apparatus)
- Brain tumor
- Cultural differences
- Decrease in circulation to brain
- Differences related to developmental age
- Environmental barriers
- Lack of information
- Physical barriers (e.g., tracheostomy, intubation)
- Physiological conditions
- Psychological barriers (e.g., psychosis, lack of stimuli)
- Side effects of medications
- Stress
- Weakening of the musculoskeletal system

ASSESSMENT FOCUS

(Refer to comprehensive assessment parameters.)
- Cardiac function
- Communication
- Neurocognition
- Respiratory function

EXPECTED OUTCOMES

The patient/family will
- Have needs met by staff members.
- Express satisfaction with level of communication ability.
- Maintain orientation.
- Maintain effective level of communication.
- Answer direct questions correctly.

SUGGESTED NOC OUTCOMES

Cognition; Communication; Communication: Expressive; Communication: Receptive; Information Processing; Client Satisfaction: Communication

INTERVENTIONS AND RATIONALES

<u>Determine:</u> Observe patient closely for cues to his or her needs and desires, such as gestures, pointing to objects, looking at items, and pantomime *to enhance understanding.* Avoid continually responding to gestures if the potential exists to improve speech *to encourage desire to improve.*

Monitor and record changes in patient's speech pattern or level of orientation. *Changes may indicate improvement or deterioration of condition.*

<u>Perform:</u> Speak slowly and distinctly in a normal tone when addressing patient and stand where patient can see and hear you. *These actions promote comprehension.*

Reorient the patient to reality: Call patient by name; tell him or her your name; give him or her background information (place, date, and time); use television or radio to augment orientation; use large calendars and communication boards (including alphabet and some common words and pictures). *These measures develop orientation skills through repetition and recognition of familiar objects.*

Use short, simple phrases and yes-or-no questions when patient is very frustrated *to reduce frustration.*

<u>Inform:</u> Instruct family members to use techniques listed above *to ease their frustration in communication with the patient.*

<u>Attend:</u> Encourage attempts at communication and provide positive reinforcement *to aid comprehension.*

Allow ample time for a response. Don't answer questions yourself if patient has ability to respond. *This improves patient's self-concept and reduces frustration.*

Repeat or rephrase questions, if necessary, *to improve communication.* Don't pretend to understand if you don't, *to avoid misunderstanding.*

Remove distractions from the environment during attempts at communication. *Reduced distractions improve comprehension.*

<u>Manage:</u> Review diagnostic test results *to determine improvement or deterioration of the disease process.* Adjust the care plan accordingly.

SUGGESTED NIC INTERVENTIONS

Active Listening; Communication Enhancement: Hearing Deficit; Communication Enhancement: Speech Deficit; Learning Facilitation; Touch

REFERENCE

Amundson, W. (2012, January). Nursing home rounds: A simple conversation can yield important clues about the health of a patient with dementia. *Minnesota Medicine, 95*(1), 26.

DEFINITION
Limitation of independent movement within the environment on foot

DEFINING CHARACTERISTICS
Impaired ability to:
- Climb stairs
- Walk on an incline or a decline
- Walk on uneven surfaces
- Walk required distances

RELATED FACTORS
- Cognitive impairment
- Deconditioning
- Depressed mood
- Environmental constraints (e.g., stairs, uneven surfaces)
- Fear of falling
- Impaired balance
- Impaired vision
- Insufficient muscle strength
- Lack of knowledge
- Limited endurance
- Musculoskeletal impairment
- Neuromuscular impairment
- Obesity
- Pain

ASSESSMENT FOCUS
(Refer to comprehensive assessment parameters.)
- Activity/exercise
- Neurocognition
- Pharmacological function
- Physical regulation

EXPECTED OUTCOMES
The patient will
- Have no evidence of complications associated with impaired walking, such as alteration in skin integrity, contractures, venous stasis, or thrombus formation.
- Maintain or improve muscle strength and joint range of motion (ROM).
- Achieve the highest level of ambulation possible (independence using wheelchair, ambulation with device, ambulation without device).
- Maintain safety during ambulation.
- Demonstrate ability to use equipment or devices safely.
- Adapt to alteration in walking.

- Participate in social and occupational activities.
- Demonstrate understanding of specific interventions related to coping with alteration in walking.
- Utilize community resources to promote and maintain the highest level of mobility.

SUGGESTED NOC OUTCOMES

Ambulation; Balance; Coordinated Movement; Endurance; Fall Prevention Behavior; Mobility; Safe Home Environment; Self-Care: Activities of Daily Living (ADLs); Joint Movement

INTERVENTIONS AND RATIONALES

<u>Determine:</u> Identify patient's level of independence using the functional mobility scale.

Communicate the findings to the staff *to provide continuity and preserve documented level of independence.*

Monitor and record daily evidence of complications related to altered walking, such as contractures, venous stasis, skin breakdown, or thrombus formation. *Patient with a history of neuromuscular dysfunction is at risk for complications.*

<u>Perform:</u> Perform ROM exercises for joints of affected limbs, unless contraindicated, at least once per shift. Progress from passive to active ROM, as tolerated, *to prevent joint contractures and muscle atrophy.*

Make sure that patient maintains anatomically correct and functional body positioning. *Proper positioning relieves pressure, thereby preventing skin breakdown and fluid accumulation in dependent extremities.* Encourage repositioning every 2 hours when patient is in bed *to decrease pressure.* Establish a turning schedule for dependent patients *to provide a method for checking on position changes.*

Implement a preambulation program (e.g., turning in bed, sitting on the side of the bed, sitting up in a chair) *to increase independence and patient's self-esteem.*

Perform the indicated medical regimen to manage or prevent complications (e.g., administration of prophylactic heparin for venous thrombosis) *to promote patient's health and well-being.*

Provide progressive ambulation up to the limits imposed by patient's condition *to maintain muscle tone and prevent complications associated with immobility.*

<u>Inform:</u> Instruct patient and family members in ambulation techniques and measures *to prevent complications to help prepare patient and family for discharge.*

Demonstrate ambulation regimen and note the date. Have patient and family members perform a return demonstration *to ensure continuity of care and use of proper technique.*

<u>Attend:</u> Encourage attendance at physical therapy sessions and reinforce prescribed activities by using the same equipment, devices, and

techniques used in therapy sessions. Request a written copy of patient's ambulation program to use as a reference. *These measures maintain continuity and help ensure patient's safety.*

Manage: Refer patient to a physical therapist for development of a program to promote walking *to assist with rehabilitation of musculo-skeletal deficits.*

Assist in identifying resources, such as a community stroke program, sports associations for the disabled, or the National Multiple Sclerosis Society, *to promote patient's reintegration into the community.*

SUGGESTED NIC INTERVENTIONS

Energy Management; Exercise Promotion: Strength Training; Exercise Therapy: Ambulation; Self-Care Assistance

REFERENCE

Shaughnessy, M., Michael, K., & Resnick, B. (2012, February). Impact of tread-mill exercise on efficacy expectations, physical activity, and stroke recovery. *Journal of Neuroscience Nursing, 44*(1), 27–35.

DEFINITION

Meandering, aimless, or repetitive locomotion that exposes the individual to harm; frequently incongruent with boundaries, limits, or obstacles

DEFINING CHARACTERISTICS

- Following behind or shadowing caregiver's locomotion
- Frequent or continuous movement from place to place, often revisiting same destinations
- Fretful or haphazard locomotion or pacing
- Inability to locate significant landmarks in a familiar setting
- Locomotion into private or unauthorized places
- Locomotion resulting in unintended leaving of a premise
- Locomotion that can't easily be dissuaded or redirected
- Persistent locomotion in search of "missing" or unattainable people or places

RELATED FACTORS

- Cognitive impairment
- Cortical atrophy
- Physiological state or need (hunger, thirst, pain, urination, constipation)
- Premorbid behavior
- Sedation
- Separation from familiar people and places
- Time of day

ASSESSMENT FOCUS

(Refer to comprehensive assessment parameters.)

- Activity/exercise
- Emotional
- Cardiac function
- Comfort
- Communication
- Coping
- Sensation/perception
- Neurocognition

EXPECTED OUTCOMES

The patient will

- Participate in physical or other _____ (specify) activities to minimize wandering behavior.
- Ambulate safely.
- Not have unplanned exits or elopements.

The patient and the family will

- Anticipate patient's wandering behavior or ambulation patterns and provide gratification before onset of wandering behavior.
- Identify factors that contribute to wandering behaviors.

SUGGESTED NOC OUTCOMES

Elopement Occurrence; Elopement Propensity Risk; Safe Wandering; Personal Safety Behavior; Safe Home Environment; Ambulation

INTERVENTIONS AND RATIONALES

Determine: Assess characteristics of wandering behavior, *to determine severity of problem and plan interventions.*

Assess reasons for specific behavior problems *to determine possible triggers for wandering behaviors.*

Determine how family members or partner handles wandering behavior *to provide a comprehensive database for planning care.*

Assess patient's hobbies and previous social, leisure, and exercise activities and patterns *to assist in planning interventions.*

Perform: Provide safe and structured daily routine (including regular exercise, walking, and range of motion exercises) and *environment to decrease wandering behavior and minimize caregiver stress.*

Avoid using physical or chemical restraints to control patient's wandering behavior. *Restraints may increase agitation, anxiety, sensory deprivation, falls, and wandering behavior.*

Check patient for hunger, thirst, discomfort, or need for toileting. *These needs may precipitate wandering.*

Inform: Instruct patient and/or family about the following:
- Use dead bolt locks on doors and keep a key accessible for quick exit *to prevent unplanned exits and facilitate entrance and exit in emergency situations.*
- Use fences and hedges around patios or yards and lock gates *to prevent unsafe exits.*
- Install electronic devices with buzzers or bells *to alert others when door or window is open.*

Attend: Encourage participation in activities (e.g., dancing) and simple household chores (e.g., raking leaves, folding laundry) *to reduce anxiety and restlessness.*

Manage: Notify neighbors, local police department, and staff in retirement communities about patient's condition. Keep a list of neighbors' names and phone numbers handy. *Awareness by others can prevent patient from becoming lost or injured.*

Utilize community resources, such as the Alzheimer's Association's Safe Return Program, *to assist in identification, location, and return of individuals with disorders characterized by wandering behaviors.*

SUGGESTED NIC INTERVENTIONS

Activity Therapy; Surveillance: Safety; Environmental Management: Safety; Home Maintenance Management; Elopement Precautions

REFERENCE

Ohayon, M. M., et al. (2012, May 15). Prevalence and comorbidity of nocturnal wandering in the U.S. adult general population. *Neurology, 78*(20), 1583–1589.

PART II

Selected Nursing Diagnoses by Medical Diagnosis

Abnormal rupture of membranes
- Deficient fluid volume
- Fear
- Hyperthermia
- Impaired individual resilience
- Readiness for enhanced child-bearing process
- Risk for bleeding
- Risk for disturbance of maternal–fetal dyad
- Risk for imbalanced fluid volume
- Risk for infection
- Risk for shock

Abortion
- Anxiety
- Complicated grieving
- Ineffective coping
- Hopelessness
- Impaired individual resilience
- Moral distress
- Readiness for enhanced coping
- Readiness for enhanced decision-making
- Risk for bleeding
- Risk for complicated grieving
- Risk for infection

- Risk for interruption of maternal–fetal dyad
- Readiness for enhanced resilience
- Risk for compromised resilience
- Risk for shock
- Situational low self-esteem

Abruptio placentae
- Acute pain
- Anxiety
- Risk for bleeding
- Complicated grieving
- Readiness for enhanced hope
- Risk for shock

Acoustic neuroma
- Chronic pain
- Disturbed sensory perception (auditory)
- Nausea
- Imbalanced nutrition: Less than body requirements
- Impaired skin integrity
- Ineffective breathing pattern
- Ineffective tissue cerebral perfusion

- Insomnia
- Readiness for enhanced knowledge
- Risk for deficient fluid volume
- Risk for electrolyte imbalance
- Risk for interruption of maternal–fetal dyad

Acquired immunodeficiency syndrome
- Caregiver role strain
- Chronic confusion
- Death anxiety
- Decisional conflict
- Defensive coping
- Deficient community health
- Grieving
- Hopelessness
- Impaired individual resilience
- Impaired memory
- Ineffective community coping
- Ineffective denial
- Ineffective protection
- Ineffective self-health management
- Ineffective sexuality patterns
- Ineffective therapeutic regimen management
- Moral distress
- Powerlessness
- Readiness for enhanced communication
- Readiness for enhanced resilience
- Readiness for enhanced self-care
- Risk for caregiver role strain
- Risk for complicated grieving
- Risk for compromised human dignity
- Risk for contamination
- Risk for infection
- Risk for loneliness
- Risk-prone health behavior
- Social isolation

Acute pancreatitis
- Acute pain
- Deficient knowledge (specify)
- Impaired comfort

- Insomnia
- Nausea
- Readiness for enhanced coping
- Risk for dysfunctional gastrointestinal motility
- Risk for electrolyte imbalance
- Risk for imbalanced fluid volume
- Risk for imbalanced nutrition: More than body requirements
- Risk for impaired liver function
- Risk for unstable glucose level
- Risk-prone health behavior

Acute renal failure
- Death anxiety
- Decreased cardiac output
- Deficient fluid volume
- Disturbed thought processes
- Dressing or grooming self-care deficit
- Excess fluid volume
- Fear
- Impaired physical mobility
- Impaired skin integrity
- Ineffective tissue perfusion (renal)
- Interrupted family processes
- Readiness for enhanced spiritual well-being
- Risk for acute confusion
- Risk for complicated grieving
- Risk for electrolyte imbalance
- Risk for imbalanced fluid volume
- Risk for ineffective renal perfusion
- Risk for infection
- Risk-prone health behavior
- Sexual dysfunction
- Disturbed sleep pattern
- Sleep deprivation
- Spiritual distress

Acute respiratory distress syndrome
- Anxiety
- Bathing or hygiene self-care deficit

- Deficient fluid volume
- Denial
- Dysfunctional ventilatory weaning response
- Fear
- Impaired comfort
- Imbalanced nutrition: Less than body requirements
- Impaired gas exchange
- Impaired skin integrity
- Impaired spontaneous ventilation
- Impaired verbal communication
- Ineffective airway clearance
- Ineffective breathing pattern
- Ineffective coping
- Ineffective tissue perfusion (cardiopulmonary)
- Insomnia
- Risk for acute confusion
- Risk for electrolyte imbalance
- Risk for ineffective cardiac tissue perfusion
- Risk for ineffective cerebral tissue perfusion
- Risk for infection
- Risk for shock
- Risk for vascular trauma
- Sleep deprivation

Acute respiratory failure
- Activity intolerance
- Death anxiety
- Decreased cardiac output
- Denial
- Disturbed sensory perception
- Disturbed thought processes
- Fear
- Impaired gas exchange
- Impaired individual resilience
- Impaired verbal communication
- Ineffective breathing pattern
- Ineffective tissue perfusion (cardiopulmonary)
- Insomnia
- Powerlessness
- Readiness for enhanced spiritual well-being

- Risk for ineffective activity planning
- Risk for acute confusion
- Risk for aspiration
- Risk for electrolyte imbalance
- Risk for ineffective cardiac tissue perfusion
- Risk for ineffective renal tissue perfusion
- Risk for infection
- Risk for shock
- Risk for suffocation
- Spiritual distress

Adrenal insufficiency
- Acute pain
- Chronic low self-esteem
- Compromised family coping
- Disturbed body image
- Disturbed personality identity
- Readiness for enhanced resilience
- Readiness for enhanced self care
- Risk for electrolyte imbalance
- Risk for imbalanced body temperature
- Risk for impaired skin integrity
- Risk for infection
- Risk-prone health behavior
- Sexual dysfunction
- Sleep deprivation

Adrenocortical insufficiency
- Risk for disproportionate growth
- Risk for infection

Affective disorders
- Anxiety
- Energy field disturbance
- Disturbed personality identity
- Disturbed sensory perception (specify)
- Disturbed thought processes
- Hopelessness
- Impaired religiosity
- Ineffective coping
- Ineffective impulse control
- Ineffective relationship

- Ineffective role performance
- Insomnia
- Readiness for enhanced coping
- Risk for loneliness
- Risk for other-directed violence
- Risk-prone health behavior
- Risk for self-directed violence
- Sexual dysfunction
- Disturbed sleep pattern
- Stress overload

Alcohol addiction and abuse
- Acute confusion
- Bathing or hygiene self-care deficit
- Defensive coping
- Deficient knowledge (specify)
- Disturbed personality identity
- Dysfunctional family processes: Alcoholism
- Functional urinary incontinence
- Imbalanced nutrition: Less than body requirements
- Impaired individual resilience
- Impaired physical mobility
- Ineffective activity planning
- Ineffective community therapeutic regimen management
- Ineffective coping
- Ineffective denial
- Ineffective family therapeutic regimen management
- Ineffective impulse response
- Insomnia
- Powerlessness
- Readiness for enhanced family processes
- Readiness for enhanced family coping
- Readiness for enhanced self-concept
- Risk for acute confusion
- Risk for compromised human dignity
- Risk for electrolyte imbalance
- Risk for imbalanced fluid volume

- Risk for impaired liver function
- Risk for poisoning
- Risk for self-directed violence
- Risk-prone health behavior
- Self-neglect
- Sexual dysfunction
- Sleep deprivation
- Spiritual distress
- Social isolation
- Stress overload

Alzheimer's disease
- Adult failure to thrive
- Anxiety
- Bathing or hygiene self-care deficit
- Bowel incontinence
- Caregiver role strain
- Chronic confusion
- Chronic low self-esteem
- Complicated grieving
- Compromised family coping
- Deficient knowledge (specify)
- Disturbed sensory perception
- Disturbed thought processes
- Functional urinary incontinence
- Grieving
- Hopelessness
- Imbalanced nutrition: Less than body requirements
- Impaired comfort
- Impaired environmental interpretation syndrome
- Impaired home maintenance
- Impaired memory
- Impaired verbal communication
- Ineffective coping
- Ineffective health maintenance
- Ineffective role performance
- Ineffective sexuality patterns
- Interrupted family processes
- Moral distress
- Readiness for enhanced knowledge

- Readiness for enhanced self-care
- Relocation stress syndrome
- Risk for caregiver role strain
- Risk for compromised human dignity
- Risk for injury
- Risk for poisoning
- Risk for trauma
- Social isolation
- Stress urinary incontinence
- Wandering

Amniotic fluid embolism

- Ineffective tissue perfusion (cardiopulmonary)
- Risk for electrolyte imbalance
- Risk for ineffective cardiac tissue perfusion
- Risk for ineffective peripheral tissue perfusion
- Risk for injury
- Risk for shock

Amputation

- Acute pain
- Anxiety
- Chronic low self-esteem
- Chronic pain
- Decisional conflict
- Deficient knowledge (specify)
- Delayed surgical recovery
- Denial
- Disturbed body image
- Disturbed personality identity
- Energy field disturbance
- Grieving
- Impaired individual resilience
- Impaired wheelchair mobility
- Impaired walking
- Ineffective activity planning
- Impaired transfer ability
- Readiness for enhanced self-care
- Readiness for enhanced hope
- Readiness for enhanced knowledge
- Risk for compromised resilience

- Risk for compromised human dignity
- Risk for injury
- Risk-prone health behavior

Amyotrophic lateral sclerosis

- Bowel incontinence
- Caregiver role strain
- Chronic low self-esteem
- Complicated grieving
- Compromised family coping
- Constipation
- Death anxiety
- Disturbed personality identity
- Dressing or grooming self-care deficit
- Dysfunctional ventilatory weaning response
- Grieving
- Hopelessness
- Impaired physical mobility
- Impaired skin integrity
- Impaired spontaneous ventilation
- Impaired verbal communication
- Impaired walking
- Impaired wheelchair ability
- Ineffective airway clearance
- Ineffective breathing pattern
- Ineffective coping
- Ineffective health maintenance
- Ineffective sexuality patterns
- Readiness for enhanced knowledge
- Risk for aspiration
- Risk for caregiver role strain
- Risk for constipation
- Risk for dysfunctional gastrointestinal motility
- Risk for electrolyte imbalance
- Risk for falls
- Risk for imbalanced fluid volume
- Risk for impaired skin integrity
- Risk for ineffective peripheral tissue perfusion

- Risk for infection
- Social isolation

Anaphylactic shock
- Decreased cardiac output
- Impaired gas exchange
- Ineffective tissue perfusion (cardiopulmonary)
- Ineffective tissue perfusion (renal)
- Ineffective tissue perfusion (cerebral)

Anemias
- Activity intolerance
- Adult failure to thrive
- Decreased cardiac output
- Fatigue
- Impaired gas exchange
- Impaired skin integrity
- Ineffective breathing patterns
- Ineffective protection
- Ineffective tissue perfusion (cardiopulmonary)
- Readiness for enhanced resilience
- Risk for infection

Angina pectoris
- Activity intolerance
- Acute pain
- Anxiety
- Deficient knowledge (specify)
- Impaired comfort
- Impaired environmental interpretation syndrome
- Ineffective denial
- Ineffective role performance
- Ineffective sexuality patterns
- Readiness for enhanced knowledge
- Risk for ineffective activity planning
- Risk for ineffective cardiac tissue perfusion
- Risk for ineffective cerebral tissue perfusion
- Risk for ineffective renal tissue perfusion
- Sedentary lifestyle
- Stress overload

Anorexia nervosa
- Anxiety
- Constipation
- Deficient fluid volume
- Disturbed body image
- Disturbed personality image
- Hyperthermia
- Imbalanced nutrition: Less than body requirements
- Impaired individual resilience
- Ineffective denial
- Ineffective impulse control
- Ineffective relationships
- Interrupted family processes
- Readiness for enhanced nutrition
- Readiness for enhanced relationship
- Readiness for enhanced sleep
- Risk for chronic low self-esteem
- Risk for constipation
- Risk for dysfunctional gastrointestinal motility
- Risk-prone health behavior
- Sleep deprivation
- Social isolation
- Spiritual distress
- Stress overload

Antisocial personality disorder
- Chronic low self-esteem
- Defensive coping
- Disturbed personal identity
- Disturbed sensory perception
- Dysfunctional family processes: Alcoholism
- Impaired home maintenance
- Impaired individual resilience
- Ineffective coping
- Ineffective role performance
- Interrupted family processes
- Readiness for enhanced relationships
- Readiness for enhanced family coping
- Risk for other-directed violence
- Risk for self-mutilation
- Risk for suicide

- Sexual dysfunction
- Social isolation

Anxiety disorder
- Anxiety
- Caregiver role strain
- Chronic low self-esteem
- Constipation
- Defensive coping
- Diarrhea
- Disturbed sensory perception
- Disturbed thought processes
- Hopelessness
- Imbalanced nutrition: More than body requirements
- Impaired home maintenance
- Ineffective denial
- Interrupted family processes
- Posttrauma syndrome
- Powerlessness
- Readiness for enhanced communication
- Readiness for enhanced coping
- Readiness for enhanced nutrition
- Readiness for enhanced self-concept
- Readiness for enhanced sleep
- Readiness for enhanced spiritual well-being
- Risk for imbalanced nutrition: Less than required
- Risk for imbalanced nutrition: More than body requirements
- Risk for impaired religiosity
- Risk for loneliness
- Risk for posttrauma syndrome
- Social isolation
- Sleep deprivation
- Stress overload

Aortic aneurysm
- Acute pain
- Excess fluid volume
- Impaired gas exchange
- Ineffective tissue perfusion (cardiopulmonary)
- Ineffective tissue perfusion (peripheral)

- Ineffective tissue perfusion (renal)
- Risk for bleeding
- Risk for electrolyte imbalance
- Risk for imbalanced fluid volume
- Risk for ineffective cerebral tissue perfusion
- Risk for shock

Aortic insufficiency
- Activity intolerance
- Decreased cardiac output
- Deficient knowledge (specify)
- Impaired gas exchange
- Ineffective tissue perfusion (cardiopulmonary)
- Risk for ineffective renal tissue perfusion

Aortic stenosis
- Activity intolerance
- Decreased cardiac output
- Deficient knowledge (specify)
- Impaired gas exchange
- Ineffective tissue perfusion (cardiopulmonary)

Appendicitis
- Acute pain
- Delayed surgical recovery
- Imbalanced nutrition: Less than body requirements
- Impaired comfort
- Risk for imbalanced fluid volume
- Risk for infection

Arterial insufficiency
- Chronic pain
- Impaired tissue integrity
- Readiness for enhanced knowledge
- Risk for ineffective peripheral tissue perfusion

Arterial occlusion
- Acute pain
- Deficient knowledge (specify)
- Disturbed sensory perception (tactile)
- Impaired comfort

- Impaired skin integrity
- Ineffective tissue perfusion (cerebral)
- Ineffective tissue perfusion (peripheral)
- Risk for ineffective peripheral tissue perfusion
- Risk-prone health behavior

Asphyxia
- Delayed growth and development
- Hypothermia
- Ineffective breathing pattern
- Ineffective gas exchange
- Risk for aspiration
- Risk for injury
- Risk for suffocation

Asthma
- Activity intolerance
- Anxiety
- Deficient knowledge (specify)
- Dressing or grooming self-care deficit
- Dry eye
- Impaired gas exchange
- Impaired oral mucous membrane
- Ineffective airway clearance
- Ineffective breathing pattern
- Ineffective coping
- Latex allergy response
- Readiness for enhanced comfort
- Readiness for enhanced family coping
- Readiness for enhanced knowledge
- Risk for compromised resilience
- Risk for infection
- Risk for latex allergy response
- Risk-prone health behavior
- Sleep deprivation
- Stress overload

Atelectasis
- Anxiety
- Bathing or hygiene self-care deficit

- Impaired gas exchange
- Impaired physical mobility
- Ineffective airway clearance
- Ineffective breathing pattern
- Impaired gas exchange
- Readiness for enhanced self-care

Attention deficit hyperactivity disorder
- Denial
- Disturbed sleep pattern
- Family therapeutic regimen management
- Ineffective activity planning
- Interrupted family processes
- Readiness for enhanced family processes
- Readiness for enhanced relationships
- Risk for delayed development
- Stress overload

Autism
- Compromised family coping
- Delayed growth and development
- Disabled family coping
- Ineffective denial
- Interrupted family processes
- Risk for delayed development
- Risk for self-mutilation

Bell's palsy
- Acute pain
- Anxiety
- Chronic low self-esteem
- Disturbed body image
- Disturbed sleep pattern
- Disturbed sensory perception (gustatory)
- Impaired comfort
- Impaired swallowing
- Impaired verbal communication
- Ineffective sexuality patterns
- Powerlessness
- Risk for compromised human dignity
- Social isolation
- Stress overload
- Unilateral neglect

Benign prostatic hypertrophy
- Deficient knowledge (specify)
- Impaired comfort
- Impaired urinary elimination
- Ineffective sexuality patterns
- Sexual dysfunction
- Urinary retention

Bipolar disorder: Depressive phase
- Chronic low self-esteem
- Constipation
- Disturbed personality identity
- Disturbed sensory perception
- Disturbed thought processes
- Feeding self-care deficit
- Hopelessness
- Imbalanced nutrition: Less than body requirements
- Ineffective coping
- Ineffective denial
- Ineffective relationships
- Ineffective health maintenance
- Insomnia
- Readiness for enhanced communication
- Readiness for enhanced coping
- Readiness for enhanced self-concept
- Risk for compromised human dignity
- Risk for ineffective activity planning
- Risk for injury
- Risk for self-directed violence
- Self-neglect
- Sexual dysfunction
- Sleep deprivation
- Social isolation
- Spiritual distress
- Stress overload

Bipolar disorder: Manic phase
- Chronic low self-esteem
- Disabled family coping
- Disturbed personality identity
- Disturbed sensory perception
- Disturbed thought processes
- Feeding self-care deficit
- Impaired home maintenance
- Impaired physical mobility
- Impaired verbal communication
- Ineffective coping
- Ineffective denial
- Ineffective impulse control
- Ineffective sexuality pattern
- Insomnia
- Risk for compromised resilience
- Readiness for enhanced family coping
- Interrupted family processes
- Risk for falls
- Risk for impaired religiosity
- Risk for injury
- Risk for other-directed violence
- Risk-prone health behavior
- Sexual dysfunction
- Spiritual distress

Bladder cancer
- Acute pain
- Fear
- Impaired tissue integrity
- Impaired urinary elimination
- Readiness for enhanced self-care
- Risk for compromised human dignity
- Risk for latex allergy response
- Overflow urinary incontinence
- Urge urinary incontinence

Blindness
- Deficient diversional activity
- Deficient knowledge (specify)
- Disturbed body image
- Disturbed sensory perception (visual)
- Fear
- Hopelessness
- Impaired physical mobility
- Ineffective self-health management
- Powerlessness

- Risk for falls
- Risk for injury
- Risk for loneliness
- Social isolation

Bone marrow transplantation
- Activity intolerance
- Complicated grieving
- Contamination
- Decreased cardiac output
- Deficient diversional activity
- Diarrhea
- Disturbed body image
- Excess fluid volume
- Grieving
- Imbalanced nutrition: Less than body requirements
- Impaired oral mucous membrane
- Impaired skin integrity
- Ineffective activity planning
- Ineffective protection
- Ineffective therapeutic management
- Risk for contamination
- Risk for electrolyte imbalance
- Risk for imbalanced fluid balance
- Risk for infection

Bone sarcomas
- Activity intolerance
- Acute pain
- Deficient knowledge
- Impaired comfort
- Impaired physical mobility
- Impaired tissue integrity
- Readiness for enhanced knowledge
- Risk for falls
- Risk for injury
- Risk for infection

Borderline personality disorder
- Chronic low self-esteem
- Disturbed personality identity
- Fear
- Impaired religiosity
- Ineffective coping
- Ineffective impulse control

- Ineffective relationships
- Risk for compromised resilience
- Risk for self-directed violence
- Risk for self-mutilation
- Social isolation

Bowel fistula
- Risk for deficient fluid volume
- Risk for infection

Bowel resection
- Anxiety
- Delayed surgical recovery
- Dysfunctional gastrointestinal motility
- Deficient knowledge
- Diarrhea
- Imbalanced Nutrition: Less than required
- Impaired skin integrity
- Risk for disturbed personal identity
- Risk for infection

Brain abscess
- Acute pain
- Decreased intracranial adaptive capacity
- Disturbed body image
- Impaired physical mobility
- Impaired skin integrity
- Ineffective sexuality patterns
- Ineffective tissue perfusion (cerebral)
- Risk for aspiration
- Risk for infection
- Risk for injury
- Risk for urge urinary incontinence

Brain tumors
- Acute confusion
- Bowel incontinence
- Constipation
- Decreased intracranial adaptive capacity
- Disturbed personality identity
- Disabled family processes
- Disturbed sensory perception
- Disturbed thought processes

- Fear
- Grieving
- Impaired environmental interpretation syndrome
- Impaired memory
- Impaired physical mobility
- Impaired tissue integrity
- Impaired urinary elimination
- Impaired verbal communication
- Ineffective coping
- Ineffective thermoregulation
- Risk for falls
- Risk for injury
- Total urinary incontinence

Breast cancer
- Acute pain
- Anxiety
- Complicated grieving
- Death anxiety
- Decisional conflict (specify)
- Deficient knowledge (specify)
- Disturbed body image
- Fear
- Grieving
- Impaired skin integrity
- Ineffective coping
- Moral distress
- Powerlessness
- Readiness for enhanced hope
- Readiness for enhanced spiritual well-being
- Readiness for enhanced resilience
- Risk for compromised human dignity
- Spiritual distress

Breast engorgement
- Acute pain
- Impaired comfort
- Impaired skin integrity
- Ineffective breastfeeding
- Readiness for enhanced breastfeeding
- Risk for infection

Bronchiectasis
- Compromised family coping
- Deficient knowledge

- Imbalanced nutrition: Less than body requirements
- Impaired gas exchange
- Ineffective airway clearance
- Ineffective breathing pattern
- Risk for electrolyte imbalance
- Risk for imbalance in fluid volume
- Risk for infection

Bulimia nervosa
- Anxiety
- Constipation
- Deficient fluid volume
- Disabled family coping
- Disturbed body image
- Hyperthermia
- Imbalanced nutrition: Less than body requirements
- Imbalanced nutrition: More than body requirements
- Impaired dentition
- Ineffective denial
- Interrupted family processes
- Powerlessness
- Risk for constipation
- Risk for electrolyte imbalance
- Risk for self-mutilation
- Risk for self-directed violence
- Sleep deprivation
- Social isolation

Burns
- Acute pain
- Constipation
- Deficient diversional activity
- Deficient fluid volume
- Disabled family coping
- Disturbed body image
- Disturbed personal identity
- Dysfunctional ventilatory weaning response
- Electrolyte imbalance
- Grieving
- Hyperthermia
- Hypothermia
- Imbalanced nutrition: Less than body requirements
- Impaired comfort
- Impaired physical mobility

- Impaired skin integrity
- Impaired spontaneous ventilation
- Ineffective breathing pattern
- Ineffective tissue perfusion (renal)
- Powerlessness
- Readiness for enhanced hope
- Readiness for enhanced self-care
- Risk for deficient fluid volume
- Risk for electrolyte imbalance
- Risk for falls
- Risk for imbalanced body temperature
- Risk for infection
- Risk for injury
- Risk for shock

Cancer
- Adult failure to thrive
- Chronic sorrow
- Death anxiety
- Deficient knowledge
- Disabled family coping
- Energy field disturbance
- Grieving
- Ineffective health maintenance
- Nausea
- Readiness for enhanced knowledge
- Readiness for enhanced religiosity
- Readiness for enhanced self-concept
- Readiness for enhanced spiritual well-being
- Risk for impaired tissue integrity
- Risk for infection
- Risk for spiritual distress

Cardiac arrhythmias
- Anxiety
- Decreased cardiac output
- Excess fluid volume
- Fear
- Ineffective sexuality patterns

- Ineffective tissue perfusion (cardiopulmonary)
- Risk for electrolyte imbalance
- Risk for imbalanced fluid volume
- Stress overload

Cardiac disease: End-stage
- Activity intolerance
- Adult failure to thrive
- Caregiver role strain
- Death anxiety
- Decisional conflict
- Decreased cardiac output
- Defensive coping
- Excess fluid volume
- Grieving
- Hopelessness
- Ineffective breathing pattern
- Ineffective coping
- Impaired physical mobility
- Risk for aspiration
- Risk for caregiver role strain
- Risk for electrolyte imbalance
- Risk for falls
- Risk for infection
- Risk for injury
- Sedentary lifestyle
- Self-care bathing, feeding, dressing, toileting deficit
- Situational low self-esteem

Cardiogenic shock
- Death anxiety
- Decreased cardiac output
- Excess fluid volume
- Fear
- Impaired gas exchange
- Ineffective breathing pattern
- Ineffective tissue perfusion (cardiac)

Carpal tunnel syndrome
- Acute pain
- Impaired physical mobility
- Ineffective tissue perfusion (peripheral)
- Risk for peripheral neurovascular dysfunction
- Sleep deprivation
- Readiness for enhanced comfort

Cataracts
- Disturbed body image
- Disturbed sensory perception (visual)
- Impaired physical mobility
- Ineffective coping
- Ineffective health maintenance
- Risk for falls
- Risk for injury

Cellulitis
- Acute pain
- Anxiety
- Deficient knowledge (specify)
- Impaired physical mobility
- Impaired skin integrity
- Risk for ineffective activity planning

Cerebral aneurysm
- Decreased intracranial adaptive capacity
- Fear
- Impaired physical mobility
- Impaired skin integrity
- Ineffective airway clearance
- Ineffective breathing pattern
- Ineffective tissue perfusion
- Risk for bleeding
- Risk for falls
- Risk for ineffective cerebral tissue perfusion
- Risk for injury
- Risk for shock

Cerebral edema
- Decreased intracranial adaptive capacity
- Impaired gas exchange
- Ineffective thermoregulation
- Risk for electrolyte imbalance
- Risk for ineffective cerebral tissue perfusion

Cerebral palsy
- Delayed growth and development
- Impaired physical mobility
- Impaired walking

- Impaired verbal communication
- Powerlessness
- Readiness for enhanced self-care
- Risk for caregiver role strain
- Risk for compromised human dignity
- Social isolation
- Toileting self-care deficit
- Total urinary incontinence

Cervical cancer
- Acute pain
- Disturbed body image
- Disturbed personal identity
- Fatigue
- Fear
- Impaired skin integrity
- Ineffective protection
- Deficient knowledge
- Risk-prone health behavior

Chemotherapy
- Constipation
- Deficient diversional activity
- Deficient fluid volume
- Diarrhea
- Disturbed sensory perception (auditory)
- Imbalanced nutrition: Less than body requirements
- Impaired gas exchange
- Impaired oral mucous membrane
- Impaired physical mobility
- Ineffective protection
- Ineffective tissue perfusion
- Nausea
- Readiness for enhanced hope
- Risk for compromised human dignity
- Risk for impaired skin integrity
- Risk for infection
- Sexual dysfunction

Chest trauma
- Dysfunctional ventilatory weaning response
- Impaired comfort

- Impaired gas exchange
- Impaired spontaneous ventilation
- Ineffective airway clearance
- Ineffective breathing pattern
- Risk for aspiration
- Risk for ineffective cardiac tissue perfusion
- Risk for shock

Child abuse
- Delayed growth and development
- Fear
- Impaired parenting
- Deficient knowledge
- Imbalanced nutrition: Less than body requirements
- Parental role conflict
- Readiness for enhanced parenting
- Risk for impaired parenting
- Risk for other directed violence
- Disturbed sleep pattern

Childbirth
- Deficient knowledge (specify)
- Ineffective childbearing process
- Interrupted family processes
- Readiness for enhanced childbearing process
- Readiness for enhanced knowledge
- Readiness for enhanced parenting
- Risk for ineffective childbearing process
- Risk for disturbed maternal–fetal dyad

Chlamydia
- Ineffective self-health management
- Ineffective sexuality patterns
- Risk for infection
- Risk-prone health behavior

Chloride imbalance
- Imbalanced nutrition: Less than body requirements

- Impaired breathing pattern
- Nausea
- Risk for electrolyte imbalance

Cholecystitis
- Acute pain
- Deficient fluid volume
- Imbalanced nutrition: Less than body requirements
- Risk for impaired liver function
- Risk for infection

Chronic bronchitis
- Activity intolerance
- Deficient knowledge (specify)
- Fatigue
- Fear
- Hopelessness
- Impaired comfort
- Impaired gas exchange
- Impaired spontaneous ventilation
- Ineffective airway clearance
- Ineffective breathing pattern
- Risk for ineffective cardiac tissue perfusion
- Risk for infection

Chronic fatigue syndrome
- Acute pain
- Disturbed sleep pattern
- Fatigue
- Hopelessness
- Powerlessness
- Readiness for enhanced therapeutic regimen management
- Social isolation
- Risk for spiritual distress

Chronic obstructive pulmonary disease
- Activity intolerance
- Adult failure to thrive
- Anxiety
- Caregiver role strain
- Compromised family coping
- Defensive coping
- Deficient fluid volume
- Deficient knowledge (specify)

- Dysfunctional ventilatory weaning response
- Fatigue
- Fear
- Hopelessness
- Imbalanced nutrition: More than body requirements
- Imbalanced nutrition: Less than body requirements
- Impaired gas exchange
- Impaired home maintenance
- Impaired oral mucous membrane
- Impaired spontaneous ventilation
- Impaired verbal communication
- Ineffective airway clearance
- Ineffective breathing pattern
- Ineffective denial
- Ineffective health maintenance
- Ineffective self-health management
- Ineffective tissue perfusion (cardiopulmonary)
- Insomnia
- Noncompliance
- Powerlessness
- Readiness for enhanced coping
- Readiness for enhanced self-health management
- Readiness for enhanced religiosity
- Risk for falls
- Risk for infection
- Risk for injury
- Risk for suffocation
- Sleep deprivation

Chronic pain
- Anxiety
- Chronic low self-esteem
- Chronic pain
- Defensive coping
- Disturbed sleep pattern
- Hopelessness
- Risk-prone health behavior
- Situational low self-esteem
- Sleep deprivation

Chronic renal failure
- Caregiver role strain
- Compromised family coping
- Death anxiety
- Deficient knowledge (specify)
- Disturbed body image
- Excess fluid volume
- Ineffective denial
- Ineffective therapeutic management
- Ineffective tissue perfusion (renal)
- Interrupted family processes
- Powerlessness
- Risk for ineffective renal perfusion
- Risk for impaired liver function
- Risk for impaired skin integrity
- Risk for infection
- Risk for vascular trauma
- Sexual dysfunction

Cirrhosis
- Compromised family coping
- Bowel incontinence
- Deficient fluid volume
- Diarrhea
- Disturbed thought processes
- Imbalanced nutrition: Less than body requirements
- Imbalanced nutrition: More than body requirements
- Ineffective breathing pattern
- Interrupted family processes: Alcoholism
- Ineffective self-health management
- Moral distress
- Nausea
- Risk for bleeding
- Readiness for enhanced religiosity
- Risk for electrolyte imbalances
- Risk for falls
- Risk for impaired liver function
- Risk for impaired skin integrity

- Risk for ineffective gastrointestinal tissue perfusion
- Risk for injury
- Risk-prone health behavior
- Self-neglect
- Stress urinary incontinence
- Total urinary incontinence

Cleft lip or palate
- Compromised family coping
- Imbalanced nutrition: Less than body requirements
- Impaired verbal communication
- Ineffective breastfeeding
- Ineffective infant feeding pattern
- Risk for aspiration
- Risk for compromised human dignity

Colic
- Disorganized infant behavior
- Impaired comfort
- Interrupted breastfeeding

Colitis
- Acute pain
- Deficient knowledge
- Deficient fluid volume
- Diarrhea
- Dysfunctional gastrointestinal motility
- Disturbed body image
- Imbalanced nutrition: Less than body requirements
- Ineffective tissue perfusion (GI)
- Risk for imbalanced body temperature
- Risk-prone health behavior

Colon and rectal cancer
- Acute pain
- Anxiety
- Constipation
- Deficient fluid volume
- Deficient knowledge (specify)
- Diarrhea
- Fear
- Impaired comfort

- Deficient knowledge
- Risk for dysfunctional gastrointestinal motility

Colostomy
- Complicated grieving
- Deficient fluid volume
- Delayed surgical recovery
- Disturbed body image
- Dysfunctional gastrointestinal motility
- Imbalanced nutrition: Less than body requirements
- Impaired skin integrity
- Ineffective sexuality patterns
- Ineffective tissue perfusion (GI)
- Readiness for enhanced hope
- Readiness for enhanced knowledge
- Readiness for enhanced self-care
- Risk for compromised human dignity
- Situational low self-esteem
- Spiritual distress

Conduct disorder
- Chronic low self-esteem
- Disturbed personal identity
- Hopelessness
- Impaired individual resilience
- Ineffective impulse control
- Interrupted family processes
- Risk for other-directed violence
- Risk for self-directed violence
- Risk for suicide

Congenital anomalies
- Disabled family coping
- Interrupted family coping
- Risk for falls
- Risk for injury
- Total urinary incontinence

Congenital heart disease
- Activity intolerance
- Decreased cardiac output
- Disturbed body image
- Ineffective breathing pattern

- Interrupted family processes
- Risk for ineffective activity planning
- Risk for disproportionate growth
- Risk for infection
- Risk for injury

Coronary artery disease
- Activity intolerance
- Acute pain
- Anxiety
- Decreased cardiac output
- Deficient knowledge (specify)
- Health-seeking behaviors
- Imbalanced nutrition: More than body requirements
- Impaired gas exchange
- Impaired home maintenance
- Ineffective sexuality patterns
- Ineffective therapeutic regimen management
- Ineffective tissue perfusion (cardiopulmonary)
- Readiness for enhanced knowledge
- Readiness for enhanced self-health management
- Risk for injury
- Risk-prone health behavior
- Sedentary lifestyle
- Stress overload

Cor pulmonale
- Activity intolerance
- Decreased cardiac output
- Excess fluid volume
- Fatigue
- Grieving
- Hopelessness
- Impaired gas exchange
- Ineffective airway clearance
- Ineffective breathing pattern
- Ineffective coping
- Risk for infection

Craniotomy
- Acute pain
- Bathing, feeding, toileting self-care deficit

- Decreased intracranial adaptive capacity
- Delayed surgical recovery
- Disturbed body image
- Disturbed sensory perception
- Disturbed sleep pattern
- Hyperthermia
- Imbalanced nutrition: Less then body requirements
- Impaired physical mobility
- Impaired skin integrity
- Ineffective airway clearance
- Ineffective breathing pattern
- Ineffective tissue perfusion (cerebral)
- Risk for falls
- Risk for infection
- Risk for injury
- Spiritual distress
- Sleep deprivation

Crohn's disease
- Acute pain
- Anxiety
- Compromised family coping
- Deficient fluid volume
- Deficient knowledge (specify)
- Diarrhea
- Disturbed body image
- Dysfunctional gastrointestinal motility
- Fear
- Imbalanced nutrition: Less than body requirements
- Impaired skin integrity
- Insomnia
- Nausea
- Noncompliance
- Readiness for enhanced hope
- Readiness for enhanced self-care
- Risk for imbalanced fluid volume
- Risk for infection
- Stress overload

Cushing's syndrome
- Activity intolerance
- Complicated grieving
- Disturbed body image

- Disturbed thought processes
- Excess fluid volume
- Hopelessness
- Imbalanced nutrition: More than body requirements
- Impaired skin integrity
- Ineffective coping
- Risk for acute confusion
- Risk for imbalanced body temperature
- Risk for imbalanced fluid volume

Cystic fibrosis
- Activity intolerance
- Caregiver role strain
- Compromised family coping
- Deficient diversional activity
- Deficient fluid volume
- Imbalanced nutrition: Less than body requirements
- Impaired gas exchange
- Ineffective activity planning
- Ineffective airway clearance
- Ineffective breathing pattern
- Parental role conflict
- Risk for delayed development
- Risk for deficient fluid volume
- Risk for imbalanced body temperature
- Risk for imbalanced fluid volume
- Risk for ineffective activity planning
- Risk for infection

Cystitis
- Acute pain
- Impaired urinary elimination
- Noncompliance
- Overflow urinary incontinence
- Risk for urge urinary incontinence
- Sleep deprivation
- Urge urinary incontinence

Deafness
- Chronic low self-esteem
- Defensive coping

- Disturbed sensory perception (auditory)
- Fear
- Impaired verbal communication
- Ineffective coping
- Readiness for enhanced coping
- Risk for falls
- Risk for injury
- Risk for trauma

Delusional disorder
- Disturbed personality identity
- Impaired home maintenance
- Risk for self-directed violence
- Risk for other directed violence
- Risk for self-mutilation

Dementia
- Activity intolerance
- Acute confusion
- Caregiver role strain
- Chronic confusion
- Disturbed sensory perception
- Disturbed thought processes
- Functional urinary incontinence
- Impaired environmental interpretation syndrome
- Impaired memory
- Impaired verbal communication
- Interrupted family processes
- Risk for loneliness
- Powerlessness
- Risk for injury
- Risk for self-directed violence
- Risk for suicide
- Self-neglect
- Social isolation
- Wandering

Depression
- Adult failure to thrive
- Caregiver role strain
- Chronic low self-esteem
- Constipation
- Deficient diversional activity
- Disturbed body image

- Disturbed personality identity
- Fatigue
- Functional urinary incontinence
- Hopelessness
- Imbalanced nutrition: More than body requirements
- Imbalanced nutrition: Less than body requirements
- Impaired home maintenance
- Ineffective coping
- Ineffective denial
- Posttrauma syndrome
- Powerlessness
- Rape-trauma syndrome
- Readiness for enhanced nutrition
- Readiness for enhanced resilience
- Readiness for enhanced hope
- Risk for compromised resilience
- Risk for constipation
- Risk for imbalanced nutrition: More than body requirements
- Risk for injury
- Risk for loneliness
- Risk for poisoning
- Risk for posttrauma syndrome
- Risk for self-directed violence
- Sexual dysfunction
- Sleep deprivation
- Social isolation
- Spiritual distress

Detached retina
- Acute pain
- Anxiety
- Disturbed sensory perception (visual)
- Risk for falls
- Risk for injury

Developmental disorder
- Disabled family coping
- Risk for impaired parent–infant–child attachment
- Risk for injury
- Risk for self-mutilation

Diabetes insipidus
- Deficient fluid volume
- Impaired oral mucous membrane
- Risk for deficient fluid volume
- Risk for imbalanced body temperature
- Risk for unstable glucose level

Diabetes mellitus
- Chronic low self-esteem
- Compromised family coping
- Constipation
- Decreased cardiac output
- Deficient knowledge (specify)
- Disturbed body image
- Disturbed sensory perception
- Grieving
- Hopelessness
- Hyperthermia
- Imbalanced nutrition: More than body requirements
- Impaired oral mucous membrane
- Impaired skin integrity
- Impaired urinary elimination
- Ineffective coping
- Ineffective health maintenance
- Ineffective sexuality patterns
- Ineffective therapeutic regimen management
- Ineffective tissue perfusion (peripheral)
- Ineffective tissue perfusion (renal)
- Interrupted family coping
- Noncompliance
- Powerlessness
- Readiness for enhanced fluid balance
- Readiness for enhanced nutrition
- Readiness for enhanced resilience
- Readiness for enhanced therapeutic regimen management
- Readiness for enhanced urinary elimination

- Risk for imbalanced fluid volume
- Risk for imbalanced body temperature
- Risk for imbalanced nutrition: More than body requirements
- Risk for impaired skin integrity
- Risk for infection
- Risk for injury
- Risk for unstable glucose level
- Risk for vascular trauma
- Risk-prone health behavior
- Self-neglect
- Social isolation

Diabetic ketoacidosis
- Deficient fluid volume
- Deficient knowledge
- Noncompliance
- Risk for acute confusion
- Risk for imbalanced body temperature
- Risk for unstable glucose level
- Risk-prone health behavior

Diarrhea
- Deficient fluid volume
- Diarrhea
- Disturbed body image
- Dysfunctional gastrointestinal motility
- Readiness for enhanced fluid balance
- Risk for electrolyte imbalance
- Risk for imbalanced fluid volume

Digoxin toxicity
- Decreased cardiac output
- Deficient knowledge (specify)
- Risk for ineffective cardiac tissue perfusion
- Risk for poisoning

Disseminated intravascular coagulation
- Decreased cardiac output
- Death anxiety

- Deficient fluid volume
- Fear
- Impaired gas exchange
- Risk for bleeding
- Risk for ineffective cardiac tissue perfusion
- Risk for shock

Dissociative disorder
- Disturbed personality identity
- Disturbed thought processes
- Impaired home maintenance
- Interrupted family processes
- Risk for self-directed violence
- Risk for other-directed violence

Diverticulitis
- Acute pain
- Constipation
- Deficient fluid volume
- Diarrhea
- Dysfunctional gastrointestinal motility
- Hyperthermia
- Imbalanced nutrition: Less than body requirements
- Risk for electrolyte imbalance

Down syndrome
- Compromised family coping
- Deficient knowledge (specify)
- Delayed growth and development
- Defensive coping
- Interrupted family processes
- Readiness for enhanced knowledge
- Readiness for enhanced self-care
- Risk for aspiration
- Risk for delayed development
- Risk for infection
- Risk for injury
- Situational low self-esteem
- Toileting self-care deficit

Drug addiction
- Acute confusion
- Adult failure to thrive
- Decisional conflict

- Defensive coping
- Deficient community health
- Disturbed personality identity
- Dysfunctional family processes: Alcoholism
- Impaired individual resilience
- Ineffective community therapeutic regimen management
- Ineffective coping
- Ineffective denial
- Ineffective family therapeutic regimen management
- Ineffective health maintenance
- Moral distress
- Risk for compromised human dignity
- Risk for falls
- Risk for injury
- Risk for impaired liver function
- Risk for poisoning
- Risk for self-directed violence
- Risk for sudden infant death syndrome
- Sexual dysfunction
- Sleep deprivation

Drug overdose
- Disturbed thought processes
- Functional urinary incontinence
- Hyperthermia
- Hypothermia
- Impaired comfort
- Impaired gas exchange
- Impaired individual resilience
- Ineffective coping
- Ineffective thermoregulation
- Risk for compromised human dignity
- Risk for poisoning
- Risk for suffocation
- Risk for self-directed violence
- Risk for suicide
- Risk for trauma

Drug toxicity
- Functional urinary incontinence
- Hyperthermia

- Hypothermia
- Impaired individual resilience
- Impaired gas exchange
- Ineffective protection
- Risk for poisoning

Duodenal ulcer
- Acute pain
- Anxiety
- Imbalanced nutrition: Less than body requirements
- Ineffective tissue perfusion (GI)
- Dysfunctional gastrointestinal motility
- Risk for shock
- Risk for ineffective gastrointestinal tissue perfusion

Ectopic pregnancy
- Acute pain
- Anxiety
- Deficient fluid volume
- Disturbed personal identity
- Fear
- Ineffective tissue perfusion (cardiopulmonary)
- Risk for electrolyte imbalance
- Risk for infection
- Risk for shock
- Situational low self-esteem

Emphysema
- Activity intolerance
- Deficient knowledge (specify)
- Fatigue
- Fear
- Hopelessness
- Imbalanced nutrition: Less than body requirements
- Impaired gas exchange
- Impaired spontaneous ventilation
- Ineffective airway clearance
- Ineffective breathing pattern
- Noncompliance
- Readiness for enhanced coping
- Readiness for enhanced decision-making

- Readiness for enhanced knowledge
- Readiness for enhanced resilience
- Readiness for enhanced sleep
- Risk for infection

Empyema
- Deficient fluid volume
- Impaired gas exchange
- Ineffective breathing pattern
- Risk for infection

Encephalitis
- Activity intolerance
- Acute pain
- Anxiety
- Constipation
- Deficient fluid volume
- Delayed growth and development
- Hyperthermia
- Impaired physical mobility
- Ineffective coping
- Ineffective thermoregulation
- Risk for infection

Endocarditis
- Activity intolerance
- Acute pain
- Anxiety
- Decreased cardiac output
- Deficient knowledge (specify)
- Excess fluid volume
- Hyperthermia
- Imbalanced nutrition: Less than body requirements
- Readiness for enhanced knowledge
- Risk for infection
- Risk for ineffective cardiac tissue perfusion

Endometrial cancer
- Acute pain
- Chronic sorrow
- Fear
- Grieving
- Impaired tissue integrity
- Ineffective protection

Endometriosis
- Anxiety
- Decisional conflict
- Deficient fluid volume
- Deficient knowledge (specify)
- Grieving
- Moral distress
- Risk for infection
- Sexual dysfunction
- Spiritual distress

Esophageal cancer
- Acute pain
- Dysfunctional intestinal motility
- Fatigue
- Fear
- Imbalanced nutrition: Less than body requirements
- Impaired individual resilience
- Impaired swallowing
- Ineffective coping
- Ineffective self-health management
- Risk for aspiration
- Risk for deficient fluid volume
- Risk for infection

Esophageal fistula
- Imbalanced nutrition: Less than body requirements
- Risk for aspiration
- Risk for deficient fluid volume

Esophageal varices
- Deficient fluid volume
- Disturbed personal identity
- Dysfunctional family processes: Alcoholism
- Imbalanced nutrition: Less than body requirements
- Moral distress
- Readiness for enhanced hope
- Risk for bleeding
- Risk for imbalanced fluid volume
- Risk for impaired skin integrity
- Risk for shock

Failure to thrive
- Deficient fluid volume
- Delayed growth and development
- Disorganized infant behavior
- Imbalanced nutrition: Less than body requirements
- Impaired parenting
- Ineffective community coping
- Risk for deficient fluid volume
- Risk for disorganized infant behavior
- Risk for impaired parenting

Fetal alcohol syndrome
- Compromised family coping
- Delayed growth and development
- Dysfunctional family processes: Alcoholism
- Ineffective community coping
- Moral distress
- Risk for delayed development
- Risk for disproportionate growth
- Disturbed sleep pattern

Food poisoning
- Acute pain
- Contamination
- Diarrhea
- Disturbed sensory perception (visual)
- Dysfunctional gastrointestinal motility
- Hyperthermia
- Impaired physical mobility
- Impaired verbal communication
- Ineffective breathing pattern
- Nausea
- Risk for contamination
- Risk for electrolyte imbalance
- Risk for imbalance of fluid volume

Fractures
- Activity intolerance
- Acute pain
- Bathing or hygiene self-care deficit

- Compromised family coping
- Deficient diversional activity
- Deficient fluid volume
- Disturbed sensory perception
- Hopelessness
- Impaired parenting
- Impaired physical mobility
- Impaired wheelchair mobility
- Impaired skin integrity
- Impaired transfer ability
- Ineffective breathing pattern
- Ineffective denial
- Risk for constipation
- Risk for disuse syndrome
- Risk for falls
- Risk for infection
- Risk for injury
- Risk for perioperative positioning injury
- Risk for peripheral neurovascular dysfunction
- Risk for trauma
- Risk-prone health behavior

Gallbladder disease
- Acute pain
- Anxiety
- Decisional conflict
- Deficient knowledge
- Delayed surgical recovery
- Fear
- Risk for infection

Gastric cancer
- Imbalanced nutrition: Less than body requirements
- Ineffective tissue perfusion (GI)
- Risk for adverse reaction to iodinated contrast media

Gastric ulcer
- Acute pain
- Anxiety
- Deficient knowledge
- Imbalanced nutrition: Less than body requirements
- Ineffective tissue perfusion (GI)
- Risk for bleeding
- Risk-prone health behavior
- Stress overload

Gastroenteritis

- Deficient fluid volume
- Diarrhea
- Dysfunctional gastrointestinal motility
- Risk for bleeding
- Risk for imbalanced fluid volume
- Risk for imbalanced body temperature

Genital herpes

- Chronic low self-esteem
- Deficient knowledge (specify)
- Hopelessness
- Ineffective community coping
- Ineffective sexuality patterns
- Impaired social interaction
- Powerlessness
- Risk for chronic low self-esteem
- Risk for infection
- Risk for loneliness
- Risk-prone health behavior
- Risk for impaired skin integrity
- Social isolation

Gestational diabetes

- Risk for infection
- Risk for imbalanced fluid level
- Risk for unstable glucose level
- Urge urinary incontinence

Gestational hypertension

- Activity intolerance
- Acute pain
- Deficient fluid volume
- Deficient knowledge (specify)
- Disturbed sensory perception (visual)
- Excess fluid volume
- Fear
- Ineffective tissue perfusion (cerebral)
- Urinary retention

Glaucoma

- Anxiety
- Deficient knowledge (specify)
- Disturbed sensory perception (visual)
- Grieving
- Hopelessness
- Risk for dry eye
- Risk for falls
- Risk for injury
- Social isolation

Glomerulonephritis

- Compromised family coping
- Excess fluid volume
- Imbalanced nutrition: Less than body requirements
- Ineffective tissue perfusion (renal)
- Risk for electrolyte imbalance
- Risk for ineffective renal perfusion
- Risk for infection

Gonorrhea

- Deficient community health
- Deficient knowledge (specify)
- Ineffective community coping
- Ineffective sexuality patterns
- Moral distress
- Noncompliance
- Risk for infection
- Risk-prone health behavior

Gout

- Activity intolerance
- Acute pain
- Deficient knowledge (specify)
- Disturbed body image
- Imbalanced nutrition: More than body requirements
- Impaired physical mobility
- Ineffective self-health management
- Noncompliance
- Risk- prone behavior

Guillain–Barré syndrome

- Activity intolerance
- Acute pain
- Anxiety
- Bathing or hygiene self-care deficit
- Bowel incontinence

- Fatigue
- Impaired gas exchange
- Impaired physical mobility
- Impaired spontaneous ventilation
- Ineffective airway clearance
- Ineffective breathing pattern
- Ineffective coping
- Powerlessness
- Risk for urge urinary incontinence

Headaches
- Acute pain
- Ineffective coping
- Insomnia
- Spiritual distress

Head injury
- Activity intolerance
- Acute confusion
- Bowel incontinence
- Chronic confusion
- Chronic sorrow
- Decreased intracranial adaptive capacity
- Deficient knowledge (specify)
- Delayed growth and development
- Disturbed sensory perception
- Disturbed thought processes
- Dressing or grooming self-care deficit
- Fear
- Impaired environmental interpretation syndrome
- Impaired gas exchange
- Impaired memory
- Impaired physical mobility
- Impaired social interaction
- Impaired swallowing
- Impaired verbal communication
- Ineffective thermoregulation
- Ineffective tissue perfusion
- Posttrauma syndrome
- Powerlessness
- Risk for activity intolerance
- Risk for aspiration
- Risk for constipation

- Risk for delayed development
- Risk for disuse syndrome
- Risk for falls
- Risk for imbalanced body temperature
- Risk for imbalanced fluid volume
- Risk for impaired parenting
- Risk for injury
- Risk for trauma
- Risk for urge urinary incontinence
- Sleep deprivation
- Total urinary incontinence
- Unilateral neglect

Head or neck cancer
- Acute pain
- Anxiety
- Disturbed body image
- Disturbed sensory perception
- Impaired oral mucous membrane
- Impaired swallowing
- Impaired tissue integrity
- Impaired verbal communication
- Ineffective airway clearance
- Situational low self-esteem
- Risk for aspiration
- Risk for imbalanced fluid volume

Heart failure
- Activity intolerance
- Acute pain
- Caregiver role strain
- Death anxiety
- Decreased cardiac output
- Deficient knowledge (specify)
- Excess fluid volume
- Fatigue
- Hopelessness
- Imbalanced nutrition: More than body requirements
- Impaired gas exchange
- Impaired home maintenance
- Ineffective airway clearance
- Ineffective breathing pattern
- Ineffective tissue perfusion

- Powerlessness
- Risk for activity intolerance
- Risk for caregiver role strain
- Risk for imbalanced fluid volume
- Risk for deficient fluid volume
- Risk for ineffective cardiac tissue perfusion
- Risk for ineffective renal tissue perfusion
- Risk for injury
- Risk for falls

Hemodialysis
- Complicated grieving
- Deficient fluid volume
- Deficient knowledge (specify)
- Disturbed body image
- Excess fluid volume
- Interrupted family processes
- Readiness for enhanced hope
- Risk for falls
- Risk for deficient fluid volume
- Risk for electrolyte imbalance
- Risk for imbalanced fluid volume
- Risk for ineffective renal tissue perfusion
- Risk for ineffective cardiac tissue perfusion
- Risk for infection
- Spiritual distress

Hemophilia
- Acute pain
- Chronic low self-esteem
- Impaired gas exchange
- Ineffective protection
- Parental role conflict
- Readiness for enhanced family coping
- Risk for bleeding
- Risk for falls
- Risk for imbalanced body temperature
- Risk for injury
- Risk for trauma
- Risk-prone health behavior

Hemorrhage
- Deficient fluid volume
- Impaired oral mucous membrane
- Ineffective thermoregulation
- Ineffective tissue perfusion (renal)
- Risk for aspiration
- Risk for bleeding
- Risk for ineffective cardiac tissue perfusion
- Risk for electrolyte imbalance
- Risk for shock

Hemorrhoids
- Acute pain
- Constipation
- Deficient knowledge (specify)
- Impaired comfort
- Impaired skin integrity

Hemothorax
- Acute pain
- Anxiety
- Deficient fluid volume
- Fear
- Impaired gas exchange
- Impaired spontaneous ventilation
- Ineffective breathing pattern
- Ineffective tissue perfusion
- Risk for bleeding
- Risk for shock

Hepatic coma
- Acute confusion
- Deficient fluid volume
- Disturbed sensory perception
- Excess fluid volume
- Imbalanced nutrition: Less than body requirements
- Impaired skin integrity
- Ineffective self-health management
- Moral distress
- Risk for acute confusion
- Risk for falls
- Risk for infection
- Risk for injury
- Risk for dysfunctional gastrointestinal motility

- Risk for electrolyte imbalance
- Risk for ineffective cerebral tissue perfusion

Hepatitis
- Deficient knowledge (specify)
- Enhanced readiness for immunization status
- Ineffective community coping
- Ineffective community therapeutic regimen management
- Nausea
- Readiness for enhanced community coping
- Risk for electrolyte imbalance
- Risk for imbalanced fluid volume

Hip fracture
- Compromised family coping
- Deficient knowledge (specify)
- Ineffective denial
- Ineffective sexuality patterns
- Powerlessness
- Risk for activity intolerance
- Risk for falls
- Risk for impaired skin integrity
- Risk for infection
- Risk for injury
- Spiritual distress

Hodgkin's disease
- Deficient knowledge
- Grieving
- Imbalanced nutrition: Less than body requirements
- Impaired physical mobility
- Impaired skin integrity
- Impaired tissue integrity
- Ineffective breathing pattern
- Ineffective oral mucous membrane
- Ineffective protection
- Risk for complicated grieving
- Risk for infection

Huntington's disease
- Bathing or hygiene self-care deficit
- Bowel incontinence

- Caregiver role strain
- Compromised family coping
- Deficient knowledge (specify)
- Hopelessness
- Impaired physical mobility
- Impaired verbal communication
- Ineffective health maintenance
- Risk for loneliness
- Moral distress
- Risk for injury
- Social isolation

Hydatidiform mole
- Acute pain
- Deficient fluid volume
- Grieving
- Risk for situational low self-esteem

Hydrocephalus
- Acute pain
- Anxiety
- Chronic low self esteem
- Compromised family coping
- Delayed growth and development
- Disturbed body image
- Ineffective coping
- Imbalanced nutrition: Less than body requirements
- Interrupted family processes
- Readiness for enhanced family processes
- Risk for impaired skin integrity
- Risk for infection
- Risk for falls

Hyperbilirubinemia
- Interrupted breastfeeding
- Neonatal jaundice
- Risk for injury
- Risk for neonatal jaundice

Hyperemesis gravidarum
- Deficient fluid volume
- Excess fluid volume
- Imbalanced nutrition: Less than body requirements

- Risk for electrolyte imbalance
- Risk for imbalanced fluid volume
- Situational low self-esteem

Hyperosmolar hyperglycemic nonketotic syndrome
- Deficient fluid volume
- Impaired skin integrity
- Ineffective tissue perfusion
- Risk for infection
- Risk for unstable glucose level

Hyperparathyroidism
- Acute pain
- Anxiety
- Deficient knowledge
- Delayed surgical recovery
- Hopelessness
- Imbalanced nutrition: Less than body requirements
- Ineffective breathing pattern
- Ineffective coping
- Risk for imbalanced body temperature
- Risk for impaired skin integrity

Hyperpituitarism
- Acute pain
- Disturbed body image
- Ineffective coping
- Risk for compromised human dignity
- Sexual dysfunction

Hypertension
- Decreased cardiac output
- Deficient knowledge (specify)
- Excess fluid volume
- Health-seeking behaviors
- Imbalanced nutrition: More than body requirements
- Impaired individual resilience
- Impaired environmental interpretation syndrome
- Ineffective denial
- Ineffective sexuality patterns
- Noncompliance (specify)
- Powerlessness

- Readiness for enhanced urinary elimination
- Risk-prone health behavior
- Risk for situational low self-esteem

Hyperthermia
- Deficient knowledge (specify)
- Hyperthermia
- Impaired oral mucous membrane
- Impaired comfort
- Ineffective thermoregulation

Hyperthyroidism
- Activity intolerance
- Decreased cardiac output
- Disturbed body image
- Disturbed thought processes
- Ineffective thermoregulation
- Insomnia
- Risk for imbalanced body temperature
- Sleep deprivation

Hypoparathyroidism
- Anxiety
- Compromised family coping
- Decreased cardiac output
- Imbalanced nutrition: Less than body requirements
- Ineffective coping
- Ineffective thermoregulation
- Risk for trauma

Hypopituitarism
- Risk for delayed development
- Risk for disproportionate growth

Hypothermia
- Deficient knowledge (specify)
- Hypothermia
- Impaired comfort
- Ineffective thermoregulation

Hypohyroidism
- Activity intolerance
- Compromised family coping
- Constipation
- Decreased cardiac output
- Disturbed body image

- Functional urinary incontinence
- Ineffective coping
- Ineffective sexuality patterns
- Ineffective thermoregulation
- Risk for delayed development
- Risk for disproportionate growth
- Risk for imbalanced body temperature
- Disturbed sleep pattern

Ileostomy
- Anxiety
- Deficient fluid volume
- Deficient knowledge
- Diarrhea
- Disturbed body image
- Fear
- Imbalanced nutrition: Less than body requirements
- Impaired skin integrity
- Ineffective sexuality patterns
- Ineffective tissue perfusion (GI)
- Risk for infection
- Risk for dysfunctional gastrointestinal motility
- Risk for situational low self-esteem

Impotence
- Deficient knowledge (specify)
- Disturbed body image
- Risk for compromised human dignity
- Sexual dysfunction
- Situational low self-esteem
- Urinary retention

Incest
- Ineffective coping
- Interrupted family processes
- Moral distress
- Posttrauma syndrome

Infertility
- Chronic sorrow
- Complicated grieving
- Deficient knowledge (specify)
- Ineffective coping

- Risk for situational low self-esteem
- Stress overload

Inhalation injuries
- Ineffective thermoregulation
- Risk for injury
- Risk for suffocation

Interstitial pulmonary fibrosis
- Activity intolerance
- Anxiety
- Deficient knowledge (specify)
- Grieving
- Impaired gas exchange
- Impaired individual resilience
- Ineffective airway clearance
- Ineffective breathing pattern
- Ineffective coping
- Insomnia
- Spiritual distress

Intestinal obstruction
- Acute pain
- Constipation
- Imbalanced nutrition: Less than body requirements
- Ineffective tissue perfusion (GI)
- Risk for aspiration
- Risk for deficient fluid volume
- Risk for dysfunctional gastrointestinal motility
- Risk for electrolyte imbalance
- Risk for imbalanced fluid volume
- Urinary retention

Intoxication
- Disturbed sensory perception
- Hypothermia
- Impaired verbal communication
- Ineffective community therapeutic regimen management
- Moral distress
- Risk for aspiration
- Risk for compromised human dignity
- Risk for falls
- Risk for injury

Joint replacement
- Acute pain
- Compromised family coping
- Deficient knowledge (specify)
- Delayed surgical recovery
- Disturbed sensory perception (kinesthetic)
- Impaired physical mobility
- Ineffective peripheral tissue perfusion
- Risk for contamination
- Risk for falls
- Risk for infection
- Risk for injury

Juvenile rheumatoid arthritis
- Acute pain
- Caregiver role strain
- Compromised family coping
- Defensive coping
- Disturbed body image
- Disturbed sensory perception (tactile)
- Grieving
- Impaired individual resilience
- Impaired physical mobility
- Ineffective health maintenance
- Ineffective role performance
- Interrupted family processes
- Risk for unstable glucose level

Kidney transplantation
- Deficient fluid volume
- Deficient knowledge (specify)
- Delayed surgical recovery
- Disturbed body image
- Ineffective protection
- Interrupted family processes
- Risk for bleeding
- Readiness for enhanced hope
- Readiness for enhanced decision-making
- Readiness for enhanced hope
- Readiness for enhanced resilience
- Risk for complicated grieving
- Risk for electrolyte imbalance
- Risk for infection

Labor and delivery
- Acute pain
- Anxiety
- Deficient knowledge (specify)
- Effective breastfeeding
- Impaired skin integrity
- Ineffective breastfeeding
- Ineffective coping
- Insufficient breast milk
- Readiness for enhanced childbearing
- Risk for bleeding
- Risk for disturbed maternal–fetal dyad
- Risk for injury
- Urinary retention

Leukemia
- Acute pain
- Grieving
- Hopelessness
- Imbalanced nutrition: Less than body requirements
- Impaired gas exchange
- Impaired oral mucous membrane
- Impaired tissue integrity
- Ineffective protection
- Ineffective tissue perfusion (cardiopulmonary)
- Ineffective tissue perfusion (renal)
- Risk for bleeding
- Risk for contamination
- Risk for falls
- Risk for imbalanced body temperature
- Risk for infection
- Risk for injury

Liver transplantation
- Anxiety
- Compromised family coping
- Defensive coping
- Deficient knowledge (specify)
- Delayed surgical recovery
- Fear
- Ineffective coping
- Ineffective protection
- Ineffective tissue perfusion (cardiopulmonary)

- Ineffective tissue perfusion (GI)
- Ineffective tissue perfusion (renal)
- Moral distress
- Risk for impaired liver function
- Risk for electrolyte imbalance
- Risk for imbalanced fluid volume
- Risk for infection
- Risk for injury

Lung abscess
- Acute pain
- Anxiety
- Impaired gas exchange
- Ineffective airway clearance
- Ineffective breathing pattern
- Ineffective coping
- Ineffective tissue perfusion (cardiopulmonary)
- Risk for imbalanced body temperature

Lung cancer
- Activity intolerance
- Death anxiety
- Fear
- Grieving
- Hopelessness
- Imbalanced nutrition: Less than body requirements
- Impaired gas exchange
- Impaired tissue integrity
- Impaired verbal communication
- Ineffective airway clearance
- Ineffective breathing pattern
- Powerlessness
- Risk for infection

Lupus erythematosus
- Acute pain
- Decreased cardiac output
- Deficient knowledge
- Fatigue
- Hyperthermia
- Imbalanced nutrition: Less than body requirements
- Impaired oral mucous membrane

- Impaired physical mobility
- Impaired skin integrity
- Ineffective coping
- Ineffective tissue perfusion
- Risk for infection
- Risk-prone health behavior

Lyme disease
- Activity intolerance
- Acute pain
- Fatigue
- Hyperthermia
- Impaired skin integrity

Lymphomas
- Death anxiety
- Disturbed sleep pattern
- Grieving
- Hopelessness
- Impaired tissue integrity
- Ineffective protection
- Readiness for enhanced decision-making
- Risk for impaired religiosity
- Risk for infection

Macular degeneration
- Activity intolerance
- Deficient knowledge
- Disturbed sensory perception (visual)
- Ineffective denial
- Powerlessness
- Readiness for enhanced hope
- Risk for caregiver role strain
- Risk for low situational self-esteem
- Risk for falls
- Risk for trauma

Malnutrition
- Imbalanced nutrition: Less than body requirements
- Ineffective community coping
- Risk for electrolyte imbalance
- Risk for injury

Maternal psychological stress
- Anxiety
- Deficient knowledge
- Ineffective breastfeeding

- Ineffective infant feeding pattern
- Ineffective role performance
- Interrupted breastfeeding
- Parental role conflict
- Risk for impaired attachment
- Risk for disturbed maternal–fetal dyad
- Risk for ineffective childbearing process
- Risk for sudden infant death syndrome
- Powerlessness

Meconium aspiration syndrome
- Ineffective breathing pattern
- Impaired gas exchange
- Impaired spontaneous ventilation
- Risk for aspiration
- Risk for injury

Melanoma
- Death anxiety
- Decisional conflict
- Defensive coping
- Disturbed body image
- Fatigue
- Hopelessness
- Impaired individual resilience
- Impaired oral mucous membrane
- Impaired skin integrity
- Powerlessness
- Spiritual distress

Ménière's disease
- Disturbed sensory perception (auditory)
- Impaired physical mobility
- Insomnia
- Nausea
- Risk for falls
- Risk for injury
- Risk for trauma

Meningitis
- Acute pain
- Bowel incontinence
- Deficient fluid volume
- Disturbed sensory perception

- Excess fluid volume
- Fatigue
- Fear
- Hyperthermia
- Ineffective airway clearance
- Ineffective breathing pattern
- Risk for imbalanced fluid volume
- Risk for infection
- Risk for injury

Menopause
- Ineffective sexuality patterns
- Insomnia
- Sexual dysfunction
- Situational low self-esteem
- Stress overload
- Risk for imbalanced body temperature

Metabolic acidosis
- Deficient knowledge (specify)
- Impaired airway clearance
- Impaired gas exchange
- Impaired oral mucous membrane
- Ineffective breathing pattern
- Risk for acute confusion
- Risk for electrolyte imbalance
- Risk for injury
- Risk for poisoning
- Risk for shock

Metabolic alkalosis
- Deficient fluid volume
- Disturbed thought processes
- Impaired oral mucous membrane
- Ineffective breathing pattern
- Risk for electrolyte imbalance
- Risk for injury

Mitral insufficiency
- Activity intolerance
- Decreased cardiac output
- Deficient knowledge (specify)
- Fatigue
- Ineffective tissue perfusion (cardiopulmonary)

Mitral stenosis
- Activity intolerance
- Decreased cardiac output
- Deficient knowledge (specify)
- Fatigue
- Ineffective tissue perfusion (cardiopulmonary)
- Risk for infection

Mood disorders
- Impaired religiosity
- Ineffective health management
- Ineffective community therapeutic regimen management
- Powerlessness
- Readiness for enhanced self-health management
- Risk for compromised resilience
- Risk for suicide
- Self-mutilation
- Social isolation
- Spiritual distress

Multiple births
- Anxiety
- Deficient knowledge (specify)
- Impaired parenting
- Ineffective coping
- Interrupted family processes
- Risk for injury
- Risk for impaired parenting
- Stress urinary incontinence

Multiple myeloma
- Activity intolerance
- Acute pain
- Excess fluid volume
- Fatigue
- Grieving
- Imbalanced nutrition: Less than body requirements
- Ineffective tissue perfusion (cerebral)
- Risk for infection

Multiple sclerosis
- Acute pain
- Bowel incontinence
- Caregiver role strain

- Chronic low self-esteem
- Death anxiety
- Deficient knowledge (specify)
- Disturbed sensory perception
- Dressing or grooming self-care deficit
- Fatigue
- Grieving
- Imbalanced nutrition: Less than body requirements
- Impaired bed mobility
- Impaired comfort
- Impaired memory
- Impaired physical mobility
- Impaired spontaneous ventilation
- Impaired urinary elimination
- Impaired wheelchair mobility
- Ineffective airway clearance
- Ineffective health maintenance
- Ineffective sexuality patterns
- Ineffective therapeutic regimen management
- Readiness for enhanced family coping
- Readiness for enhanced spiritual well-being
- Risk for activity intolerance
- Risk for caregiver role strain
- Risk for infection
- Risk for spiritual distress
- Risk for urge urinary incontinence
- Risk-prone health behavior

Multisystem trauma
- Anxiety
- Bathing or hygiene self-care deficit
- Deficient fluid volume
- Dysfunctional ventilatory weaning response
- Ineffective tissue perfusion
- Impaired spontaneous ventilation
- Powerlessness
- Risk for electrolyte imbalance
- Risk for ineffective cardiac tissue perfusion

- Risk for ineffective cerebral tissue perfusion
- Risk for infection
- Risk for suffocation
- Risk for trauma

Muscular dystrophy
- Caregiver role strain
- Deficient knowledge (specify)
- Disturbed sensory perception (kinesthetic)
- Feeding self-care deficit
- Hopelessness
- Impaired physical mobility
- Impaired transfer ability
- Impaired swallowing
- Ineffective health maintenance
- Readiness for enhanced family coping
- Risk for caregiver role strain
- Risk for urge urinary incontinence
- Risk-prone health behavior

Myasthenia gravis
- Bowel incontinence
- Chronic low self-esteem
- Dressing or grooming self-care deficit
- Dysfunctional ventilatory weaning response
- Fatigue
- Fear
- Impaired gas exchange
- Impaired physical mobility
- Impaired verbal communication
- Ineffective airway clearance
- Readiness for enhanced self-care
- Risk for urge urinary incontinence

Myocardial infarction
- Activity intolerance
- Acute pain
- Anxiety
- Compromised family coping
- Death anxiety
- Decreased cardiac output

- Health-seeking behaviors
- Ineffective coping
- Ineffective denial
- Ineffective role performance
- Ineffective sexuality patterns
- Ineffective tissue perfusion
- Readiness for enhanced spiritual well-being
- Readiness for enhanced relationships
- Risk for ineffective cardiac tissue perfusion
- Risk for spiritual distress
- Risk-prone health behavior
- Sedentary lifestyle
- Sexual dysfunction
- Situational low self-esteem
- Sleep deprivation
- Spiritual distress

Neonatal asphyxia
- Compromised family coping
- Delayed growth and development
- Hypothermia
- Ineffective breathing pattern
- Risk for aspiration
- Risk for injury
- Risk for sudden infant death syndrome
- Risk for suffocation
- Risk for sudden infant death syndrome

Neonatal hyperbilirubinemia
- Interrupted breastfeeding
- Neonatal jaundice
- Risk for neonatal jaundice

Neurologic impairment (neonatal)
- Compromised family coping
- Ineffective infant feeding pattern
- Disorganized infant behavior
- Readiness for enhanced organized infant behavior
- Risk for disorganized infant behavior

Neuromuscular trauma
- Impaired skin integrity
- Impaired swallowing
- Overflow urinary incontinence
- Posttrauma syndrome
- Risk for aspiration
- Risk for constipation
- Risk for disuse syndrome
- Unilateral neglect

Nutritional deficiencies
- Imbalanced nutrition: Less than body requirements
- Impaired skin integrity
- Risk for impaired parenting
- Risk for infection

Obesity
- Imbalanced nutrition: More than body requirements
- Readiness for enhanced nutrition
- Readiness for enhanced self-concept
- Risk for constipation
- Risk for impaired skin integrity
- Situational low self-esteem
- Stress urinary incontinence

Obsessive-compulsive disorder
- Anxiety
- Compromised family coping
- Decisional conflict
- Disturbed personal identity
- Impaired home maintenance
- Ineffective coping
- Ineffective denial
- Insomnia
- Risk for impaired religiosity
- Risk for injury
- Risk for spiritual distress
- Risk for self-directed violence
- Risk for other-directed violence
- Risk for suicide
- Self-mutilation
- Sleep deprivation
- Social isolation

Organic brain syndrome
- Adult failure to thrive
- Impaired verbal communication
- Risk for deficient fluid volume
- Wandering

Osteoarthritis
- Activity intolerance
- Acute pain
- Compromised family coping
- Deficient knowledge (specify)
- Disturbed body image
- Dressing or grooming self-care deficit
- Imbalanced nutrition: More than body requirements
- Impaired home maintenance
- Impaired physical mobility
- Impaired wheelchair ability
- Ineffective health maintenance
- Ineffective self-health management
- Risk for injury
- Risk for falls
- Risk for injury

Osteomyelitis
- Acute pain
- Disturbed body image
- Impaired coping
- Impaired physical mobility
- Impaired skin integrity
- Impaired tissue integrity
- Ineffective coping
- Ineffective tissue perfusion (specify)
- Risk for infection
- Risk for injury
- Risk for falls

Osteoporosis
- Deficient knowledge (specify)
- Disturbed body image
- Fear
- Ineffective denial
- Ineffective self-health management
- Ineffective sexuality patterns

- Loneliness
- Nutrition imbalanced: Less than body requirements
- Powerlessness
- Risk for falls
- Risk for injury
- Risk for trauma
- Risk-prone health behaviors
- Self-neglect
- Social isolation

Ovarian cancer
- Constipation
- Death anxiety
- Fear
- Grieving
- Imbalanced nutrition: Less than body requirements
- Impaired tissue integrity
- Ineffective coping
- Ineffective protection
- Nausea
- Powerlessness
- Readiness for enhanced hope
- Readiness for enhanced resilience
- Readiness for enhanced spiritual well-being
- Risk for falls
- Spiritual distress
- Urinary retention

Panic disorder
- Anxiety
- Chronic low self-esteem
- Deficient knowledge (specify)
- Fear
- Impaired individual resilience
- Ineffective coping
- Insomnia
- Powerlessness
- Risk for posttrauma syndrome
- Sleep deprivation
- Risk for spiritual distress

Paralysis
- Autonomic dysreflexia
- Bowel incontinence
- Caregiver role strain
- Complicated grieving

- Compromised family coping
- Disuse syndrome
- Hopelessness
- Impaired bed mobility
- Impaired physical mobility
- Impaired skin integrity
- Impaired walking
- Ineffective coping
- Ineffective health maintenance
- Ineffective role performance
- Ineffective sexuality patterns
- Powerlessness
- Reflex urinary incontinence
- Risk for caregiver role strain
- Risk for impaired skin integrity

Parkinson's disease
- Activity intolerance
- Bowel incontinence
- Caregiver role strain
- Chronic low self-esteem
- Compromised family coping
- Death anxiety
- Deficient knowledge (specify)
- Disturbed body image
- Disturbed sensory perception (tactile)
- Feeding self-care deficit
- Grieving
- Hopelessness
- Imbalanced nutrition: Less than body requirements
- Impaired home maintenance
- Impaired individual resilience
- Impaired physical mobility
- Impaired transfer ability
- Ineffective breathing pattern
- Ineffective coping
- Ineffective health maintenance
- Ineffective role performance
- Ineffective sexuality patterns
- Loneliness
- Powerlessness
- Readiness for enhanced therapeutic regimen management
- Risk for aspiration
- Risk for caregiver role strain

- Risk for compromised human dignity
- Risk for injury
- Risk for falls
- Risk for loneliness
- Risk for urge urinary incontinence
- Social isolation

Pelvic inflammatory disease
- Acute pain
- Deficient fluid volume
- Ineffective sexuality pattern
- Risk for infection
- Risk-prone health behavior
- Sexual dysfunction

Pericarditis
- Activity intolerance
- Acute pain
- Anxiety
- Decreased cardiac output
- Deficient knowledge
- Ineffective tissue perfusion (cardiopulmonary)
- Risk for ineffective cardiac tissue perfusion
- Risk for infection
- Risk for shock

Perinatal trauma
- Delayed growth and development
- Decisional conflict
- Hypothermia
- Impaired gas exchange
- Impaired spontaneous ventilation
- Risk for injury
- Risk for ineffective cardiac tissue perfusion
- Risk for ineffective cerebral tissue perfusion
- Risk for ineffective renal tissue perfusion
- Risk for shock
- Risk for vascular trauma

Peripheral vascular disease
- Activity intolerance
- Acute pain

- Deficient diversional activity
- Deficient knowledge (specify)
- Impaired physical mobility
- Impaired skin integrity
- Impaired tissue integrity
- Ineffective self-health management
- Risk for falls
- Risk for impaired skin integrity
- Risk for ineffective peripheral tissue perfusion
- Risk for vascular trauma
- Risk for infection
- Risk for injury
- Risk for peripheral neurovascular dysfunction
- Risk-prone health behavior

Peritoneal dialysis
- Caregiver role strain
- Defensive coping
- Deficient fluid volume
- Deficient knowledge (specify)
- Disabled family coping
- Disturbed body image
- Excess fluid volume
- Imbalanced nutrition: Less than body requirements
- Impaired individual resilience
- Interrupted family processes
- Risk for electrolyte imbalance
- Risk for infection
- Risk for injury

Peritonitis
- Acute pain
- Anxiety
- Decreased cardiac output
- Deficient fluid volume
- Nausea
- Risk for electrolyte imbalance
- Risk for ineffective gastrointestinal tissue perfusion
- Risk for ineffective cardiac tissue perfusion
- Risk for ineffective renal tissue perfusion
- Risk for imbalanced fluid volume

- Risk for infection
- Risk for shock

Personality disorders
- Decisional conflict
- Deficient knowledge
- Disturbed personal identity
- Impaired individual resilience
- Interrupted family processes
- Loneliness
- Risk for loneliness
- Risk for self-directed violence
- Risk for suicide
- Sexual dysfunction
- Social isolation

Phobic disorder
- Anxiety
- Disturbed personal identity
- Fear
- Hopelessness
- Ineffective coping
- Powerlessness
- Risk for compromised resilience
- Risk for loneliness
- Social isolation

Placenta previa
- Anxiety
- Fear
- Ineffective denial
- Risk for disturbed maternal–fetal dyad
- Risk for situational low self-esteem

Pleural effusion
- Acute pain
- Dysfunctional ventilatory weaning response
- Hyperthermia
- Impaired gas exchange
- Ineffective breathing pattern
- Risk for infection

Pleurisy
- Acute pain
- Fatigue
- Impaired gas exchange
- Ineffective breathing pattern

Pneumonia
- Bathing or hygiene self-care deficit
- Feeding and toileting self-care deficit
- Deficient fluid volume
- Imbalanced nutrition: Less than body requirements
- Impaired gas exchange
- Impaired physical mobility
- Impaired spontaneous ventilation
- Impaired verbal communication
- Ineffective airway clearance
- Ineffective breathing pattern
- Ineffective tissue perfusion (cardiopulmonary)
- Readiness for enhanced sleep
- Risk for aspiration
- Risk for electrolyte imbalance
- Risk for imbalanced fluid volume
- Risk for infection

Pneumothorax
- Anxiety
- Ineffective breathing pattern
- Fear
- Impaired gas exchange
- Acute pain
- Ineffective tissue perfusion (cardiopulmonary)
- Impaired spontaneous ventilation

Poisoning
- Contamination
- Delayed growth and development
- Disturbed sensory perception
- Ineffective tissue perfusion (renal)
- Nausea
- Risk for aspiration
- Risk for bleeding
- Risk for injury
- Risk for poisoning
- Risk for shock

Polycystic kidney disease
- Acute pain
- Anxiety
- Defensive coping
- Deficient knowledge (specify)
- Fear
- Ineffective tissue perfusion (renal)
- Interrupted family processes
- Moral distress
- Risk for infection

Polycythemia vera
- Acute pain
- Disturbed sensory perception (visual)Fatigue
- Impaired gas exchange
- Impaired skin integrity
- Ineffective breathing pattern
- Risk for bleeding
- Risk for injury

Postpartum hemorrhage
- Anxiety
- Deficient fluid volume
- Ineffective tissue perfusion
- Risk for bleeding
- Risk for ineffective renal tissue perfusion
- Risk for shock

Posttraumatic stress disorder
- Ineffective impulse control
- Ineffective relationships
- Defensive coping
- Disabled family coping
- Disturbed personal identity
- Disturbed sensory perception
- Hopelessness
- Ineffective activity planning
- Interrupted family processes

Posttrauma syndrome
- Powerlessness
- Risk for loneliness
- Risk for posttrauma syndrome
- Risk for other-directed violence
- Risk for self-directed violence
- Risk for self-mutilation

- Risk for suicide
- Situational low self-esteem
- Sleep deprivation

Pregnancy
- Anxiety
- Deficient knowledge (specify)
- Impaired tissue integrity
- Ineffective coping
- Ineffective tissue perfusion (peripheral)
- Interrupted family processes
- Readiness for enhanced childbearing
- Readiness for enhanced fluid balance
- Readiness for enhanced relationships
- Risk for constipation

Premature labor
- Anxiety
- Deficient knowledge (specify)
- Effective breastfeeding
- Impaired parenting
- Ineffective coping
- Risk for disturbed maternal–fetal dyad
- Risk for infection
- Situational low self-esteem

Premature rupture of membranes
- Risk for infection

Prematurity
- Compromised family coping
- Delayed growth and development
- Disorganized infant behavior
- Hypothermia
- Imbalanced nutrition: Less than body requirements
- Impaired verbal communication
- Ineffective breastfeeding
- Ineffective breathing pattern
- Ineffective infant feeding pattern
- Ineffective thermoregulation
- Interrupted breastfeeding

- Readiness for enhanced parenting
- Risk for aspiration
- Risk for delayed development
- Risk for disorganized infant behavior
- Risk for disturbed maternal–fetal dyad
- Risk for impaired parent–infant–child attachment
- Risk for sudden infant death syndrome

Pressure ulcers
- Imbalanced nutrition: Less than body requirements
- Impaired physical mobility
- Impaired skin integrity
- Impaired tissue integrity
- Ineffective protection
- Risk for deficient fluid volume
- Risk for infection

Prolapsed intervertebral disc
- Acute pain
- Impaired physical mobility
- Powerlessness
- Reflex urinary incontinence
- Urinary retention

Prostate cancer
- Acute pain
- Chronic sorrow
- Deficient knowledge
- Impaired skin integrity
- Impaired tissue integrity
- Risk for situational low self-esteem
- Sexual dysfunction
- Urinary retention

Prostatectomy
- Acute pain
- Disturbed body image
- Ineffective protection
- Ineffective role performance
- Impaired skin integrity
- Risk for infection
- Urinary retention

Pseudomembranous colitis
- Deficient fluid volume
- Diarrhea
- Impaired skin integrity
- Ineffective tissue perfusion (cardiopulmonary)
- Ineffective tissue perfusion (GI)
- Ineffective tissue perfusion (renal)
- Risk for bleeding
- Risk for electrolyte imbalance

Psoriasis
- Deficient knowledge
- Disturbed body image
- Impaired skin integrity
- Powerlessness
- Risk for imbalanced body temperature
- Social isolation
- Risk for infection

Pulmonary edema
- Activity intolerance
- Bathing or hygiene self-care deficit
- Decreased cardiac output
- Dysfunctional ventilatory weaning response
- Excess fluid volume
- Fear
- Impaired gas exchange
- Impaired verbal communication
- Ineffective airway clearance
- Ineffective breathing pattern
- Ineffective tissue perfusion (cardiopulmonary)
- Risk for ineffective cardiac tissue perfusion
- Risk for ineffective cerebral tissue perfusion
- Risk for ineffective renal tissue perfusion

Pulmonary embolus
- Acute pain
- Anxiety
- Activity intolerance
- Decreased cardiac output

- Deficient fluid volume
- Impaired gas exchange
- Impaired verbal communication
- Ineffective breathing pattern
- Ineffective tissue perfusion (cardiopulmonary)
- Risk for ineffective cardiac tissue perfusion

Pyelonephritis
- Acute pain
- Excess fluid volume
- Impaired physical mobility
- Risk for infection
- Risk for electrolyte balance
- Risk for imbalanced fluid volume

Pyloric stenosis
- Acute pain
- Imbalanced nutrition: Less than body requirements
- Risk for aspiration
- Risk for imbalanced body temperature

Radiation therapy
- Acute pain
- Deficient fluid volume
- Diarrhea
- Imbalanced nutrition: Less than body requirements
- Impaired oral mucous membrane
- Impaired physical mobility
- Impaired tissue integrity
- Ineffective protection
- Nausea
- Sexual dysfunction
- Rape
- Anxiety
- Complicated grieving
- Fear
- Posttrauma syndrome
- Rape-trauma syndrome
- Risk for compromised human dignity
- Risk for thermal injury
- Situational low self-esteem
- Social isolation

Raynaud's disease
- Deficient knowledge (specify)
- Disturbed sensory perception (tactile)
- Impaired tissue integrity
- Ineffective tissue perfusion (peripheral)
- Risk for impaired skin integrity
- Risk for ineffective peripheral tissue perfusion

Renal calculi
- Acute pain
- Ineffective denial
- Risk for infection
- Urinary retention

Renal cancer
- Acute pain
- Deficient fluid volume
- Risk for electrolyte balance
- Risk for imbalanced fluid volume

Renal disease: End-stage
- Caregiver role strain
- Chronic low self-esteem
- Decisional conflict
- Defensive coping
- Excess fluid volume
- Grieving
- Hopelessness
- Ineffective coping
- Ineffective denial
- Ineffective role performance
- Ineffective sexuality patterns
- Risk for caregiver role strain
- Risk for disuse syndrome
- Risk for infection
- Risk for poisoning
- Risk for spiritual distress
- Spiritual distress

Respiratory distress syndrome
- Dysfunctional weaning response
- Impaired gas exchange
- Impaired spontaneous ventilation
- Ineffective airway clearance

- Ineffective breathing pattern
- Ineffective thermoregulation
- Risk for infection

Reye's syndrome
- Decreased intracranial adaptive capacity
- Delayed growth and development
- Hyperthermia
- Impaired physical mobility
- Ineffective thermoregulation

Rheumatoid arthritis
- Activity intolerance
- Acute pain
- Deficient knowledge (specify)
- Disturbed body image
- Dressing or grooming self-care deficit
- Impaired physical mobility
- Impaired skin integrity
- Impaired transfer ability
- Ineffective coping
- Ineffective denial
- Ineffective health maintenance
- Ineffective protection
- Ineffective therapeutic regimen management
- Insomnia
- Risk for disuse syndrome
- Risk for falls
- Risk for ineffective activity planning
- Risk for injury
- Risk-prone health management
- Sexual dysfunction

Salmonella
- Constipation
- Diarrhea
- Hyperthermia
- Nausea
- Risk for imbalanced fluid volume
- Risk for dysfunctional gastrointestinal motility
- Risk for electrolyte imbalance
- Risk for imbalanced fluid volume

- Risk for infection
- Urinary retention

Sarcoidosis
- Activity intolerance
- Acute pain
- Decreased cardiac output
- Disturbed body image
- Impaired gas exchange
- Ineffective breathing pattern

Schizophrenia
- Anxiety
- Bathing or hygiene self-care deficit
- Caregiver role strain
- Disturbed personal identity
- Disturbed sensory perception
- Dysfunctional family processes
- Functional urinary incontinence
- Hopelessness
- Impaired home maintenance
- Impaired social interaction
- Interrupted family processes
- Ineffective coping
- Ineffective therapeutic family regimen management
- Ineffective health maintenance
- Ineffective relationships
- Ineffective role performance
- Interrupted family processes
- Insomnia
- Risk for caregiver role strain
- Risk for injury
- Risk for poisoning
- Risk for self-directed violence
- Risk for suicide
- Sexual dysfunction
- Social isolation

Seizure disorders
- Anxiety
- Chronic low self-esteem
- Delayed growth and development
- Disturbed sensory perception (tactile)

- Impaired environmental interpretation syndrome
- Impaired memory
- Ineffective airway clearance
- Ineffective breathing pattern
- Ineffective coping
- Ineffective therapeutic management
- Risk for delayed development
- Risk for falls
- Risk for injury
- Risk for spiritual distress
- Risk for trauma
- Risk-prone health behavior
- Social isolation
- Self-neglect

Self-destructive behavior
- Anxiety
- Chronic low self-esteem
- Ineffective denial
- Risk for poisoning
- Risk for self-directed violence
- Risk for self-mutilation

Sepsis
- Acute confusion
- Acute pain
- Diarrhea
- Dysfunctional ventilatory weaning response
- Hyperthermia
- Hypothermia
- Nausea
- Imbalanced nutrition: Less than body requirements
- Impaired spontaneous ventilation
- Ineffective thermoregulation
- Risk for ineffective cardiac tissue perfusion
- Risk for ineffective renal perfusion
- Risk for shock

Sexual assault
- Posttrauma syndrome
- Rape-trauma syndrome
- Risk for self-directed violence
- Risk for suicide

Shaken baby syndrome
- Disabled family coping
- Impaired parenting
- Interrupted family processes
- Risk for impaired parenting
- Risk for ineffective cerebral tissue perfusion
- Risk for impaired attachment
- Risk for injury
- Risk for other-directed violence

Shock
- Decreased cardiac output
- Deficient fluid volume
- Impaired gas exchange
- Impaired oral mucous membrane
- Impaired spontaneous ventilation
- Ineffective airway clearance
- Ineffective tissue perfusion (cardiopulmonary)
- Ineffective tissue perfusion (cerebral)
- Ineffective tissue perfusion (renal)
- Risk for electrolyte imbalance
- Risk for infection

Sickle cell anemia
- Acute pain
- Impaired gas exchange
- Impaired physical mobility
- Ineffective protection
- Ineffective tissue perfusion (peripheral)
- Ineffective tissue perfusion (renal)

Sjögren's syndrome
- Acute pain
- Disturbed sensory perception (gustatory)
- Risk for dry eye
- Impaired oral mucous membrane

Spina bifida
- Bowel incontinence
- Impaired skin integrity

- Latex allergy response
- Risk for physical immobility
- Risk for latex allergy response
- Urinary incontinence

Spinal cord defects
- Chronic low self-esteem
- Delayed growth and development
- Impaired urinary elimination
- Overflow urinary incontinence
- Readiness for enhanced family coping
- Risk-prone health behavior
- Total urinary incontinence

Spinal cord injury
- Activity intolerance
- Autonomic dysreflexia
- Bathing or hygiene self-care deficit
- Bowel incontinence
- Chronic pain
- Chronic sorrow
- Complicated grieving
- Constipation
- Deficient diversional activity
- Deficient knowledge (specify)
- Delayed growth and development
- Disturbed body image
- Disturbed sensory perception
- Fear
- Hopelessness
- Impaired physical mobility
- Impaired spontaneous ventilation
- Impaired transfer ability
- Impaired urinary elimination
- Ineffective airway clearance
- Ineffective health maintenance
- Ineffective sexuality patterns
- Ineffective therapeutic regimen management
- Moral distress
- Posttrauma syndrome
- Powerlessness

- Readiness for enhanced communication
- Readiness for enhanced therapeutic regimen management
- Reflex urinary incontinence
- Risk for autonomic dysreflexia
- Risk for constipation
- Risk for delayed development
- Risk for disuse syndrome
- Risk for impaired skin integrity
- Risk for infection
- Risk for trauma
- Risk for urge urinary incontinence
- Risk-prone health behavior
- Sleep deprivation
- Social isolation
- Total urinary incontinence
- Urinary retention

Spinal tumor
- Autonomic dysreflexia
- Bowel incontinence
- Chronic low self-esteem
- Disturbed sensory perception (kinesthetic)
- Dressing or grooming self-care deficit
- Impaired physical mobility
- Impaired urinary elimination
- Ineffective breathing pattern
- Reflex urinary incontinence
- Risk for autonomic dysreflexia
- Risk for impaired skin integrity
- Risk for injury
- Risk for urge urinary incontinence
- Sexual dysfunction
- Situational low self-esteem
- Total urinary incontinence

Spouse abuse
- Anxiety
- Defensive coping
- Deficient knowledge (specify)
- Fear

- Hopelessness
- Posttrauma syndrome
- Powerlessness
- Rape-trauma syndrome
- Readiness for enhanced hope
- Readiness for enhanced knowledge
- Readiness for enhanced parenting
- Readiness for enhanced power
- Readiness for enhanced self-concept
- Readiness for enhanced self-health management
- Risk for other-directed violence
- Risk for suicide
- Stress overload

Streptococcal throat
- Acute pain
- Hyperthermia
- Impaired oral mucous membrane
- Risk for infection

Stroke
- Acute confusion
- Bathing or hygiene self-care deficit
- Bowel incontinence
- Caregiver role strain
- Chronic confusion
- Chronic sorrow
- Compromised family coping
- Constipation
- Death anxiety
- Decreased intracranial adaptive capacity
- Deficient knowledge (specify)
- Disturbed body image
- Disturbed sensory perception (tactile)
- Fatigue
- Functional urinary incontinence
- Hopelessness
- Imbalanced nutrition: More than body requirements

- Imbalanced nutrition: Less than body requirements
- Impaired bed mobility
- Impaired environmental interpretation syndrome
- Impaired gas exchange
- Impaired home maintenance
- Impaired memory
- Impaired physical mobility
- Impaired social interaction
- Impaired swallowing
- Impaired urinary elimination
- Impaired verbal communication
- Impaired walking
- Ineffective airway clearance
- Ineffective breathing pattern
- Ineffective health maintenance
- Ineffective sexuality patterns
- Ineffective thermoregulation
- Ineffective tissue perfusion (cerebral)
- Interrupted family processes
- Powerlessness
- Readiness for enhanced family processes
- Risk for activity intolerance
- Risk for aspiration
- Risk for caregiver role strain
- Risk for compromised human dignity
- Risk for disuse syndrome
- Risk for impaired skin integrity
- Risk for injury
- Risk for poisoning
- Situational low self-esteem
- Sleep deprivation
- Social isolation
- Stress urinary incontinence
- Total urinary incontinence
- Unilateral neglect

Suicidal behavior
- Anxiety
- Chronic low self-esteem
- Disturbed personal identity
- Ineffective denial

- Readiness for enhanced spiritual well-being
- Risk for poisoning
- Risk for self-directed violence
- Risk for self-mutilation

Tendinitis
- Acute pain
- Activity intolerance
- Impaired physical mobility
- Ineffective role performance

Testicular cancer
- Acute pain
- Death anxiety
- Disturbed body image
- Fear
- Hopelessness
- Powerlessness
- Sexual dysfunction
- Risk for situational low self-esteem

Thoracic surgery
- Acute pain
- Deficient fluid volume
- Fatigue
- Fear
- Impaired gas exchange
- Ineffective airway clearance
- Ineffective breathing pattern
- Risk for bleeding
- Risk for infection
- Risk for perioperative position injury

Thrombophlebitis
- Acute pain
- Impaired gas exchange
- Impaired skin integrity
- Ineffective tissue perfusion (peripheral)
- Risk for impaired skin integrity
- Risk for infection
- Risk for injury
- Risk for vascular trauma

Tracheoesophageal fistula
- Imbalanced nutrition: Less than body requirements
- Risk for aspiration

Tracheostomy
- Imbalanced nutrition: Less than body requirements
- Impaired skin integrity
- Impaired verbal communication

Transient ischemic attacks
- Acute confusion
- Disturbed sensory perception (tactile)
- Impaired environmental interpretation syndrome
- Impaired memory
- Ineffective tissue perfusion (cerebral)
- Risk for bleeding
- Risk for ineffective cerebral tissue perfusion

Trauma
- Death anxiety
- Disabled family coping
- Disturbed sensory perception (auditory)
- Energy field disturbance
- Risk for bleeding
- Risk for self-directed violence
- Risk for shock

Trigeminal neuralgia
- Acute pain
- Anxiety
- Deficient knowledge (specify)
- Imbalanced nutrition: Less than body requirements

Tuberculosis
- Deficient community health
- Deficient knowledge
- Fatigue
- Fear
- Impaired dentition
- Impaired gas exchange
- Ineffective airway clearance
- Ineffective breathing pattern
- Ineffective community coping
- Risk for infection
- Risk for loneliness
- Social isolation

Urinary calculi
- Acute pain
- Anxiety
- Impaired urinary elimination
- Ineffective tissue perfusion (renal)
- Readiness for enhanced urinary elimination
- Risk for infection

Urinary diversion
- Acute pain
- Constipation
- Disturbed personal identity
- Grieving
- Impaired skin integrity
- Ineffective breathing pattern
- Ineffective sexuality patterns
- Risk for Infection
- Sexual dysfunction

Urinary incontinence
- Anxiety
- Functional urinary incontinence
- Impaired skin integrity
- Overflow urinary incontinence
- Reflex urinary incontinence
- Social isolation
- Stress urinary incontinence
- Total urinary incontinence

Urinary tract infection
- Acute pain
- Impaired urinary elimination
- Readiness for enhanced urinary elimination
- Risk for infection

- Risk for urge urinary incontinence
- Stress urinary incontinence
- Urge urinary incontinence

Uterine prolapse
- Disturbed body image
- Stress urinary incontinence
- Risk for situational low self-esteem

Uterine rupture
- Acute pain
- Deficient fluid volume
- Ineffective tissue perfusion (cardiopulmonary)
- Ineffective tissue perfusion (cerebral)
- Ineffective tissue perfusion (renal)
- Risk for bleeding
- Risk for electrolyte imbalance
- Risk for shock

Vascular insufficiency
- Impaired tissue integrity
- Risk for peripheral neurovascular dysfunction

Viral hepatitis
- Deficient fluid volume
- Imbalanced nutrition: Less than body requirements
- Impaired skin integrity
- Risk for impaired skin integrity
- Risk for infection
- Social isolation

APPENDICES

CLASS	OBJECTIVE DATA
Functional domain	
Activity/exercise	Functional mobility status: 0 = completely independent 1 = requires use of equipment or device 3 = requires help from another person and equipment or device 4 = dependent, doesn't participate in activity
Comfort	Muscle tone: listless to rigid Autonomic responses: pulse rate, diaphoresis, blood pressure, respiratory rate. Behavior changes: loss of consciousness (LOC), increased irritability, lethargy, or aggression; elderly and young children can manifest pain in behavior changes.
Growth and development	Height/weight—compare to pediatric growth grid: Concern if child has $\uparrow\downarrow$ 2 SD on the CDC Growth Chart Bone/Tooth development Developmental Exam (DDS II)
Nutrition	Weight (compare to normal chart) Laboratory studies: Serum albumin, glucose: infant 60–105 Children and adults 70–115. Bilirubin total: normal adults 0.1–1.2 mg/dL 0- to 1-day-old: <6 mg/dL 1- to 2-day-old: <12mg/dL 3- to 5-day-old <12mg/dL Breast exam: sore or bleeding nipples, engorgement, signs of infection, signs of oxytocin release
Self-care	Self-care status: score separately for bathing, hygiene, dressing, grooming, feeding, and toileting 0 = completely independent 1 = requires use of equipment or device 3 = requires help from another person and equipment or device 4 = dependent, doesn't participate in activity
Sexuality	Use of antihypertensives, neuroleptics, sedatives, tranquilizers, or sexual enhancing drugs
Sleep/rest	
Values/beliefs	

*Ralph, S. (2009). *Assessment Parameters Based on Taxonomy of Nursing Practice.*
Copyright by Author, Hamilton, VA.
Dochterman, J. M., & Jones, D. A. (Eds.). (2003). Unifying nursing languages:
The harmonization of NANDA, NIC, and NOC. Washington, DC: NursesBooks.org.

Usual activity level, daily schedule, usual exercise patterns

Reports of inability to carry out activities of daily living (ADLs) or instrumental activities of daily living (IADLs); overwhelming lack of energy (thyroid studies: abnormalities in thyroid hormone levels can manifest in decreased energy levels)

Characteristics of pain: location, duration, time of day when pain is most severe, sources of relief

Placement on pain scale 1–10 with 10 being most severe; for children: faces scale

Use of pain medications (including prescription/and over-the-counter/illegal)

Growth history; genetic factors, lead screening, Sexual Maturation Index Scale for Adolescents; Signs of puberty for girl as early as 8 and boy 9; concern if no signs of puberty in girls 13 and boys 14

Daily food intake, usual dietary patterns, food preferences, food allergies, changes in weight, dentures (proper fit). Report of difficulty breastfeeding or incomplete emptying (normal weight gain key in assessing nutritional status for infants and children). Infants should reach birth weight by 2 weeks, double birth weight by 6 months, triple birth weight by 1 year, and 4 × birth weight by 2.5 years; slow weights gain 2–3 lb a year normal until adolescence.

BMI: concern if greater than 10 kg/m^2

Report of difficulty or inability to carry some one or more ADLs

Perception of sexual identity; sexuality status: changes in sexual behavior, usual patterns of sexuality, sexual dysfunction, impotence, vaginismus, decreased or increased libido, dyspareunia, premature ejaculation

Description of sleep patterns, usual sleep routines, expression of tiredness or lack of being rested after sleep, use of sleep-disturbing drugs, usual activity and work patterns, sleep environment

Pain: medications, alcohol consumption, depression, caffeine intake, and stress affect sleep

Sleep apnea: enlarged tonsils in young children; in older children and adults obesity may be a finding for sleep apnea

Spiritual status, including religious affiliation, current perception of faith and religious practices, spiritual beliefs linked to current distress, change in usual spiritual practices, relationship between spiritual beliefs and everyday living, unmet spiritual needs (meaning and purpose, love and relatedness, forgiveness)

(Continued)

CLASS	OBJECTIVE DATA
Physiological Domain	
Cardiac function	Cardiovascular status: heart rate and rhythm; skin color, temperature, and turgor; jugular vein distension, hepatojugular reflux, heart sounds, blood pressure, peripheral pulses, electrocardiogram, results of echocardiogram
Elimination	Gastrointestinal (GI) status: stool characteristics, bowel sounds, abdominal distension Genitourinary status: characteristics of urine, palpation of bladder, results of intravenous pyelogram, electrolytes, blood urea nitrogen [BUN], creatinine level, urinalysis, intake and output, mucous membranes, urine specific gravity
Fluid and electrolytes	Fluid and electrolyte status, weight, intake and output, urine specific gravity, skin turgor, mucous membranes, results of laboratory studies (hemoglobin [Hgb]/hematocrit [Hct]—overhydration or dehydration; Hct ↑dehydration ↓ decreased if the person has been rehydrated too rapidly or is retaining fluid. Hct should be 3 times the Hgb. Serum electrolytes, BUN, urinalysis, arterial blood gas [ABGs]), characteristics of stool, vomiting, nasogastric drainage, blood loss
Neurocognition	Neurological status, LOC, orientation to person, place, and time, pupillary response, sensory status, motor status. Mental status, abstract thinking, insight, judgment, recent and remote memory; Mini Mental Status Examination
Pharmacological function	
Physical regulation	Vital signs (blood pressure, temperature, pulse, respirations); signs of inflammation or allergic responses; skin status, color, temperature, and turgor. Tactile sensations in upper and lower extremities, motor nerve function, peripheral pulses (compare bilaterally using the following scale: 0 = absent, 1 = weak, barely palpable, 2 = weak, diminished, 3 = slightly weak, easily located, 4 = normal, easily located), vascular status (capillary refill time, blanching, skin temperature, and skin color)
Reproduction	
Respiratory function	Respiratory status, rate and depth of respirations, symmetry of chest expansion, use of accessory muscles, palpation for fremitus, percussion of lung fields, auscultation for breath sounds, ABG levels: When the PCO_2 and HCO_3 increase and decrease together the imbalance is metabolic. When the PCO_2 and HCO_3 move in opposite directions think respiratory: metabolic together respiratory apart; pulse oximetry; results of chest x-ray, cough, characteristics of sputum; results of pulmonary function studies and sputum cultures; presence or absence of gag and swallow reflexes; artificial airway, ventilator settings

History of valvular disorder, congenital heart disease or myopathy, myocardial infarction, congestive heart failure, shortness of breath, frequent respiratory infections red flag for undiagnosed cardiac conditions in children

Bowel: usual elimination patterns, change in bowel patterns, reports of constipation or diarrhea, history of laxative, suppositories, or enema use, history of GI disorder

Urinary: history of urinary tract disorder (renal calculi, infection, trauma, surgery), elderly and infants may only have behavioral changes to indicate urinary tract infection (UTI); night time bed wetting in an older or previously toilet-trained child can indicate UTI, usual voiding pattern, report of urine leakage or retention, use of incontinence aids, perception of bladder fullness

History of renal, cardiac, GI disorders, burns, diabetes mellitus, use of diuretics or rehydration fluid instead of water for imbalances when indicated

History of spinal cord trauma, head trauma, alcoholism delirium, stroke, transient ischemic attacks; description of symptoms, headache, nasal congestion, blurred vision, chest pain, diaphoresis and flushing above the level of the spinal cord injury

List all medications (prescribed, over-the-counter, and illicit drugs) and responses. Changes in LOC, balance, and behavior can indicate drug toxicity

History of allergic responses to food, drugs, or other irritants (especially latex). Facial and extremity swelling, difficulty breathing, rashes, may indicate reaction

Elevated eosinophils indicate allergic response; exposure to heat or cold. History of burns, fractures or trauma, mechanical (cast, brace, etc.) or vascular obstruction

Maternal history. Number of pregnancies, live births, abortions, or miscarriages. History of contraceptive use, sterilization procedures, fertility problems

History of respiratory disorder, use of respiratory medications (for asthma, bronchitis, emphysema, interstitial lung disease, pneumonia); smoking history

(Continued)

CLASS	OBJECTIVE DATA
Physiological Domain (*Continued*)	
Sensation/perception	Auditory status, ear position, size and symmetry, tympanic membrane (cerumen, color of canal, deformities, intactness or tension, landmarks), results of audiometric evaluation (Rinne, Weber, Schwabach, and speech and noise tests), use of hearing aid
	Gustatory: taste sensation, including change from baseline, ability to differentiate sweet, salty, sour, and bitter tastes; changes in weight or smell
	Kinesthetic: motor coordination and muscular strength, flaccidity or atrophy; perception of body part location and changes in position
	Olfactory: olfactory status, nosebleeds, foul taste in mouth, sneezing, postnasal drip, dry or sore mouth or throat, excessive tearing, facial pain, eye pain
	Tactile: impaired tactile perception (tingling, pain, numbness; response to sharp and dull stimuli, signs of bruises, cuts, scrapes, or other injury)
	Visual: visual status, corneal reflex, extraocular movements, fields of gaze, inspection of lid and eyeball, ophthalmoscopy, palpation of lid and eyeball, pupil size and accommodation, tonometry, use of glasses, contact lenses or intraocular implants, visual acuity (near and distant), visual fields
Tissue integrity	Oral: oral status, gums, lips, tongue, mucous membranes, signs of salivary dysfunction, teeth
	Skin: integumentary status, color, elasticity, hygiene, lesions, moisture, sensation, quantity and distribution of hair, texture, turgor, pressure ulcer (place, stage, size, characteristics), CBC, Hgb/Hct, serum albumin, blood coagulation studies, serum electrolytes, mobility status, urinary or bowel incontinence
Psychosocial Domain	
Behavior	
Communication	Speech patterns, judgment, thoughts, perception of reality, memory, characteristics of speech (coherence of topics, logic and relevance of responses, volume, voice tone and modulation, presence of speech defects such as stuttering, fast or slow speech, slurred speech, dysarthria, garbled speech, echolalia, aphasia, dysphasia), orientation, mood, affect, gender and age; use of communication aids

Auditory: history of ear disorders, trauma, surgery; perception of auditory ability; use of
adaptive auditory aids (lip reading, gestures, signing). Delayed development of speech and
language may indicate hearing loss. Gentamycin and aspirin toxicity can lead to hearing
loss. Bacterial meningitis strong link to hearing loss. Tip of the ears not matching the outer
canthus of the eye, equal low set ears can be indicative of mental retardation and congenital
syndromes. Skin tags and sinus on the auricle may be linked to kidney structural defects.

Gustatory: history of vitamin or mineral deficiency, neurologic or oral disorders, chemotherapy,
or radiation therapy; medication history (antidepressants such as clomipramine, antineoplastic
agents, penicillamine, captopril, lithium, interferon alfa-2a, levamisole, zidovudine)

Kinesthetic: history of cerebral palsy, multiple sclerosis, muscular dystrophy, spinal disorders;
use of safety devices

Olfactory: history of nasal disease or allergy, intranasal drug abuse, surgery or trauma;
use of phenothiazines, estrogen, metronidazole, antineoplastics, prolonged use of nasal
decongestants or topical anesthetics. Frequent sinus infections and colds can alter sense
of smell. Altered sense of smell can also indicate CNS damage

Tactile: history of chemotherapy, alcohol use, medications such as clomipramine, ceftizomine,
amiodarone hydrochloride, dichlorphenamide, guanadrel, anistreplase, interferon alfa-2b,
zidovudine

Visual: history of eye disorders, trauma, surgery. Strabismus normal up to six months of age.
Children's vision is about 20/30 until 7–8 years of age. May develop near sightedness after
puberty due to physiological change in the lens shape.

Oral: dental health history, tooth development, frequency of dental visits, frequency of
brushing and flossing, history of malnutrition, anorexia, bulimia, infections, allergies, lead
poisoning, rubella, caries, extractions, bridges, braces, dentures.

Skin: history of skin problems, trauma, lesions (color, borders, elevation, and bleeding),
surgery, chronic metabolic or systemic disease, immunocompromised, renal or hepatic
disease, radiation or chemotherapy.

Trauma that does not fit history may indicate abuse.

Bruises that are on soft tissue areas, in a pattern, may indicate abuse.

Anticoagulants and antiseizure medications may cause bruising

Patient's understanding of health problem and treatment plan, past history with health care
providers, participation in health care planning and decision making; recognition and
realization of potential growth, health, autonomy

Developmental history of communication patterns, knowledge of difference among passive,
assertive, and aggressive responses. Infants through nonverbal cues. Direct communication
at parent.

Toddlers: direct communication at parents initially, talk at eye level with the child use
play and simple speech

School-age: concrete thinkers, take speech literally. Direct the communication at them. Simple
language with few analogies.

(Continued)

CLASS	OBJECTIVE DATA
Psychosocial Domain (*Continued*)	
Coping	Evidence of physical injuries, laboratory studies (pregnancy test, tests for sexually transmitted diseases)
Emotional	Symptoms of anxiety, depression (Depression Screening tool) HEADSS screening tool for adolescents
Knowledge	Learning ability (affective, cognitive, and psychomotor domains), developmental stage, demonstrated skills in managing health problems, memory, mental status, orientation
Roles/relationships	Family genogram, caregiver's age sex, level of education, occupation, general health, nationality, area of residence Infant's status: muscle tone, reflexes, lethargy, irritability, seizures, tremors; Brazelton Neonatal Behavioral Assessment Scale, Dubowitz Maturity Scale, Bayley Scales of Infant Development
Self-perception	Musculoskeletal status, contractures, subluxation, muscle atrophy, pain, deformity
Environmental Domain	
Health care system	
Populations	Community demographics, including age and sex distribution, ethnic groups, racial groups, education and income level Prevalence of health problems, availability of health care services Other data: drug and alcohol abuse, automobile accidents, homicides, suicides, domestic violence, burglaries, teenage pregnancy, sexually transmitted diseases, low-birth weight infants, incidence of congenital abnormalities
Risk management	Toxicology results, LOC, mental status, presence of dangerous products

Adolescents: communicate with them in private and with parent. Want honesty. Expect both child-like and adult like behavior. Don't use adolescent's language. May resist authority figures.

Need to use appropriate interpreter; do not use untrained personnel or family members to communicate.

Allow elderly people time to reminisce about past.

Speak slowly to allow for auditory processing.

Do not yell at a hearing impaired patient.

Face patient when speaking.

Patient's perception of health problem, coping mechanisms, problem-solving ability, decision-making competencies, relationships, family system, self-worth, patterns of coping with loss, experiences with relocation

Health status, support systems, expressed concerns about impending death, history of loss, changes in appetite, sleep and eating patterns, alcohol consumption

Changes in work or school performance, activity level or libido, expression of emptiness, loneliness, low self-esteem, overwhelmed

Health status, educational level, cultural status, requests for information; demonstrated understanding of material

Family status, including roles of family members, effects of illness on patient's family, family's understanding of patient's illness, ability to meet needs of patient, quality of relationships

Cultural status, including affiliation with racial, ethnic, or religious groups

Parental status, including level of education, knowledge of growth and development, stability of relationship

Infant's status, Including sleep patterns, prematurity, developmental disorder

Parent–child interaction

Verbal and nonverbal responses to actual (burns, surgery-amputation, mastectomy, laryngectomy), or perceived change in body structure and function

Patient's experiences with the health care system

Health history: accidents, adolescents most at risk for injury.

2- to 5-years-olds most at risk for poisoning and drowning. Allergies, exposure to pollutants, falls, hyperthermia, hypothermia, poisoning, seizures, trauma, sensory–perceptual changes Support systems, financial resources

DOMAIN

I. Functional domain includes diagnoses, outcomes, and interventions to promote basic needs.	II. Physiological domain includes diagnoses, outcomes, and interventions to promote optimal biophysical health.

Classes includes diagnoses, class outcomes, and interventions that pertain to:

Activity/exercise: Physical activity, including energy conservation and expenditure.	**Cardiac function:** Cardiac mechanisms used to maintain tissue profusion.
Comfort: A sense of emotional, physical, and spiritual well-being and relative freedom from distress.	**Elimination:** Process related to secretion and excretion of body wastes.
Growth and development: Physical, emotional, and social growth and development milestones.	**Fluid and electrolyte:** Regulation of fluid/ electrolytes and acid base balance.
Nutrition: Processes related to taking in, assimilating, and using nutrients	**Neurocognition:** Mechanisms related to the nervous system and neurocognitive functioning, including memory, thinking and judgment.
Self-care: Ability to accomplish basic and instrumental ADLs	**Pharmacological function:** Effects (therapeutic and adverse) of medications or drugs and other pharmacologically active products.
Sexuality—Maintenance or modification of sexual identity and patterns.	**Physical regulation:** Body temperature, endocrine, and immune system responses to regulate cellular processes.
Sleep/rest: The quantity and quality of sleep, rest, and relaxation patterns.	**Reproduction:** Processes related to human procreation and birth.
Values/beliefs: Ideas, goals, perceptions, spiritual, and other beliefs that influence choices or decisions.	**Respiratory function:** Ventilation adequate to maintain ABGs within normal limits. **Sensation/perception:** Intake and interpretation of information through the senses, including seeing, hearing, touching, tasting, and smelling. **Tissue integrity:** Skin and mucous membrane protection to support secretion, excretion, and healing.

This structure is in the public domain and can be freely used without permission; neither the structure nor a modification can be copyrighted by any person, group, or organization; any use of the structure should acknowledge the source. From Dochterman, J. M., & Jones, D. A. (Eds.). (2003). *Unifying Nursing Language: The Harmonization of NANDA, NIC, and NOC.* Washington, DC: NursingBooks.Org.

III. Psychosocial domain includes diagnoses, outcomes, and interventions to promote optimal mental and emotional health and social functioning.

IV. Environmental domain includes diagnoses, outcomes, and interventions to promote and protect the environmental health and safety of individuals, systems, and communities.

Behavior: Actions that promote, maintain, or restore health.

Health care system: Social, political, and economic structures and processes for the delivery of health care services.

Communication: Receiving, interpreting, and expressing spoken, written, and nonverbal messages.

Populations: Aggregates of individuals, or communities having characteristics in common.

Coping: Adjusting or adapting to stressful events.

Risk management: Avoidance or control of identifiable health threats.

Emotional: A mental state or feeling that may influence perceptions of the world.

Knowledge: Understanding skill in applying information to promote, maintain, and restore health.

Roles/relationships: Maintenance and/or modification of expected social behaviors and emotional connectedness with others.

Self-perception: Awareness of one's body and personal identity.

Appendix C: Action Intervention Types

TYPE	DEFINITION	EXAMPLES
Determine	Finding out or establishing	Assess, monitor, observe, evaluate
Perform	Doing a task	Hygiene, insert, position, change, feed
Inform	Telling about something	Describe, explain, teach
Attend	Being concerned about	Assist, relate
Manage	Being in charge of or bringing order	Organize, refer, obtain

Adapted from *International Classification for Nursing Practice by International Council of Nurses*, 2005, p. 130, Geneva, Switzerland. Examples are not exhaustive.

Index